Qìgōng Meditation

Small Circulation

Don't be afraid!

不用害怕！

Dare to challenge.....

敢於挑戰.....

Dare to accept.....

敢於接受.....

Dare to dream.....

敢於夢想.....

- Dare to emerge from the traditional matrix -

- be free from spiritual bondage -

"The philosopher should be a man willing to listen to every suggestion, but determined to judge for himself. He should not be biased by appearances, have no favorite hypothesis, be of no school, and in doctrine have no master. He should not be a respecter of persons, but of things. Truth should be his primary object. If to these qualities be added industry, he may indeed hope to walk within the veil of the temple of Nature."

—Michael Faraday (1791–1867)

Qìgōng Meditation

Small Circulation

Second Edition

The Foundation of Spiritual Enlightenment

Dr. Yáng, Jwìng-Mǐng

YMAA Publication Center
Wolfeboro, NH. USA

YMAA Publication Center
PO Box 480
Wolfeboro, NH 03894
1-800-669-8892 www.ymaa.com info@ymaa.com

ISBN 9781594399176 (print)
ISBN 9781594399183 (ebook)
ISBN 9781594399190 (hardcover)

This book set in EB Garamond and Avenir.

First edition edited by Keith Brown and David Silver
Second edition copyedit by Doran Hunter
Cover design by Axie Breen
Photos by YMAA Publication Center unless otherwise noted.

20220831

Publisher's Cataloging in Publication

Names: Yang, Jwing-Ming, 1946-
Title: Qìgōng meditation small circulation : the foundation of spiritual enlightenment / Dr. Yáng, Jwìng-Mǐng.
Description: Second edition. | Wolfeboro, NH USA : YMAA Publication Center, [2022] | Revises the 2006 first edition. | Text in English, with some Chinese characters included. | Includes bibliographical references, translation and glossary of Chinese terms, and index.
Identifiers: ISBN: 9781594399176 (paperback) | 978194399190 (hardcover) | 9781594399183 (ebook) | LCCN: 2022944102
Subjects: LCSH: Qi gong. | Qi (Chinese philosophy) | Meditation. | Qi gong--Therapeutic use. | Breathing exercises--Therapeutic use. | Mind and body. | Well-being. | Longevity. | Spirituality. | Taoist philosophy. | Buddhist philosophy. | BISAC: HEALTH & FITNESS / Longevity. | HEALTH & FITNESS / Tai Chi. | BODY, MIND & SPIRIT / Healing / Energy (Qigong, Reiki, Polarity) | SELF-HELP / Meditations.
Classification: LCC: RA781.8 .Y363 2022 | DDC: 613.7/148--dc22

Printed in Canada.

FSC www.fsc.org MIX Paper from responsible sources FSC® C103567

Contents

CHAPTER 4. FIVE REGULATINGS

PART III. SMALL CIRCULATION MEDITATION

CHAPTER 5. THEORETICAL ROOT OF SMALL CIRCULATION MEDITATION

CHAPTER 6. EMBRYONIC BREATHING

CHAPTER 7. IMPORTANT POINTS IN MEDITATION

CHAPTER 8. SMALL CIRCULATION MEDITATION PRACTICE

Dedication

To my friend whom I can't forget
Mr. Wolfgang Pastore

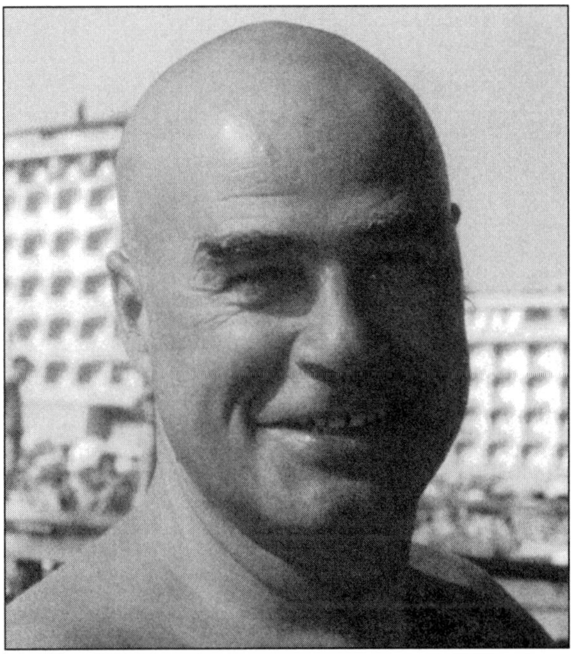

Editor's Note

David Silver

Master Yáng, Jwìng-Mǐng has made it his life's purpose to research and translate all of the available ancient documents pertaining to the subjects of Qìgōng and Internal Cultivation. His extensive scientific background, paired with his training in Soft (Tàijíquán, 太極拳), Hard (Long Fist, 長拳), and Soft-Hard (White Crane, 白鶴) martial arts, empowers him with a comprehensive insight on the subjects of human physiology, universal electromagnetic energy, and the relationship between them.

Ancient Buddhist, Daoist, Qìgōng, and martial arts documents are often fragments, each discussing a certain aspect of its training, from the author's unique perspective based on his or her experience and contemplation. These documents are truly among the most precious artifacts of human history, sometimes passed down in the form of songs and poems, transmitted from teacher to student. Because many documents are only a piece of the puzzle, Qìgōng and Meditation are frequently misunderstood, or passed down in an incomplete form. In an effort to preserve this accumulated knowledge, most of Master Yáng's works are written as stand-alone documents, offering readers worldwide a complete overview to the subject matter, as he works toward a "Unified Theory" of Qìgōng.

Several chapters in this book offer information discussed in Master Yáng's previous works. If you have truly assimilated this information already, you are encouraged to move on to later chapters. However, as Master Yáng's tireless research continues, his insight expands, and it may benefit the reader to humbly read each chapter and again immerse oneself entirely in the subject, starting with its general concepts and theories. Master Yáng is fond of scolding his students for neglecting fundamental training, saying "Don't be a Jedi too soon."

Many cultural and spiritual centers have been destroyed in times of war. It is impossible to know how much knowledge, and how many written works, have been lost forever. It is impossible to know what the future holds for humanity, what humanity holds for itself, or how much of today's scientific and spiritual information will survive.

I share Master Yáng's hope that the interrelated subjects of Qìgōng, meditation, and human bioelectricity will continue to be researched and will become an important focus of scientific, medical and spiritual study. In 100 or 500 years, the situation on Earth (and other planets) will be so different that it is nearly impossible to conceive. We must hope that by then things will have changed for the better; that humanity has rediscovered its common spirituality, reopened our third eye, and created a balanced and peaceful global society.

If not, I hope someone finds this book.

David Silver
Boston, April 2005

Foreword

Thomas G. Gutheil, MD

"Qìgōng is a science of inner feeling which relates to spiritual cultivation."

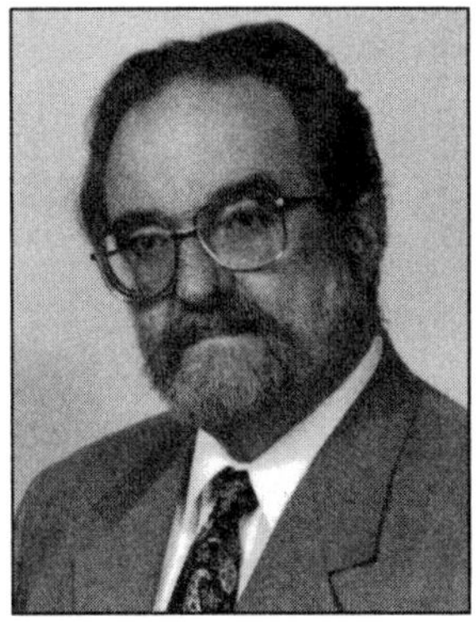

This definition may strike the Western reader as somewhat strange, since it fuses an Eastern concept of biologic energy and the idea of science, together with feeling and spirituality—concepts which are usually quite separate in Western thinking. But the very essence of Qìgōng is its union of physical, mental and spiritual issues into one discipline.

Western medicine is just beginning to explore the role of meditation in various forms as a legitimate adjunct to other approaches. The concept known as mindfulness, in which meditation consists of focus on breathing and the attempt to empty the mind of linear thought, is one such modern application. Though not as popular as it once was, transcendental mediation represents another form. Tàijí, sometimes described as moving meditation, is, of course, one of the oldest forms but one which is enjoying a modern resurgence, even in alternative medicine where it is used to aid with a number of medical problems such as high blood pressure and ulcers. Yoga has also been practiced, sometimes in conjunction with mindfulness practice, to achieve some of the same states of tranquility. Finally, in the scientific community, studies of the so-called relaxation response represent another form that this method may take in current practice. Producing results ranging from feelings of inner harmony and tranquility to actual decreases in blood pressure, these techniques have gradually found a place in popular awareness and fields of healing.

In this work Dr. Yáng, Jwìng-Mǐng continues his astonishingly productive life-long endeavor of unearthing hidden, secret, lost, and otherwise unavailable ancient Chinese texts and translating them for the world of readers. The present book also takes its place in a series of works that explore almost every aspect of Qìgōng from its roots to its practical applications (see bibliography). Moreover, the present volume represents an updating of understanding of the fundamental principles of Qìgōng since publication of the predecessor volumes.

Based on the foundation of Internal Elixir Qìgōng practice, this book takes the reader to the next level of spiritual cultivation. Moving from an overview of the topic, Master Yáng takes the reader through meditation training; then the specifics of Small Circulation, and then a look toward the future development of the subject.

While retaining the colorful and highly metaphoric language of the original texts, Dr. Yáng makes the complex subject accessible and useful to the interested reader or practitioner. A helpful glossary furthers this accessibility. The thoughtful reader may thus gain a deep understanding of the basic sciences of this aspect of Qìgōng practice.

Thomas G. Gutheil, M.D.
Harvard Medical School

Preface (Original 2006 Edition)

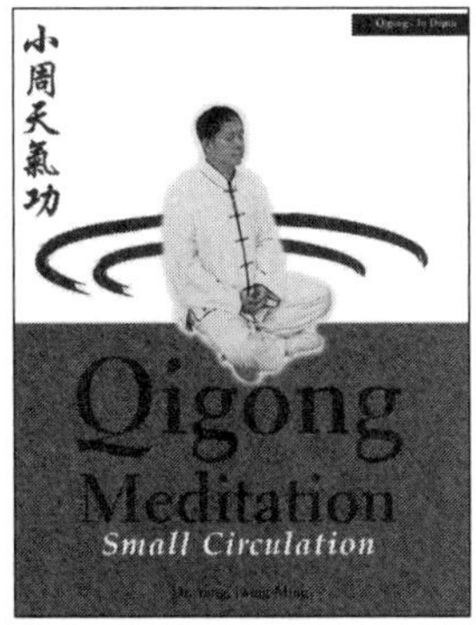

First edition, as published in 2006.

Several friends have asked how I found time and energy to achieve proficiency in three Chinese martial arts styles, at the same time obtaining my master's degree in physics and Ph.D. in mechanical engineering. The main reason I could achieve each goal I set was that I learned how to concentrate through meditation. I have practiced and studied meditation since I was seventeen. I could relax whenever I was tense, and ponder profoundly when I needed to. Meditation brought me another world—the world of spiritual awareness, which enabled me to build up self-confidence, wisdom and a better understanding of the world.

Small Circulation Meditation (Small Cyclic Heaven or Microcosmic Meditation, Xiǎozhōutiān Jìngzuò, 小周天靜坐) has been well known for centuries throughout the East, including China, India, Indo-China, Korea, and Japan. According to ancient documents from Buddhist and Daoist monasteries, if one practices correctly under a master's guidance, it might take only 90 days to learn to circulate Qì in the Small Circulation path of the Conception and Governing Vessels. But I did not achieve this goal until I was 24 because I was young and did not know the correct theory and technique. Documentary information was sparse, so I asked my White Crane and Tàijíquán masters. Due to lack of personal teaching experience, they refused to guide me. They simply advised me not to continue because of the danger involved. I could not calm down my mind to practice, due to my school work and martial arts training. From the ages of 15 to 19, in addition to school work, I trained Tàijíquán in the early morning, and White Crane every evening. My meditation practice suffered as a result.

I finished my M.S. degree of science at Táiwān University. I was 23. Information was revealed to the public on meditation, and I could finally understand some theory. Then I was drafted into the Air Force as a military physics teacher. I had much time and little pressure, so I could calm my mind and put all my understanding into practicing every day for the whole year. I completed the Small Circulation path that summer, continuing until I married at age 27.

Being married, my life was very different and difficult, and my meditation was disrupted. I came to the United States in 1974 for Ph.D. study. I practiced a little but could not advance further due to the new environment and the pressure of studies. I only used meditation to calm my troubled mind. The following year, my wife arrived to join me from Táiwān, and in the year that followed, we lost our first child. Again I stopped meditating. I was sad and disappointed. Meditation had been part of my life and now I could not continue. After graduating with my Ph.D. from Purdue in 1978, my first son was born, then my daughter, followed by my second son. The financial pressure of supporting the family was so great, I almost forgot the pleasure and peace meditation could bring. But though I could not practice, I did not give up, and started collecting Qìgōng documents. Around 1980, many hidden Qìgōng documents started to be revealed. I studied them and deepened my understanding of the subject.

To follow my dream, I resigned from my engineering job in 1984 and dedicated my effort to writing and study. Life was great and the pressure of work was gone, but the financial reality of supporting my family worried me so much I often could not sleep at night. I fell ill in the spring of 1984. Without health insurance, I did not see a doctor. One of my students, studying as a medical doctor, visited me and told me I had had pneumonia for nearly two months and was near death. My dentist brother in Táiwān sent me some antibiotics, and two weeks later my recurrent fever was disappearing. Three months later I published my first Qìgōng book, *Chì Kūng—Health and Martial Arts*. The new edition is called *Qìgōng for Health and Martial Arts*. Surprisingly, this book started to bring some income, and I could smile again.

Since 1984, I had continued to read, study, and research. More books and ancient documents were revealed in Táiwān and mainland China. The second half of the 1980s became the most joyful of my life, as many more hidden documents were revealed. The most valuable to me were the secret classics, *Yìjīnjīng* (*Muscle/Tendon Changing*, 易筋經) and *Xǐsuǐjīng* (*Marrow/Brain Washing*, 洗髓經), said to have been written by Dámó (達摩) around 500 CE in the Shàolín monastery. These classics are very profound. To many Qìgōng practitioners, their theory remains obscure, but to me they were the most precious knowledge I had ever received.

Studying them, I discovered the missing part of Qìgōng practice, its Yīn side. Part of the Yìjīnjīng (Yáng side) secret had previously been revealed through Shàolín martial arts, but not the Xǐsuǐjīng (Yīn side). These two classics are two sides, Yīn and Yáng, of the same Qìgōng training, and both are required to reach enlightenment or Buddhahood. Yìjīnjīng builds up and circulates Qì throughout the body to strengthen it (Yáng side). Xǐsuǐjīng leads accumulated Qì from the Real Lower Dāntián (Zhēn Xiàdāntián, 真下丹田) to the bone marrow, and also up to nourish the brain cells for spiritual enlightenment (Yīn side).

To accumulate abundant Qì for Yìjīnjīng and Xǐsuǐjīng training, Small Circulation Meditation must first be practiced. This is the foundation of Internal Elixir Qìgōng (Nèidān Qìgōng, 內丹氣功) without which Qì would be too weak to build up physical strength or to nurture spiritual enlightenment.

To fully comprehend the theory and training in these documents, I had to devote all my effort to it. This meant writing books about it. Through translating the documents, I was forced to ponder the meaning of every word. It also forced me to find related information with which to unravel the knots. My efforts came to fruition with publication of the books, *The Root of Chinese Qìgōng*, and *Qìgōng—The Secret of Youth* (previously *Muscle/Tendon Changing and Marrow/Brain Washing Chì Kūng*).

Since 1984, countless Qìgōng documents, written by hundreds of ancient Qìgōng experts during the last four thousand years, have been compiled and published in mainland China. This has been a source of deep joy to me. I feel so lucky to have been born at this time, not only with access to these documents, but having a strong scientific background to analyze and understand them. Due to enhanced communication between East and West, great interest in this art of internal energy has also been aroused in Western society.

The more books I have written, the deeper I have understood this art. My mission in life is to present my Qìgōng knowledge in Western languages. All my children have grown up now, and my financial situation is stable. I resumed meditation practice in 1992, and can apply my understanding of Qìgōng theory in my practice. For the rest of my life, I plan to enjoy reading and understanding these Qìgōng documents, the fruits of four thousand years of human feeling and spiritual cultivation. This will make my life meaningful and happy.

I have taught Small Circulation in the USA since 1981. After more than 20 years of teaching experience, I have modified some traditional practice methods to make them safer and more suitable for practitioners in modern society. In this book, I share these methods with you. However, any book can only offer an opinion from the writer's point of view. You are the one who must collect more books, read and comprehend them, and finally arrive at a consistent scientific theory and method of practice, suitable to your lifestyle.

This book deals with vital new subject matter, including updated information and insights concerning subjects covered in earlier books. It focuses on profound discussion of the theory and practice of Small Circulation. Traditional training methods and modified ones are compared and analyzed. As long as you remain humble, and read and ponder carefully and sincerely, you should reach the goal of Small Circulation without risk. You should also discuss the subject with experienced practitioners.

The first part of the book reviews the general concepts and theory of Qìgōng. In the second part, traditional meditation training, procedures, and theory are summarized, to show how traditional Qìgōng meditators reached the goal of enlightenment. The third part discusses the theory and practice of Small Circulation, especially Embryonic Breathing (Tāixí, 胎息), the root of all Internal Elixir Qìgōng practice. More than 100 ancient documents discuss this important subject. For a deeper discussion of this subject, refer to my previous book, *Qìgōng Meditation—Embryonic Breathing*. In Part IV, we discuss the relevance of the subject matter to society.

Dr. Yáng, Jwìng-Mǐng

Publisher's Note on the 2nd Edition

This 2nd edition includes pinyin with tonal marks, a new Chinese character font (Biau-Kai), and selected illustration enhancements.

An important contribution to this new edition is the use of tonal marks on the pinyin. Pinyin is the current standard for Romanizing Chinese characters so they can be read by non-Chinese speaking readers. By adding tonal marks to the Romanized Chinese words (pinyin), we can have a guide for properly pronouncing these words.

Before we can begin learning how to pronounce pinyin words, we must recognize some common differences in how some letters sound.[1]

ü Start pronouncing "ee" in English and then round your lips to pronounce "oo".
q Pronounced like "ch" in chin.
x Pronounced like a blend of "she" and "he".
z Pronounced like "ds" in kids.
c Pronounced like "ts" in bats.
zh Pronounced like "ger" in germ.
ch Pronounced like "chur" in church.
sh Pronounced like "sur" in sure.
er Pronounced like "ar" in are.
i When i follows z, c, s, it sounds like "zz": zzz, czz, szz.
When i follows zh, ch, sh, r, it sounds like "rr": zhrr, chrr, shrr, rrr.

There are primarily four tonal categories written in pinyin.[2]

1. mā 媽 (mom). Begins high and stays high.
2. má 麻 (hemp). Begins at mid-range and ends high.
3. mǎ 馬 (horse). Begins mid-range, dips low, ends mid-range.
4. mà 罵 (scold). Begins high and ends low.

There are many websites offering guides for the pronunciation of Chinese words and how to interpret and pronounce pinyin words with the tonal marks. We encourage readers to explore these valuable online tools. Some are provided below for your reference.

https://dictionary.hantrainerpro.com/
https://en.wikipedia.org/wiki/Pinyin
https://ymaa.com/publishing/spoken-chinese-glossary

1 https://www.mandarintutor.com/resources/pinyinintro
2 https://www.duchinese.net/blog/learn-to-read-chinese-tones/

Part I

Foundations

CHAPTER 1

General Concepts

1-1. Introduction (Jièshào, 介紹)

Qìgōng study and practice have become very popular since being introduced into Western society in the 1970s. However, many problems still remain:

1. Only a few books explain Qìgōng scientifically, bringing scientific theory and ancient experience together. So many people are still skeptical about Qìgōng science.
2. Few scholars and scientific researchers are willing to spend effort pursuing and verifying this Qìgōng science. Qìgōng is a newcomer to Western society, and few convincing scientific results are reported in scholarly studies and papers.
3. Many people are still in traditional and religious bondage, preventing them from opening their minds to another spiritual culture. Qìgōng is a science of inner feeling and spiritual cultivation. If one cannot or dares not jump out of the traditional matrix, one cannot accept this science which has been studied by Chinese and Indian society for more than four thousand years.
4. Few qualified Qìgōng practitioners can read, understand, and accurately translate the abundant ancient Qìgōng documents. I estimate that less than 1 percent of the ancient documents have been translated into Western languages. Most have been hidden in Buddhist and Daoist monasteries and only revealed in recent decades.
5. Many Qìgōng practitioners have used Qìgōng as a tool to abuse and mislead their followers. This has led people into superstitious belief and blind worship, making scientific scholars doubt the truth of Qìgōng practice.

Chinese Qìgōng derives from more than four thousand years of experience in healing and prevention of disease, and in spiritual cultivation. Four major schools have emerged: medical, scholar, religious, and martial. Qìgōng is one major essence of Chinese culture which cannot be separated from its people.

Western science has developed from its focus on the material world. That which can only be felt is considered unscientific; inner feeling and development are ignored. But to the Chinese, feeling is a language which allows mind and body to communicate, extending beyond the body to communicate with nature (heaven and earth) or Dào (道). This feeling has been studied and has become the core of Chinese culture, and is especially cultivated in Buddhist and Daoist society, where the final goal is to attain spiritual enlightenment, or Buddhahood. Through more than two thousand years of study and practice, this cultivation has reached such a high level that it cannot yet be interpreted by material science. I believe it will take some time to break through this barrier and for Western scientists to accept this concept.

From my more than four decades of Qìgōng practice, and from studying many ancient documents, I am confident at last that I have derived and understood the map of this Qìgōng science. As long as a "Dào searcher" (Xúndàozhě, 尋道者) is willing to study this map, even without guidance from a qualified master, one should still be able to stay on the correct path of study.

I have interpreted this map in several books:

1. *The Root of Chinese Qìgōng*. This book establishes a firm foundation for understanding Chinese Qìgōng.
2. *The Essence of Shàolín White Crane*. This is a martial Qìgōng book, and the theory is complete. However, the manifestation of this theory is in the White Crane style.
3. *Qìgōng—The Secret of Youth*. This book interpreted the crucial ancient classics, *Muscle/Tendon Changing* and *Marrow/Brain Washing Qìgōng (Yìjīnjīng, Xǐsuǐjīng*, 易筋經・洗髓經), passed down by the Indian monk Dámó (達摩), around 500 CE.
4. *Qìgōng Meditation—Embryonic Breathing* discusses Internal Elixir Qìgōng (Nèidān, 內丹). Embryonic breathing (Tāixí, 胎息) is a key practice in building and maintaining abundant inner energy. Without this practice as a foundation, the achievement of Internal Elixir would be shallow.

The practices described in these four books build a firm foundation for Internal Elixir Qìgōng (Nèidān Qìgōng, 內丹氣功), making it possible for the next step in spiritual cultivation, Small Circulation, to be understood.

In this book, I introduce Small Circulation in four parts. Part I introduces and summarizes general Qìgōng knowledge of Small Circulation. Part II discusses traditional training procedures for Small Circulation and Enlightenment. Part III introduces Small Circulation training methods, while Part IV lists questions which remain to be answered someday. My next area of research will be on the topics of Grand Circulation and Spiritual Enlightenment Meditation, published as *Qìgōng—Grand Circulation for Spiritual Enlightenment*.

1-2. What Is Qì and What Is Qìgōng? (Héwèi Qì? Héwèi Qìgōng? 何謂氣？何謂氣功？)

We first discuss the general concept of Qì, through both the traditional understanding and the modern scientific paradigms and concepts explaining Qìgōng.

A General Definition of Qì (Qì Zhī Yībān Dìngyì, 氣之一般定義)

Qì is the energy or natural force which fills the universe. The Chinese believe in Three Powers (Sāncái, 三才) of the universe: Heaven (Tiān, 天), Earth (Dì, 地) and Man (Rén, 人). Heaven (the sky or universe) has Heaven Qì (Tiānqì, 天氣), the most important of the three, consisting of forces exerted by heavenly bodies, such as sunshine, moonlight, gravity, and energy from the stars. Weather, climate, and natural disasters are governed by Heaven Qì (Tiānqì, 天氣). Every energy field strives to stay in balance, so when the Heaven Qì loses its balance, it tries to rebalance itself through wind, rain, and even tornadoes and hurricanes, which enable Heaven Qì to achieve a new energy balance.

Earth Qì (Dìqì, 地氣) is controlled by Heaven Qì. Too much rain forces a river to flood or change its path, but without rain, vegetation will die. The Chinese believe Earth Qì is made up of lines and patterns of energy, as well as the earth's magnetic field and the heat concealed underground. These energies must also be in balance, otherwise disasters such as earthquakes occur. When Earth Qì is balanced and harmonized, plants grow and animals thrive.

Finally, each individual person, animal, and plant has its own Qì field, which always seeks balance. Losing Qì balance, an individual sickens, dies, and decomposes. All natural things, including mankind and our Human Qì (Rénqì, 人氣), are determined by the natural cycles of Heaven Qì and Earth Qì. Throughout the history of Qìgōng, people have been most interested in Human Qì and its relationship with Heaven Qì and Earth Qì.

In China, Qì is also defined as any energy which demonstrates power and strength, be it electricity, magnetism, heat, or light. Electric power is called Electric Qì (Diànqì, 電氣), and heat is called Heat Qì (Rèqì, 熱氣). When a person is alive, his body's energy is called Human Qì (Rénqì, 人氣).

Qì also expresses the energy state of something, especially of living things. The weather is called Heaven Qì (Tiānqì, 天氣) because it indicates the energy state of the heavens. When something is alive it has Vital Qì (Huóqì, 活氣), and when dead it has Dead Qì (Sǐqì, 死氣) or Ghost Qì (Guǐqì, 鬼氣). When a person is righteous and has the spiritual strength to do good, he is said to have Normal Qì or Righteous Qì (Zhèngqì, 正氣). The spiritual state or morale of an army is called its Energy State (Qìshì, 氣勢).

Qì can represent energy itself, or else the state of the energy. It is important to understand this when you practice Qìgōng, so your mind is not channeled into a narrow understanding of Qì, limiting your future understanding and development.

A Narrow Definition of Qì (Qì Zhī Xiáyì, 氣之狹義)

Now let us look at how Qì is defined in Qìgōng society today. Among the Three Powers, the Chinese have been most concerned with Qì affecting health and longevity. After four thousand years emphasizing Human Qì, now when people mention Qì they usually mean Qì circulating in our bodies.

In ancient Chinese medical and Qìgōng documents, the word Qì was written "炁 " This character consists of two words, "旡" on top, which means "nothing", and "灬" at the bottom, which means "fire." So Qì was originally written as "no fire." In ancient times, physicians and Qìgōng practitioners attempted to balance the Yīn and Yáng Qì circulating in the body, so there was "no fire" in the internal organs. Each internal organ needs a specific amount of Qì to function properly. If it receives an improper amount (usually too much, which makes it too Yáng or on fire) it starts to malfunction, in time causing physical damage. The goal of Qìgōng was to attain a state of "no fire," which eventually became the word Qì.

But in more recent publications, the Qì of "no fire" has been replaced by the word "氣," again constructed of two words, "气" which means "air," and "米" which means "rice." Later practitioners realized that post-birth Qì is produced by breathing in air and consuming food. Air is called "Kōngqì" (空氣), literally "Space Energy."

For a long time, people debated what type of energy circulates in our bodies. Many believed it to be heat, others electricity, while others again assumed it was a mixture of heat, electricity, and light. This debate continued into the 1980s, when the concept of Qì gradually became clear. Today, science postulates that, with the possible exception of gravity, there is actually only one type of energy in the universe, namely electromagnetic energy. Líght and heat are also manifestations of electromagnetic energy. The Qì in our bodies is actually bioelectricity, and our bodies are a living electromagnetic field. Thus, the Qì is affected by our thoughts, feelings, activities, the food we eat, the quality of the air we breathe, our lifestyles, the natural energy that surrounds us, and also the unnatural energy which modern technology inflicts upon us.

The following scientific formula represents the major biochemical reaction in our body:

$$\text{glucose} + 6O_2 \longrightarrow 6CO_2 + 6H_2O$$

$$\Delta G^{o\prime} = -686 \text{ Kcal}$$

→ Heat
Líght
Bioelectricity (Qì)

As you can see, rice is glucose, oxygen is air, and bioelectricity is Qì.

A General Definition of Qìgōng (Qìgōng Zhī Yībān Dìngyì, 氣功之一般定義)

In China, the word "Gōng" (功) is often used instead of "Gōngfū" (Kūng Fū, 功夫), meaning energy and time. Any study or training which requires energy and time to achieve is called Gōngfū. It can be applied to any special skill or study requiring time, energy, and patience. Qìgōng is a science which studies the energy in nature. The main difference between this energy science and Western energy science is that Qìgōng focuses on the inner energy of human beings, while Western energy science pays more attention to the energy outside the human body. When you study Qìgōng, it is worthwhile to consider the modern scientific point of view, and not restrict yourself to traditional beliefs.

The Chinese have studied Qì for thousands of years, recording information on the patterns and cycles of nature in books such as the *Yìjīng* (易經, 1122 BCE), which describes the natural forces of Heaven (Tiān, 天), Earth (Dì, 地), and Man (Rén, 人). These Three Powers (Sāncái, 三才) manifest as Heaven Qì, Earth Qì, and Human Qì, with their definite rules and cycles. The rules are unchanging, while the cycles return to repeat themselves. The *Yìjīng* applies these principles to calculate changes in natural Qì, through a process called the Eight Trigrams (Bāguà, 八卦). From the Eight Trigrams are derived the 64 Hexagrams. The *Yìjīng* was probably the first book describing Qì and its variations in nature and man. The relationship of the Three Natural Powers and their Qì variations were later discussed extensively in the book *Theory of Qì's Variation* (*Qìhuàlùn*, 氣化論).

Understanding Heaven Qì is very difficult, and was especially so in ancient times. But since natural cycles recur, accumulated experience makes it possible to trace the natural patterns. Understanding the rules and cycles of Heavenly Timing (Tiānshí, 天時) helps describe changes in the seasons, climate, weather, and other natural occurrences. Many of these routine patterns and cycles are caused by the rebalancing of Qì. Various natural cycles recur every day, month, or year, while others return only every twelve or sixty years.

Earth Qì forms part of Heaven Qì. From understanding the rules and structure of the earth, you understand the process whereby mountains and rivers are formed, plants grow and rivers move, and also where it is best to build a house and which direction it should face to be a healthy place to live. In China, Geomancy Teachers (Dìlǐshī, 地理師), or Wind Water Teachers (Fēngshuǐshī, 風水師), make their living this way. The term Wind Water (Fēngshuǐ, 風水) is used because the location and character of wind and water are the most important factors in evaluating a location. These experts use the accumulated body of geomantic knowledge and the *Yìjīng* to help make important decisions such as where and how to build a house, where to bury the dead, and how to rearrange homes and offices to be better and more prosperous places in which to live and work.

Human Qì has been studied most thoroughly, encompassing many different aspects. The Chinese believe Human Qì is affected and controlled by Heaven Qì and Earth Qì, and that they in fact determine your destiny. By understanding the relationship between nature and people, and also Human Relations (Rénshì, 人事), you may predict wars, the destiny of a country, a person's desires and temperament, and even their future. The people who practice this profession are called Calculate Life Teachers (Suànmìngshī, 算命師).

However, the greatest achievement in the study of Human Qì is in regard to health and longevity. Since Qì is the source of life, if you understand how Qì functions and know how to regulate it correctly, you may live a long and healthy life. As a part of nature, you are channeled into its cycles, and it is in your best interest to follow the way of nature. This is the meaning of Dào (道), which can be translated as the Natural Way.

Many different aspects of Human Qì have been researched, including acupuncture, massage, herbal treatment, meditation, and Qìgōng exercises. Their use in adjusting Human Qì flow has become the root of Chinese medical science. Meditation and moving Qìgōng exercises are used to improve health and cure certain illnesses. Daoists and Buddhists also use meditation and Qìgōng exercises in their pursuit of enlightenment.

In conclusion, the study of any of the aspects of Qì, including Heaven Qì, Earth Qì, and Human Qì, should be called Qìgōng. However, since the term is usually used today only in reference to the cultivation of Human Qì through meditation and exercises, we will conform to this narrower definition.

A Narrow Definition of Qìgōng (Qìgōng Zhī Xiáyì, 氣功之狹義)

The narrow definition of Qì is the energy circulating in the human body. Qìgōng studies and trains the Qì circulating in the body. Qìgōng includes how our bodies relate to Heaven Qì and Earth Qì, and the overlapping fields of acupuncture, herbal treatment, martial arts Qìgōng, Qìgōng massage and exercises, and religious enlightenment Qìgōng.

In ancient times, Qìgōng was called "Tǔnà" (吐納), meaning to "utter and admit," referring to its focused breathing. Qìgōng depends on correct breathing. Zhuāngzi (莊子) said, "Blowing to breathe, utter the old and admit the new. The bear's natural movement, and the bird's extending (of the neck), are all for longevity. This is favored by those living as long as Péng, Zǔ (彭祖), who practice Dǎoyǐn (導引, guide and lead), and nourish the shape (cultivate the body)."[1] Péngzǔ was a legendary Qìgōng practitioner during the reign of emperor Yáo (堯, 2356 BCE), said to have lived for 800 years. Qìgōng was also called Dǎoyǐn, meaning to use the mind and physical movement to guide and lead Qì circulation. The movements imitate natural movements of animals such as bears and birds. A famous medical Qìgōng set passed down from that time is called The Five Animal Sports (Wǔqínxì, 五禽戲), which imitates the movements of the tiger, deer, bear, ape, and bird.

Qìgōng defines twelve major channels (Shíèrjīng, 十二經) in the body, branching into many secondary channels (Luò, 絡), similar to the blood circulatory system. The primary channels are like arteries and veins, while the secondary ones are like capillaries. The Twelve Primary Qì Channels are also like rivers, while the secondary channels are like streams flowing into and out of the rivers. Qì is distributed throughout the body through this network which connects the extremities to the internal organs, and the skin to the bone marrow. The internal organs of Chinese medicine do not necessarily correspond to the physical organs as understood in the West, but rather to a set of clinical functions related to the organ system.

The body also has Eight Vessels (Bāmài, 八脈), called strange meridians (Qíjīng, 奇經), that function like reservoirs and regulate the Qì circulation. The famous Chinese Daoist medical doctor Lǐ, Shí-Zhēn (李時珍) described them in his book, *The Study of Strange Meridians and Eight Vessels* (*Qíjīng Bāmài Kǎo*, 奇經八脈考): "The regular meridians (Twelve Primary Qì Channels) are like rivers, while the strange meridians (Eight Vessels) are like lakes. When the Qì in the regular meridians is abundant and flourishing, they overflow into the strange meridians."[2]

When Qì in the eight reservoirs is full and strong, so is the Qì in the rivers. Stagnation in any channel leads to irregularity in the Qì flow to the extremities and organs, and illness may develop. Every channel has its own particular Qì flow, its strength affected by your mind, the weather, time of day, food you have eaten, and even your mood. In dry weather, Qì in the lungs tends to be more positive and Yáng than in wet weather. When you are angry, the Qì flow in your liver channel will be irregular. Qì strength in different channels varies throughout the day in a regular cycle, and at any particular time one channel is strongest. For example, between 11 am and 1 pm the Qì flows most strongly in the heart channel. The Qì level of the same organ differs from one person to another. For more detail on the relationship of the Qì flow and time of day, refer to the YMAA book, *Qìgōng for Health and Martial Arts*.

When Qì flow in the twelve channels is irregular, the eight reservoirs regulate it back to normal. When one experiences a sudden shock, Qì in the bladder becomes deficient. The reservoir immediately regulates it to recover from the shock, unless the reservoir Qì is also deficient, or if the shock is too great. Then, the bladder contracts, causing urination.

A sick person's Qì tends to be either too positive (excess Yáng, 陽) or too negative (deficient Yīn, 陰). A Chinese physician would prescribe herbs to adjust the Qì, or else insert acupuncture needles at various points to adjust the flow and restore balance. The alternative is to practice Qìgōng, using physical and mental exercises to adjust the Qì.

In Scholar society, Qìgōng is defined differently, focusing on regulating disturbances of the Emotional Mind into a state of calm. This relaxes the body and enables Qì to rebalance and circulate smoothly, so mental and physical health may be attained.

In Daoist and Buddhist society, Qìgōng is the method to lead Qì from the Lower Dāntián (下丹田), or elixir field, to the brain for spiritual enlightenment or Buddhahood. This place in the abdomen stores Qì like a bioelectric battery. (We will discuss the

Dāntián in detail in section 2-3.) Religious Qìgōng is considered the highest and most rigorous level of Chinese Qìgōng training.

In martial arts society, Qìgōng is the theory and method of manifesting Qì to energize the physical body to its maximum efficiency and power. Martial arts Qìgōng originated from religious Qìgōng, especially Muscle/Tendon Changing and Marrow/Brain Washing Qìgōng (Yìjīnjīng and Xǐsuǐjīng, 易筋經、洗髓經), and the profoundest level of martial arts Qìgōng training is the same as that of religious Qìgōng, namely spiritual enlightenment.

1-3. Categories of Qìgōng (Qìgōng Zhī Fēnlèi, 氣功之分類)

I would like to discuss the scope of human Qìgōng, and the traditional concept of Nèidān (內丹, Internal Elixir) and Wàidān (外丹, External Elixir), to clarify the differences between the styles of Qìgōng practice around the world.

A. Scope of Qìgōng Practice—Physical and Mental (Qìgōng Liànxí Zhī Guīfàn, 氣功練習之規範)

If we trace Qìgōng history back to before the Chinese Qín and Hàn Dynasties (255 BCE–223 CE, 秦、漢), we find the origin of many Qìgōng practices in dancing. Dancing exercises the body and maintains it in a healthy condition. Matching movement with music harmonizes the mind, either to energize it or calm it down. This Qìgōng dancing was later passed to Japan during the Hàn Dynasty, and became the very elegant, slow, and refined dancing still practiced today in the Japanese Royal Court.

African and Native American dancing, in which the body is bounced up and down, also loosens the joints and improves Qì circulation. Any activity which regulates Qì circulation in the body, even jogging or weightlifting, may be regarded as Qìgōng. Aspects of this include the food we eat, the air we breathe, and even our emotions and thoughts.

In Figure 1-1, the vertical axis to the left represents Qì use by the physical body (Yáng), and the right vertex that of the mind (Yīn). The more to the left an activity is represented, the more physical effort and the less mental effort is needed. This can be aerobics, dancing, walking, or jogging in which the mind is used less than the body. This does not require special training, and is classified as secular Qìgōng. At the mid-point of the graph, mental and physical activity are combined in equal measure. This would be the slow-moving Qìgōng commonly practiced, in which the mind is used to lead Qì in coordination with movement. With slow, relaxed movements, the Qì led by the mind may reach deeper into the ligaments, marrow, and internal organs. Deep internal feeling can lead Qì there significantly. Tàijí, White Crane, Snake, and Dragon are typical systems of Qìgōng, cultivated intensively in Chinese medical and martial arts societies.

At a deeper level of practice, the mind becomes critically important. It is actively involved while you are in deep relaxation. This is cultivated primarily by scholars and religious Qìgōng practitioners. There may be some physical movement in the lower abdomen, but the main focus is cultivating a peaceful and neutral mind, and pursuing the final goal of spiritual enlightenment. This practice includes Sitting Chán (坐禪) (i.e., Zen), Embryonic Breathing (Tāixí Jìngzuò, 胎息靜坐), Small Circulation (Xiǎozhōutiān, 小周天), Grand Circulation (Dàzhōutiān, 大周天), and Brain Washing Enlightenment Meditation (Xǐsuǐgōng, 洗髓功).

Different Qìgōng practices aim for different goals. For a long, happy life, you need health of mind and body. The best Qìgōng for health is at the middle of our model, to regulate both body and mind. You may practice the Yīn side through still meditation, and the Yáng side through physical activity. This balances Yīn and Yáng, and abundant Qì may be accumulated and circulated.

From this we may conclude:

1. Any activity able to improve Qì circulation is Qìgōng.
2. Qìgōng which emphasizes the physical aspect will improve physical strength and Qì circulation, conditioning the muscles, tendons, and ligaments.

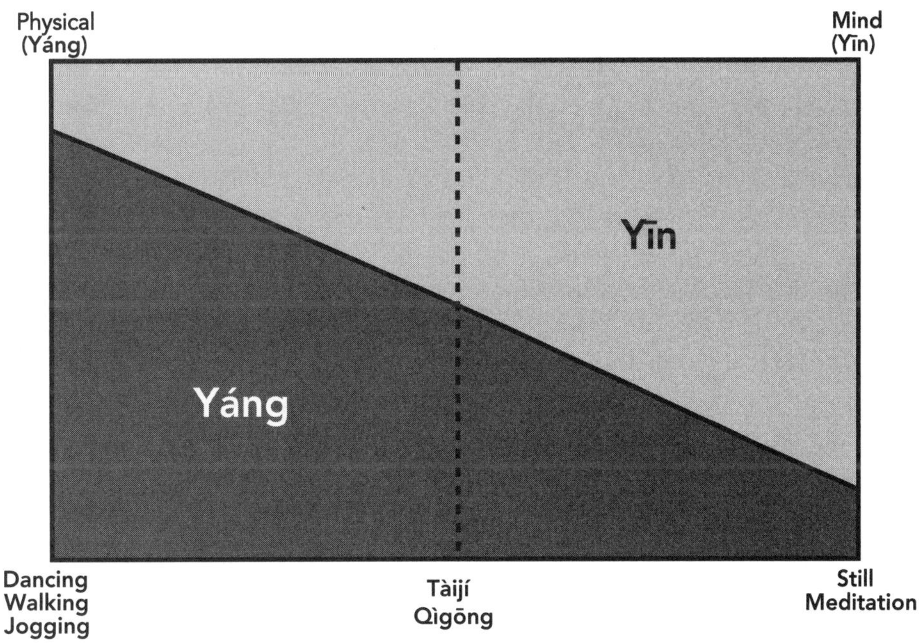

Figure 1-1. The Range of Defined Qìgōng

3. Qìgōng activating both the physical and the mental can reach deeper, enhancing physical strength and Qì circulation. By coordinating the relaxed physical body with a concentrated mind, Qì may circulate deep inside the joints, internal organs, and even the bone marrow.
4. Qìgōng which focuses on achieving a profound meditative state may, however, neglect physical movement, causing physical strength to degenerate.

External and Internal Elixirs (Wàidān and Nèidān, 外丹與內丹)

Qìgōng practices can be divided according to their training theory and methods into two general categories, Wàidān (外丹, External Elixir) and Nèidān (內丹, Internal Elixir). Understanding the differences between them gives you an overview of Qìgōng practice.

Wàidān (External Elixir, 外丹). Wai means external, and Dān means elixir. External here means the skin and surface of the body, and also the limbs, as opposed to the torso at the center of the body, which includes the vital organs. Elixir is the life-prolonging substance for which Chinese Daoists searched for millennia. They first thought it was something physical which could be prepared from herbs or from chemicals purified in a furnace. After thousands of years of experimentation, they found the elixir within, namely, Qì circulating in the body. To prolong your life, you must develop the elixir in your body, cultivating, protecting, and nourishing it.

In Wàidān Qìgōng practice, you exercise to build Qì in your arms and legs. When enough Qì accumulates there, it flows through the Twelve Primary Qì Channels clearing obstructions and into the center of the body to nourish the organs. A person who works out, or has a physical job, is generally healthier than one who sits around all day.

Massage, acupuncture, and herbal treatment are all Wàidān practices. Massaging the body produces Qì, stimulating the cells to a more energized state. Qì is raised and circulation enhanced. After a massage you are relaxed, and the higher levels of Qì in the muscles and skin flow into the torso and internal organs. This is the theoretical foundation of Tuīná (push and grab, 推拿) Qìgōng massage. Acupuncture may also enhance Qì, regulating the internal organs.

Any stimulation or exercise that generates a high level of Qì in the limbs or at the surface of the body, which then flows into the center of the body, can be classified as Wàidān (Figure 1-2).

Nèidān (Internal Elixir, 內丹). Nei means internal. Nèidān means to build up the elixir internally, inside the body instead of in the limbs, in the vessels rather than the channels. Whereas in Wàidān, Qì is built up in the limbs or skin then moved into the body through the primary Qì channels, Nèidān exercises build up Qì inside the body and lead it out to the limbs (Figure 1-3). This is accomplished by special breathing techniques

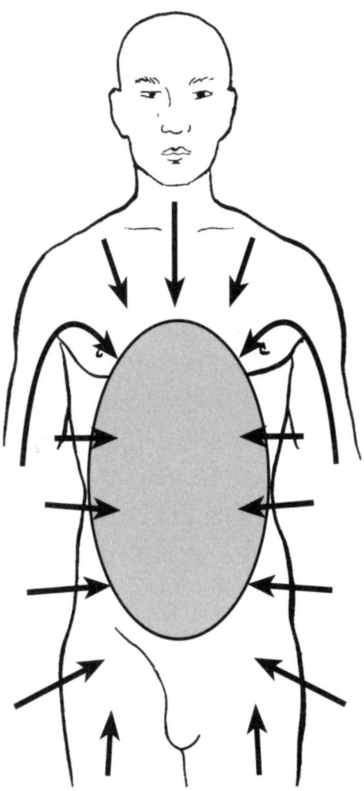

Figure 1-2. External Elixir (Wàidān)

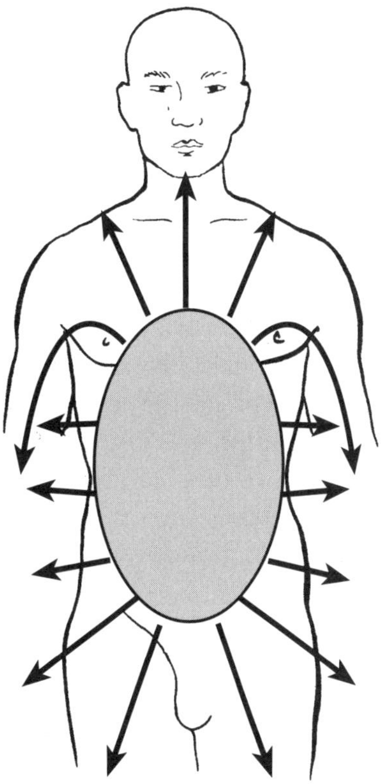

Figure 1-3. Internal Elixir (Nèidān)

during meditation. First, one builds abundant Qì in the Lower Dāntián, the bioelectric battery, then leads it to the Eight Vessels for storage. Then Qì in the Twelve Primary Channels can be regulated smoothly and efficiently.

Nèidān is more profound than Wàidān, and is more difficult to understand and practice. Traditionally, Nèidān Qìgōng practices were passed down more secretively than Wàidān, especially at the highest levels such as Marrow/Brain Washing, which were passed down to only a few trusted disciples.

Schools of Qìgōng Practice (Qìgōng Liànxí Zhī Ménpài, 氣功練習之門派)

Qìgōng has four major categories according to the purpose of training: A. curing illness, B. maintaining health, C. enlightenment or Buddhahood, and D. martial arts. Most styles serve more than one of these purposes. For example, Daoist Qìgōng aims for longevity and enlightenment, but you need to maintain good health and cure sickness. Knowing the history and principles of each category helps understand their essence more clearly.

Medical Qìgōng—for Healing. In ancient China, most emperors respected scholars and their philosophy. Doctors were not highly regarded, because they made their diagnosis by touching the patient's body, which was considered characteristic of the lower social classes. Although doctors were commonly looked down upon, they quietly passed down the results of their research to following generations. Of all the groups studying Qìgōng in China, doctors have been at it the longest. Since the discovery of Qì circulation in the human body about four thousand years ago, Chinese doctors have devoted major efforts to study it, developing acupuncture, acupressure, and herbal treatment.

Many Chinese doctors also created sets of Qìgōng for maintaining health or curing specific illnesses. Doing only sitting meditation with breathing, as in scholar Qìgōng or Buddhist Chán meditation, is not enough to cure illness, and they believed in using movement to increase Qì circulation. Although a calm and peaceful mind is important for health, exercising the body is more important. They learned through practice that people who exercised properly got sick less often, and their bodies degenerated less quickly than people who just sat around. Specific movements increase Qì circulation in specific organs, and are used to treat specific illnesses and restore normal function.

Some movements are similar to the way certain animals move. For an animal to survive in the wild, it must instinctively protect its body, especially accumulating its Qì and preserving it. We humans have lost many of these instincts over time, as we have been separating ourselves from nature.

A typical, well-known set of such exercises is Wǔqínxì (Five Animal Sports, 五禽戲), created nearly two thousand years ago by Huátuó (華佗), though some say it was by Jūnqiàn (君倩). Another famous set is Bāduànjǐn (八段錦), The Eight Pieces of Brocade. It was developed by Marshal Yuè, Fēi (岳飛) during the Southern Sòng Dynasty (1127–1280 CE, 南宋), who was a soldier and scholar rather than a doctor.

Before physical damage manifests in an organ, there is first an abnormality in Qì circulation. Excess Yīn or Yáng is the root of illness and organ damage. In a specific channel, abnormal Qì circulation leads to organ malfunction. If the condition is not corrected, the organ degenerates. The best way to heal is to adjust and balance the Qì before there is any physical problem, and this is the major goal of acupuncture and acupressure treatment. Herbs and special diets also help regulate the Qì.

As long as the illness is limited to Qì stagnation and there is no physical organ damage, Qìgōng exercises can be used to readjust Qì circulation and treat the problem. But if the sickness is already so serious that the organs have started to fail, the situation is critical and specific treatment is necessary. This can be acupuncture, herbs, or even an operation. Ulcers, asthma, and even certain kinds of cancer are often treated effectively with simple exercises.

Over thousands of years of observing nature, Qìgōng practitioners went even deeper. Qì circulation changes with the seasons, so they helped the body during these periodic adjustments. In each season different organs have characteristic problems. For example, at the beginning of autumn, the lungs adapt to breathing colder air, making them susceptible to colds. Other organs are also affected by seasonal changes, and by one another. Focusing on these seasonal Qì disorders, they developed movements to speed up the body's adjustment. These sets were originally created to maintain health, and later were also used for curing sickness.

Scholar Qìgōng—for Maintaining Health. Before the Hàn Dynasty (206 BCE–221 CE, 漢朝), two major scholar societies arose. One was founded by Confucius (551–479 BCE, Kǒngzǐ, 孔子) during the Spring and Autumn Period (722–484 BCE, Chūnqiū, 春秋). His philosophy was popularized and expanded by Mencius (372–289 BCE, Mèngzǐ, 孟子) during the Warring States Period (403–222 BCE, Zhànguó, 戰國). Scholars who practice his philosophy are called Confucians (Rújiā, 儒家). Their basic philosophy consists of Loyalty (Zhōng, 忠), Filial Piety (Xiào, 孝), Humanity (Rén, 仁), Kindness (Ài, 愛), Trust (Xìn, 信), Justice (Yì, 義), Harmony (Hé, 和) and Peace (Píng, 平). Humanity and human feelings are the main subjects, and Confucian philosophy is the root of much of Chinese culture.

The second major scholar society was Daoism (Dàojiā, 道家), established by Lǎozi (老子) in the 6th century BCE. His classic, the *Dào Dé Jīng* (道德經, *Classic on the Virtue of the Dào*), describes human morality. During the Warring States Period, his follower Zhuāngzhōu (莊周) wrote a book called *Zhuāngzi* (莊子), which led to the forming of another strong branch of Daoism. Before the Hàn Dynasty, Daoism was considered a branch of scholarship. However, in the East Hàn Dynasty (25–168 CE, 東漢), traditional Daoism was combined with Buddhism (which was newly imported from India) by Zhāng, Dào-Líng (張道陵), and began to be treated as a religion. Daoism before the Hàn Dynasty should be considered scholarly Daoism rather than religious.

With regard to Qìgōng, both schools emphasized maintaining health and preventing disease. Many illnesses are caused by mental and emotional excesses. When one's mind is disturbed, the organs do not function normally. For example, depression may cause stomach ulcers and indigestion. Anger may cause the liver to malfunction. Sadness may lead to stagnation and tightness in the lungs, and fear can disturb the normal functioning of the kidneys and bladder. To avoid illness, you need to balance and relax your thoughts and emotions. This is called Regulating the Mind (Tiáoxīn, 調心).

Both schools emphasize gaining a peaceful mind through meditation. In still meditation, the primary training is getting rid of thoughts, clearing the mind. As the flow of thoughts and emotions slows down, you feel mentally and emotionally neutral, leading to self-control. In this state of "no thought" you even relax deep down into your internal organs, and your Qì circulation is smooth and strong.

This still meditation is very common in Chinese scholar society, which focuses on regulating the mind, body, and breath, so Qì flows smoothly and sickness may be averted. Their training is called Xiūqì (修氣), which means cultivating Qì. This is very different from the religious Daoist Qìgōng, called Líànqì (練氣), meaning "to train Qì to make it stronger."

Qìgōng documents from Confucians and Daoists are mainly limited to maintaining health. Their aim is to follow natural destiny and maintain health. This is quite different from that of religious Daoists after the East Hàn Dynasty, who believed one's destiny could be changed. They believed it possible to train your Qì to make it stronger, and to extend your life. Scholar society maintained that "in human life, seventy is rare."[3] Few common people in ancient times reached seventy as a result of the harsh conditions. They also said, "peace with Heaven and delight in your destiny" (Āntiān Lèmìng, 安天樂命), and "cultivate the body and await destiny" (Xiūshēn Sìmìng, 修身俟命). Compare this with the philosophy of the later Daoists, who said, "one hundred and twenty means dying young."[4] They proved by example that life can be extended, and destiny resisted and overcome.

Religious Qìgōng for Enlightenment or Buddhahood. Religious Qìgōng, though not as popular as other categories in China, has achieved the greatest accomplishments of all categories of Qìgōng. It was kept secret in the monasteries, and only revealed to seculars, or laypeople, in the last century.

It comprises mainly Daoist and Buddhist Qìgōng. The main purpose of their training is striving for enlightenment or Buddhahood. They seek to rise above normal human suffering and escape from the cycle of continual reincarnation. They believe all human suffering is caused by the seven passions and six desires (Qīqíng Líùyù, 七情六慾). The seven passions are happiness (Xǐ, 喜), anger (Nù, 怒), sorrow (Āi, 哀), joy (Lè, 樂), love (Ài, 愛), hate (Hèn, 恨), and desire (Yù, 慾). The six desires are the six sensory pleasures of the eyes, ears, nose, tongue, body, and mind. If you are bound to them, you will reincarnate after death. To avoid this, they train to be spiritually independent of the body, and of physical attachments and circumstances. Thereby they enter the heavenly kingdom and gain eternal peace. This rigorous training is called Unification of Heaven and Man (Tiānrén Héyī, 天人合一). It is extremely difficult to achieve in the everyday world, so practitioners generally shun society and move into the solitude of the mountains, where they can concentrate all their energies on spiritual cultivation.

Religious Qìgōng practitioners train to strengthen internal Qì, to nourish their spirit (Shén, 神) until it can survive the death of the body. Marrow/Brain Washing Qìgōng training enables them to lead Qì to the brain, where the spirit resides, and to raise the brain cells to a higher energy state. This training used to be restricted to only a few advanced priests in China and Tibet. Over the last two thousand years, Tibetan and Chinese Buddhists, and the religious Daoists, have followed the same principles to become the three major religious schools of Qìgōng training.

This religious striving toward enlightenment or Buddhahood is recognized as the highest and most difficult level of Qìgōng. Many practitioners reject the rigors of this religious striving, and practice Marrow/Brain Washing Qìgōng solely for longevity. It was these people who eventually revealed the secrets of Marrow/Brain Washing to the outside world, as described in *Qìgōng—The Secret of Youth*.

Martial Qìgōng—for Fighting. Chinese martial Qìgōng developed from Dámó's *Muscle/Tendon Changing and Marrow/Brain Washing Qìgōng Classic (Yìjīnjīng, Xǐsuǐjīng*; 易筋經，洗髓經), written in the Shàolín Temple (Shàolínsì, 少林寺) during the Líáng Dynasty (502–557 CE, 梁朝). Shàolín monks training this Qìgōng improved their health and greatly increased their martial power and effectiveness. Since then, many martial styles have developed further Qìgōng sets, and many martial styles have been created based on Qìgōng theory. Martial artists have played a major role in Chinese Qìgōng society.

When Qìgōng theory was first applied to martial arts, it was used to increase the power and efficiency of the muscles. The mind which is generated from clear thinking (Yì, 意) leads Qì to the muscles to energize them to function more efficiently. The average person generally uses his muscles at about 40 percent efficiency. Training a strong Yì to lead Qì to the muscles effectively, one may energize the muscles to a higher level, increasing fighting effectiveness.

Acupuncture theory enabled fighting techniques to reach even more advanced levels. Martial artists learned to attack vital cavities, disturbing the enemy's Qì flow to cause injury and death. Central to this is understanding the route and timing of Qì circulation in the body, to strike the cavities accurately and to the correct depth. These techniques are called Diǎnxuè (點穴, Pointing Cavities) or Diǎnmài (點脈, Pointing Vessels).

While most martial Qìgōng practices also improve the practitioner's health, there are some which, although they build up some special skill useful for fighting, also damage the practitioner's health. An example of this is Iron Sand Palm (Tiěshāzhǎng, 鐵砂掌). Although it builds amazing destructive power, it can also harm your hands and affect the Qì circulation in the hands and internal organs.

Many martial styles have developed from Dámó's 6th-century Qìgōng theory and methods. They can be roughly divided into external and internal styles. The external styles emphasize building Qì in the limbs for physical martial techniques, following the practices of Wàidān Qìgōng. The concentrated mind is used during the exercises to energize the Qì. This significantly increases muscular strength and the effectiveness of the martial techniques. Qìgōng trains the body to resist punches and kicks, by leading Qì to energize the skin and the muscles, enabling them to resist a blow without injury. This training is called Iron Shirt (Tiěbùshān, 鐵布衫) or Golden Bell Cover (Jīnzhōngzhào, 金鐘罩). Martial styles which use Wàidān training are called external styles (Wàijiā, 外家). Hard Qìgōng training is called Hard Gōng (Yìnggōng, 硬功). Shàolín Gōngfū is a typical example of a style using Wàidān martial Qìgōng.

Although Wàidān Qìgōng increases the martial artist's power, training the muscles can cause overdevelopment, leading to energy dispersion (Sàngōng, 散功). To prevent this, when an external martial artist reaches a high level of external training he will start training internal Qìgōng, which specializes in curing the energy dispersion problem. "The external styles are from external to internal and from hard to soft."[5]

By contrast, Internal Martial Qìgōng is based on the theory of Nèidān. Qì is generated in the torso instead of the limbs, and later led to the limbs to increase power. To lead Qì to the limbs, the techniques must be soft and muscle use kept to a minimum. Nèidān martial training is much more difficult than Wàidān. For more detail refer to the book, *Tai Chi Chuan Martial Power*.

Several internal martial styles were created in the Wǔdāng (武當山) and Éméi (峨嵋山) Mountains. Popular ones are Tàijíquán (太極拳), Bāguàzhǎng (八卦掌), Líùhé Bāfǎ (六合八法) and Xíngyìquán (形意拳). Even internal martial styles, called Soft Styles, must sometimes use muscular strength while fighting. Utilizing strong power in a fight requires Qì to manifest externally, using harder, more external techniques. "Internal styles are from internal to external and from soft to hard."[6]

Although Qìgōng is widely studied in Chinese martial society, the main focus is on increasing fighting ability rather than on health. Good health is considered a by-product of training. Only recently has health started receiving greater attention in martial Qìgōng, especially in the internal martial arts.

1-4. Theory of Yīn and Yáng, Kǎn and Lí (Yīn/Yáng Kǎn/Lí Zhī Lǐlùn, 陰陽坎離之理論)

The most important concepts in Qìgōng practice are the theories of Yīn and Yáng, and of Kǎn and Lí. These two different concepts have become confused in Qìgōng society, even in China. If you understand them clearly, you have grasped an important key to Qìgōng practice.

What Are Kǎn and Lí?

The terms Kǎn (坎) and Lí (離) occur frequently in Qìgōng documents. In the Eight Trigrams, Kǎn represents Water while Lí represents Fire. Kǎn and Lí training has long been of major importance to Qìgōng practitioners.

Although Kǎn-Lí and Yīn-Yáng are related, Kǎn and Lí are not Yīn and Yáng. Kǎn is Water, which cools your body down and makes it more Yīn, while Lí is Fire, which warms your body and makes it more Yáng. Kǎn and Lí are the methods or causes, while Yīn and Yáng are the results. When Kǎn and Lí are adjusted correctly, Yīn and Yáng are balanced and interact harmoniously.

Qìgōng practitioners believe your body is always too Yáng, unless you are sick or have not eaten for a long time. Excess Yáng leads the body to degenerate and burn out, causing aging. Using Water to cool down your body, you can slow the aging process and lengthen your life. Qìgōng practitioners improve the quality of Water in their bodies, and reduce the quantity of Fire. You should always keep this subject at the top of your list for study and research. If you earnestly ponder and experiment, you will grasp the trick of adjusting them.

Water and Fire represent many things in the body. First, Qì is classified according to Fire or Water. When your Qì is not pure, causing your body to heat up and your mind to become unstable (Yáng), it is classified as Fire Qì (Huǒqì, 火氣). The Qì which is pure and can cool your physical and spiritual bodies, making them more Yīn, is Water Qì (Shuǐqì, 水氣). Your Qì should never be purely Water. It may cool down the Fire, but should never quench it, which would signify death.

Fire Qì agitates and stimulates the emotions, generating from them the Emotional Mind called Xīn (心), which is considered the Fire mind or Yáng mind. On the other hand, the mind that Water Qì generates is calm, steady and wise. It is called Yì (意), and considered to be the Water mind or Wisdom Mind. If your spirit is nourished primarily by Fire Qì, although your spirit may be high, as a Yáng spirit it will be scattered and confused. If the spirit is nourished and raised up mainly by Water Qì, it will be a firm, steady Yīn mind. When your Yì governs your Xīn effectively, your will, as strong emotional intention, can be firm.

Your Qì is the main cause of the Yīn and Yáng of your body, mind and spirit. To regulate Yīn and Yáng, you need to regulate Water and Fire Qì at their source.

To analyze Kǎn and Lí and adjust them efficiently, apply modern science to marry the past and the present, and to give birth to the future. The reliance of modern medicine on drugs is the worst way to cure illness or gain health. The best way is to solve the problem at its root. Ancient China did not have our modern medical chemistry, and had to develop other ways to adjust the body's Water and Fire. We could learn much from them. For example, many arthritis patients today rely on medicine to reduce pain. While this may offer temporary relief from pain, it does not cure the problem. When the medicine is gone, the pain resumes. Chinese medical Qìgōng cures arthritis by rebuilding the strength of the joints. Patients increase Qì circulation with slow, easy exercises, and massage to strengthen the joints. These practices readjust the Yīn and Yáng balance, allowing the body to repair the damage and increase the strength of the joints. This approach addresses the root of the problem.

Nevertheless, many modern medical practices conform to Kǎn and Lí theory. Fever is treated by applying medicine and ice cubes to reduce the temperature. Ice cubes are used to reduce swelling caused by injuries. Whether you follow ancient or modern medicine, the basic theory of healing remains the same, namely adjustment of Kǎn and Lí. Medical chemistry has brought us much that is marvelous, but also many problems.

The key is understanding the circulation of Qì, or bioelectricity, in the body. Regulating it strengthens the body and maintains health, allowing doctors to correct irregular

Qì even before the appearance of physical symptoms, and increasing the quality and duration of life.

The Keys to Kǎn and Lí Adjustment

Here we discuss how Kǎn and Lí relate to your breathing, mind and spirit, and the keys to regulating them in Qìgōng practice. Combining them, we construct a secret key which leads to the Qìgōng treasure.

Kǎn and Lí of Breathing. In Qìgōng, breathing is considered a strategy to lead the Qì. Directing your breath, you may lead Qì to the skin or marrow. Breathing slowly can calm the Qì flow, while rapid breathing can invigorate it. When you are excited, your body is Yáng, and you exhale longer than you inhale. This leads Qì to the skin, where excess Qì dissipates through sweat. When you are sad your body is Yīn, and you inhale longer than you exhale. This preserves Qì by leading it inward, and you feel cold. Through breathing you adjust the body's Yīn and Yáng, so breathing has Kǎn and Lí.

Inhaling is a Water (Kǎn) activity, because you lead Qì inward to store it in the bone marrow. This reduces Guardian Qì (Wèiqì, 衛氣) and the Qì in the muscles and tendons, calming the body's Yáng. Exhaling is a Fire (Lí) activity because it brings Qì out to the muscles, tendons and skin to energize them, making the body more Yáng, and enhancing Guardian Qì. When the body is more Yáng than its surroundings, its Qì is dissipated.

Yīn and Yáng should be balanced so your body functions harmoniously. The trick is using breathing strategies. Usually inhalation and exhalation should be equal. When you are excited your body is too Yáng, so you may inhale longer and deeper to calm your mind and lead Qì in, to make it more Yīn.

Exhalation leads Qì to the skin and to the five extremities (the crown, the two Láogōng (P-8, 勞宮) cavities at the center of the palms, and the two Yǒngquán (K-1, 湧泉) cavities near the centers of the soles), to exchange with your surroundings. Inhalation leads Qì deep inside your body to reach the internal organs and marrow. Table 1-1 summarizes how different breathing strategies affect Yīn and Yáng in their various manifestations.

Kǎn and Lí of the Mind. According to Chinese tradition, one has two minds: Xīn (心) and Yì (意). Xīn means heart, the mind generated by emotional disturbance, or Emotional Mind. The Chinese word Yì comprises three characters. The top one means establish (Lì, 立), the middle one means speaking (Yuē, 曰), and the bottom one means heart (Xīn, 心). That means the Emotional Mind is under control as you establish communication with your heart. Yì can be translated as Wisdom Mind. Xīn makes you excited and disturbs your emotions, making your body Yáng, so it is considered Lí. Yì makes you calm, peaceful and able to think clearly (Yīn), so it is considered Kǎn.

In Qìgōng training, the mind is the general who directs the battle, decides on fighting strategy (breathing), and directs the movement of the soldiers (Qì). As a general, you

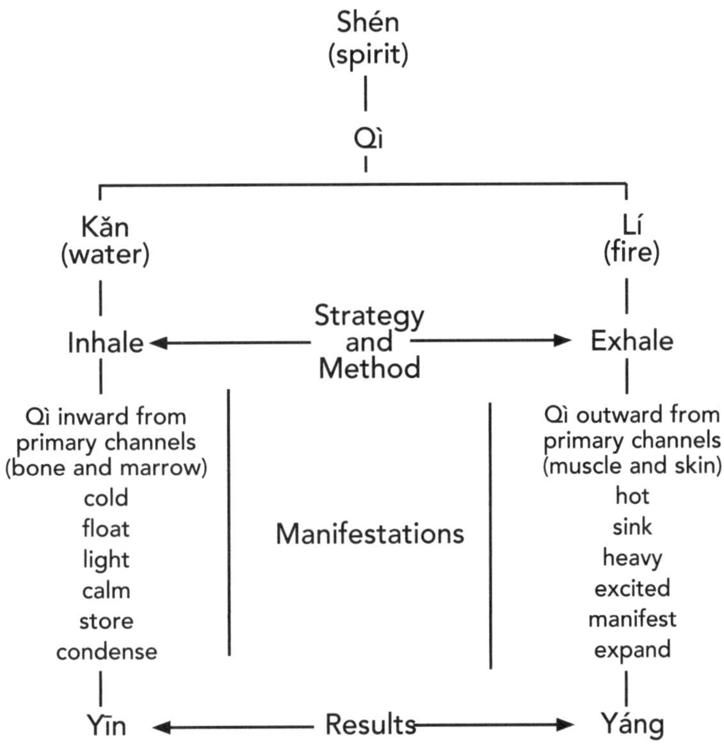

Table 1-1. The Effects of Breathing on the Body's Yīn and Yáng in their Various Manifestations

control your Xīn (Emotional Mind) and use your Yì (Wisdom Mind) to judge the situation and decide on the proper strategy.

In Qìgōng, your Yì dominates the situation and generates an idea. This idea generates and executes the strategy (breathing), and is the force moving the Qì. When your mind is excited and energized, the strategy (breathing) is more offensive (emphasizing exhalation) and Qì circulation is more vigorous and expansive. This aggressive mind is considered a Fire mind, making your body more Yáng. When the strategy is more defensive (emphasizing inhalation), Qì circulation will be calmer and more condensed. A calm or depressed mind is a Water mind, since it makes your body more Yīn.

The mind's Kǎn and Lí are more important than breathing, since the mind determines the strategy. Regulating mind and breathing are the two basic techniques for controlling your body's Yīn and Yáng. Regulating mind and breathing cannot be separated. When the mind is regulated, so can the breathing, and when breathing is regulated, the mind enters a deeper level of calm.

Kǎn and Lí of the Shén. Now let's consider the most decisive element in winning a battle: the Shén (Spirit). Shén is the morale of the general's officers and soldiers. There are many cases throughout history of armies winning battles against great odds because the morale of their soldiers was high.

It is the same in Qìgōng training, where the Shén determines how successful your Qìgōng practice will be. Your Yì, the general who makes the strategy, must be concerned with raising up the fighting morale (Shén) of the soldiers (Qì). When morale is high the soldiers are led efficiently and strategy is executed effectively.

Using Yì to raise Shén is the primary key to successful Qìgōng training. Shén is the headquarters which governs Qì, together with the Yi. Yì and Shén are closely related and cannot be separated.

When Yì is energized, Shén is also raised. You want to raise up your Shén but not get it excited. When Shén is raised, strategy is carried out effectively, but if Shén is excited, the body becomes too Yáng, which is not desirable in Qìgōng practice. When you practice Qìgōng, you want to keep your Shén high at all times, to govern the strategy and the Qì. This enables you to regulate Kǎn and Lí.

Shén is the control tower which adjusts Kǎn and Lí, but does not have Kǎn and Lí itself. Some practitioners consider raised Shén to be Lí (Fire) and calm Shén to be Kǎn (Water).

Now, let us draw a few important conclusions from this discussion:

- Kǎn (Water) and Lí (Fire) are not Yīn and Yáng. Kǎn and Lí are methods which regulate Yīn or Yáng.
- Qì itself is only a form of energy and does not have Kǎn and Lí. When Qì is excessive or deficient, it can make the body too Yáng or too Yīn.
- When you adjust Kǎn and Lí in the body, the mind is the first concern. The mind can be Kǎn or Lí. It determines the strategy (breathing) for withdrawing Qì (Kǎn) or expanding it (Lí).
- Breathing has Kǎn and Lí. Inhaling is Kǎn as it makes the body more Yīn, while exhaling, which makes the body more Yáng, is Lí.
- Shén does not have Kǎn and Lí. Shén is the key to making the adjustment of Kǎn and Lí effective.

The Keys to Adjusting Kǎn and Lí

The keys to Kǎn and Lí adjustment are mentioned repeatedly in the ancient documents. The first key is that Shén and Breathing mutually rely on each other. The second key is that Shén and Qì mutually combine.

Shén and Breathing Mutually Dependent (Shénxí Xiāngyī, 神息相依). Breathing is the strategy which directs Qì in various ways, controlling and adjusting Kǎn and Lí, which in turn control the body's Yīn and Yáng. Shén is the controlling influence which makes strategy work most efficiently. Shén governs strategy directly, and controls Kǎn and Lí and the body's Yīn and Yáng indirectly. The success of your Kǎn and Lí adjustment depends upon your Shén.

When Shén matches respiration, it leads Qì directly to condense and expand in the most efficient way. Shén must match the breathing for it to be raised up or calmed down, and the breathing must rely on Shén to make the strategy work. It seems Shén and breathing are dependent on each other and cannot be separated. This training is called Shénxí Xiāngyī, which means Shén and breathing depend on each other. When Shén and breathing match each other, it is called Shénxí (神息) or spirit breathing, because it seems your Shén is actually doing the breathing.

Shénxí Xiāngyī is a technique in which, when Shén and breathing are united, Shén controls the Qì directly.

Shén and Qì Mutually Combine (Shénqì Xiànghé, 神氣相合). When Shén and breathing match each other as one, the Qì is led directly, so Shén and Qì become one. This is called Shénqì Xiànghé, which means Shén and Qì mutually harmonized. Shén governs Qì directly and efficiently. Harmony of Shén and Qì is the result of Shén and breathing being mutually dependent.

Dámó believed that to have a long and peaceful life, Shén and Qì must coordinate and harmonize with each other. He said, "If one does not keep mother (Qì) and son (Shén) together, though Qì breathes internally, Shén is labored and craves the external, so Shén is always debauched and dirty and thus not clear. If Shén is not clear, original harmonious Qì will disperse gradually, and they cannot be kept together."[7] The spirit is very important, and regulating Shén is one of the highest levels of Qìgōng practice. To reach a high level of harmony, first regulate your Emotional Mind, which is hard to achieve in secular society.

1-5. Qìgōng and Health (Qìgōng Yǔ Jiànkāng, 氣功與健康)

When we discuss the relationship between Qìgōng practice and health, we should first define health. There are two aspects of health, the Yáng side of physical health which can be seen, and the Yīn side of mental health which can only be felt. More than half of today's sickness is caused by mental problems such as depression, stress, and mental fatigue. There are several reasons:

1. Due to our changing social structure, the pressure of living in today's society is greater than ever. Our modern lifestyle only started in the 20th century. Before then, industry did not heavily dominate the social structure, and many people lived as farmers. The struggle of living in a society demanding more

money and material enjoyment dominates our thinking and generates great pressure. In a few short decades, we have become slaves to money. We have lost the original lifestyle which connected us with nature and spiritual feeling. We are facing a revolution which is changing the old life style to the new one, generating many mental problems.

2. Medical science has advanced to a high level and controls most common illnesses, but is still limited to the Yáng side of understanding. It lacks interest in and knowledge of the bioenergetic aspect of body, mind, and spirit. Because of this, we miss half of human science, and are unable to solve several problems and illnesses. We cannot effectively cure problems such as cancer and AIDS. Also, lacking understanding of our mental and spiritual center, we cannot solve mental illness. Many scientists believe that we understand less than 12 percent of the function of the brain.
3. Due to the decline of religious belief, seculars have lost their guide in understanding the meaning of life. This is because knowledge of the general public has increased, and religious dogma is questioned more seriously than ever. Religious authorities cannot offer an educational program which is persuasive to the new open-minded generation. Most churches still preach with methods used for thousands of years. This is very unfortunate, since many people have become lost in today's new society. Many Westerners cannot find new meaning in their lives from traditional religion, so turn to Eastern religions and philosophy, hoping to find answers and peace.
4. Internal cultivation, such as meditation, has been largely ignored. Many people build up a facade in order to hide their true selves from others. We lie and hide our fears and guilty feelings deep in our subconscious mind. Going to confession (Western way), or removing our mask through meditation (Eastern way), were traditional ways of releasing pent-up emotions and balancing our feelings. Today, many people have lost these two most powerful methods of relieving mental imbalance induced by suppressed emotions and feelings of guilt.

Our mental condition is closely related to our health. Many diseases are caused by mental imbalance, which results in disharmonious Qì circulation in the body. To have good health you need a strong body, but also a healthy mind. Qìgōng for healing and for maintaining health is based on this concept.

To maintain physical strength, Qìgōng exercises which condition the muscles, tendons, ligaments, and bones were developed. Before Dámó (483 to 536 CE, 達摩), many exercises were developed by doctors to regulate sickness and facilitate healing. Dámó brought a different concept as recorded in the *Muscle/Tendon Changing Classic*

(*Yìjīnjīng*, 易筋經). Since then, based on this training, countless Wàidān Qìgōng styles were created.

Meditation was developed by different schools to regulate the mind into peace and harmony. Meditation not only brings a peaceful mind, but also builds up abundant Qì to circulate in the body, through the Qì channels and vessels.

Modern medical science has improved health and extended lives significantly. But today's scientific achievement is still in its infancy. Many new problems have arisen due to the new social structure and environment. The pressure generated in today's society has caused many mental problems, and many new diseases have emerged. For example, the increase of breast cancer is caused by going against the course of nature. Even fifty years ago, many women could expect to bear at least ten children. There was a constant Qì exchange between mothers and babies. Today we control birth and most women will not bear more than three babies in their lifetime. Qì is trapped in the breast area and generates cancer cells. We should understand one important thing. The body we have now has developed through millions of years of evolution. It is impossible for us to fit into the new lifestyle created only in the last few decades.

Similarly, lower back pain is caused by lack of exercise. Physical labor was the traditional way of maintaining strength and health, but now machines have replaced most of it, and naturally, the torso degenerates rapidly. Again, common knee problems are generated by lack of walking, which was required in society until fifty years ago. Automobile transport has caused degeneration of our knees.

Other than that, human sperm production has decreased significantly over the last two decades, caused by our new lifestyle.[8] Traditionally, people went to bed shortly after sunset and woke up at dawn. Our bodies adapted to nature over millions of years. In our new lifestyle we often do not go to bed before midnight. According to Qìgōng theory, the Qì in our bodies manifests as physical action during daytime. Qì nourishes our brain and sexual organs through the spinal cord at night. If we go to sleep by 9 pm, it takes two to three hours of natural breathing during sleep to lead Qì from the surface to nourish deep inside. By midnight it is ready to nourish the brain and sexual organs. Brain energy is recharged, and sperm and sexual hormones are produced. The modern lifestyle has introduced a new time schedule which precludes the natural production of hormones. Naturally, production of sperm has decreased over the last two decades.If it continues in this way, the problem will be even more significant and serious.

Countless other problems have been generated by new products which cause material and energetic pollution. Through lack of understanding of human energy and its vulnerability to this pollution, we live in a world at great risk of physical and mental imbalance. To solve these problems, we must first achieve awareness before we can awaken others. Profound and significant study and research needs to be conducted and acted upon.

1-6. Qìgōng and Longevity (Qìgōng Yǔ Chángshòu, 氣功與長壽)

To many secular people, longevity means long life, without regard to health or the meaning of life. Most of the people today want to live long physically, even though they are in pain mentally. Longevity is important to them, not happiness.

Others search for the meaning of life to make longevity more meaningful. They look for a way to extend physical life and at the same time keep mental peace in harmony with the physical body. For them, Qìgōng for longevity was developed.

To religious Daoists, longevity is considered very important and crucial to reaching enlightenment. They believe it takes many lifetimes to reach enlightenment to be reunited with the Dào. They believe, as do the Buddhists, that the physical body is only born for the spirit to reside in temporarily for further spiritual cultivation. The physical body has no further purpose or meaning. To Buddhists, the physical body is unimportant and they often ignore its condition, emphasizing only the cultivation of the mind and the spirit. But Daoists believe that if you live longer in each lifetime, you will have more time for spiritual cultivation, and need not reincarnate as many times before reaching enlightenment. So they take good care of the physical body. So to some religious people, the meaning of longevity is to provide a longer time for spiritual cultivation.

Then what are the keys or requirements to reach longevity? How do we reach this goal? These questions have been asked in every human generation. Now let us summarize some key points of longevity from past human experience.

Key points:

1. **The balance and harmony of the Qì body (Yīn) with the physical body (Yáng).** When there is balance and harmony of Yīn and Yáng, excess energy is minimized. Health is maintained and longevity reached through a healthy lifestyle and by keeping Yīn and Yáng in balance through Qìgōng training.
2. **Follow the way of the Dào,** adjusting your body to fit in with natural cycles such as the time of day and the change of the seasons. Avoid artificial material or energetic pollution.
3. **Understand the physical body and Qì body scientifically.** Through this we can find a way to slow down the aging process and find the key to attaining spiritual enlightenment.

These concepts were also discussed in medical Qìgōng society. One of the oldest medical classics, *Yellow Emperor's Inner Classic: Simple Questions* (*Huángdì Nèijīng. Sùwèn*, 黃帝內經・素問), said: "The ancient people who knew the Dào modeled themselves after Yīn and Yáng, matched the ways of nature, controlled their eating and drinking, lived with regularity, did not labor without knowing their limit, and so were able keep the shape (body) and the Shén (spirit) together. Therefore, they end their heaven years (the age granted by heaven) completely and pass hundred years, then gone."[9] For a healthy body, concern yourself with the harmony of Yīn and Yáng and follow the Natural Way. Only then can you reach longevity.

Let us summarize how we reach these goals with Qìgōng.

Physical Body:

1. **Keep the bone marrow clean.** The majority of blood cells are produced by the bone marrow. Once we reach thirty, the bone marrow starts to degenerate rapidly and quality and quantity of blood production decreases. Blood cells carry nutrients, oxygen, and the Qì required to replace old cells with new ones. Without enough healthy blood cells, cell replacement stagnates and degeneration of the body sets in.
   Degeneration of bone marrow results from deficiency of Qì. Without abundant Qì, blood production from bone marrow is slow and deficient. Bone marrow washing Qìgōng teaches how to lead Qì to the bone marrow, as described in the book, *Qìgōng—The Secret of Youth*.
2. **Maintain health of the body, especially the torso.** For health and longevity, we need physical and mental health. Without a strong healthy body, even though you have abundant energy, you still cannot manifest this energy into physical form.
   A healthy physical body depends on the condition of your torso, especially the spine. Through the spinal cord our brain controls the whole body. Any spinal problem disturbs the smooth control by your brain. Along the spine there are two Qì vessels, one being the spinal cord itself (Thrusting Vessel, Chōngmài, 衝脈), and the other being outside the spine, just beneath the skin (Governing Vessel, Dūmài, 督脈). They distribute Qì to the central nervous system and out to the limbs. If your spine is healthy, Qì circulation will not be stagnant. Most blood cells are produced in the spinal marrow and the pelvis. When Qì circulates abundantly, degeneration of bone marrow is slowed, and production of healthy blood cells maintained.
3. **Provide the best quality food and air for cell replacement.** Approximately one trillion cells in our bodies die each day. To replace them, we must provide good quality food and air, or else the new cells will be unhealthy and we will age faster. Deep breathing is one of the main keys to keeping cells healthy.
4. **Boost hormone production in the body.** Hormones (Original Essence) act as catalysts to expedite a smooth metabolism. When hormone production slows down, cell replacement does too, and our bodies degenerate faster.

Qì and the Mind:

1. **Accumulate Qì at the Real Lower Dāntián, which produces elixir Qì and also stores it.** From this energy center, Qì is distributed throughout the body. The Lower Dāntián has a similar structure to the brain, with the capacity for memory.[10,11] They are connected through the spinal cord and the central nervous system, where electric conductivity is highest and resistance is lowest. Though there are two brains, their function can be considered as one. The lower brain can store bioelectricity. When the mind generates an idea (EMF, electromotive force), Qì is led to the body for action. When the Qì stored at the Real Lower Dāntián is abundant, the life force is strong; otherwise we are weak and die young. We discuss this subject in more detail in Chapter 2.
2. **Accumulate Qì in the Eight Vessels.** With an abundant level of Qì in the Lower Dāntián, distribute it to the Eight Vessels, or Qì reservoirs, and regulate it in the Twelve Primary Qì Channels, or Qì rivers. Small Circulation meditation is one of the most important ways to increase Qì and circulate it. For more information on channels and vessels, refer to section 2-2.
3. **Circulate Qì smoothly in the Twelve Primary Qì Channels.** Only when Qì is distributed everywhere smoothly can the cells in the body obtain proper Qì nourishment and our life force be strong. To reach this goal, balance exercise (Yáng) with relaxation (Yīn).
4. **Maintain an emotionally neutral state.** In Chinese scholar Qìgōng, regulating the Emotional Mind is most important. Aging is caused by imbalance of Qì distributed in the body, caused in part by emotional disturbance. Set yourself free from emotional bondage to live peacefully and harmoniously.
5. **Raise the spirit of vitality.** When your spirit is high, your life force is strong. To raise the spirit of vitality, having stored abundant Qì at the Real Lower Dāntián, lead it up to the brain to nourish the spirit. This raises the spirit and leads to enlightenment.
6. **Understand the meaning of life.** Analyze your life and try to understand its meaning. Without understanding, you are rudderless and confused, leading to depression and low spirits. When you have a goal in life, your thinking and activities are meaningful.

Possible Modern Methods for Longevity

This summarizes how Qìgōng relates to longevity. If we borrow the knowledge and experience of the past, we may find a modern, scientific path to longevity. Here are a few suggestions for today's medical scientists.

Physically:

1. **Investigate the human "Body Electric."** Study the electric properties of the body to understand its electric circuitry. This will pinpoint Qì imbalances and stagnation, and enable external electromagnetic fields to correct them. Then we could prevent sickness before it manifests. In just fifty years, every household will have a scanner to scan the body's energetic condition and correct it. We will be able to preserve physical strength significantly.
2. **Maintain proper hormone level.** Artificial hormones can meet our maintenance requirements. Many people already extend their lives with artificial human growth hormone.[12–15]
3. **Maintain blood production in the bone marrow.** Abundant Qì supply to the marrow is necessary. In the future we will clean the bone marrow using external electromagnetic intervention. We will have plenty of healthy blood cells to carry oxygen, Qì, and nutrients everywhere for cell replacement.
4. **Slow down the cell aging process.** Invent a machine or energy chamber to slow down the aging process of the cells, to extend life.
5. **Increase Qì storage in the Real Lower Dāntián.** In the future, we may find a mechanical way to enhance Qì storage in the Real Lower Dāntián; First to condition the battery itself, and then charge it externally.

Mentally:

1. **Humbly learn from ancient experiences which offer guidelines for the future.** They have shown what is possible and where the problem may be. If our scientific dignity ignores this accumulated experience, we may repeat their mistakes. One who is wise remembers both past successes and failures.
2. **Make life meaningful.** Many people have no meaning in their lives, making them depressed and unhealthy. To direct them we must establish nonreligious spiritual centers, where they can meditate and recognize the spiritual role of their existence. Through meditation, the mind can be clear and peaceful, providing an environment for self-recognition. This is the first step to self-understanding and the path of spiritual enlightenment, and their minds will direct them to the right path in life.

3. **Raise up the spirit of vitality.** When one recognizes oneself, one will see how to fit into this society, and raise up the spirit of vitality. Using scientific methods to activate more brain cells and open the third eye, we may be able to shorten the path to enlightenment. Our spirit of vitality will be high, the most important invisible factor in longevity.

Longevity and Spiritual Cultivation

According to Buddhism, one may need hundreds or even thousands of lifetimes to cultivate the spirit, and see the true nature of reality, in order to reach enlightenment. In each life, one might improve only a little. Before one is twenty years old, one starts to feel one's spiritual identity, the first step to spiritual recognition. Throughout life, one collects information and experience, filters them, and finally understands their meaning. The spirit learns new ideas. If you die in your twenties you have only a few years for cultivation. The best time for spiritual cultivation begins from the age of thirty, when one has a few advantages for spiritual cultivation:

1. **Understanding the world better.** By this age, one has been educated and has experienced the world. One may adjust their circumstances and become serious about spiritual life.
2. **Better financial situation.** With financial security, the mind is calmer, and not trapped in the circle of daily survival, so it can focus more on the spiritual than the material side.
3. **Better mental preparation.** By thirty, one is more mature both mentally and spiritually, and more ready for spiritual cultivation.
4. **A more logical mind.** By age thirty, one's knowledge and judgment have developed logical thinking, which is crucial for correct spiritual development. Spiritual cultivation guided by imagination can only lead you away from the true nature of reality, and into deeper bondage of emotional confusion.

The longer you live, the more time for cultivation and development of your spiritual understanding to a higher level. If you die young, you have only a short time for cultivation, and progress will be limited in this lifetime.

1-7. Qìgōng and Spiritual Enlightenment (Qìgōng Yǔ Shéntōng, 氣功與神通)

Even though both Western and Eastern cultures have experienced and documented the existence of the spirit in the past, neither has been able to explain it clearly and satisfactorily. What, then, is the spirit? How do we define it? Since I am more familiar with Chinese concepts from the Buddhist and Daoist point of view, I will focus on their concept and understanding.

The ancient Chinese concept originated with *The Book of Changes* (*Yìjīng*, 易經), believing there are two poles or dimensions coexisting in space. One is called Yīn space (Yīnjiān, 陰間) and the other Yáng space (Yángjiān, 陽間). When these two poles or spaces coexist, Yīn and Yáng energy interact and exchange, from which process life is derived. The first derivation is spiritual life, and from this physical life is formed. Once physical lives are generated, spiritual lives can reside in them, uniting the Yīn spiritual body and Yáng physical body. The universe is alive, bearing both spiritual and physical existence at the same time. Every life formed or generated from this Yīn-Yáng space follows the patterns of nature and is a small universe within itself. It is said, "The universe is a large heaven and earth, man is a small heaven and earth."[16] Each life, even insects and animals, has its own heaven and earth.

In space, there are millions of universes, and within each there are millions of galaxies. Within each galaxy there are countless solar systems. Scientists postulate that our universe may be shaped like an egg with two poles (Figure 1-4).[17] It is believed that life derives from the energy interaction of these two poles.

We also have two poles in our bodies to sustain our lives. Since ancient times, the Chinese have known the body has two poles: one called the Real Lower Dāntián, at the the center of gravity, and the other called the Upper Dāntián, in the brain where the spirit resides. These two poles are related to each other. When energy in the Lower Dāntián is abundant, the spirit in the Upper Dāntián will be high. Since ancient times Daoists have searched for ways of building up abundant Qì in the Real Lower Dāntián. Today's science now recognizes that we have two brains, one in the head and the other in our gut.[10,11] This conforms to ancient experience.

What, then, is the spirit? The spirit is the true nature, or Dào (Tàijí), of this universe. It is the essential energy from which lives are derived. It is the origin of all living beings. Dào may be what is called God in Western society. Líke the universe, we also have this spirit within us.

Our Original Spirit, before birth, is pure and truthful. But after birth, our environment conditions us and we construct a conscious mind. We enter the bondage of emotional mud, and experience pain and happiness in life.

Daoists and Buddhists believe that to promote the spirit to a higher level, we must be born in physical form and borrow the body's sense organs to collect information about nature. This process generates confusion, but after filtering information through the Wisdom Mind, we gradually understand nature. To stimulate the spirit to learn and become aware, we lie, cheat, commit mistakes, experience pleasure and pain, and stay trapped in emotional bondage. Slowly and gradually, through emotional stimulation, we learn to be smart and truthful, and to keep a neutral mind. This is the path of returning our spirit to the neutral state, of unification with the natural spirit; since nature does not have this emotional bondage. You may reach the level of unification of heaven and man (Tiānrén Héyī, 天人合一), and will not reincarnate again, having gained eternal spiritual life.

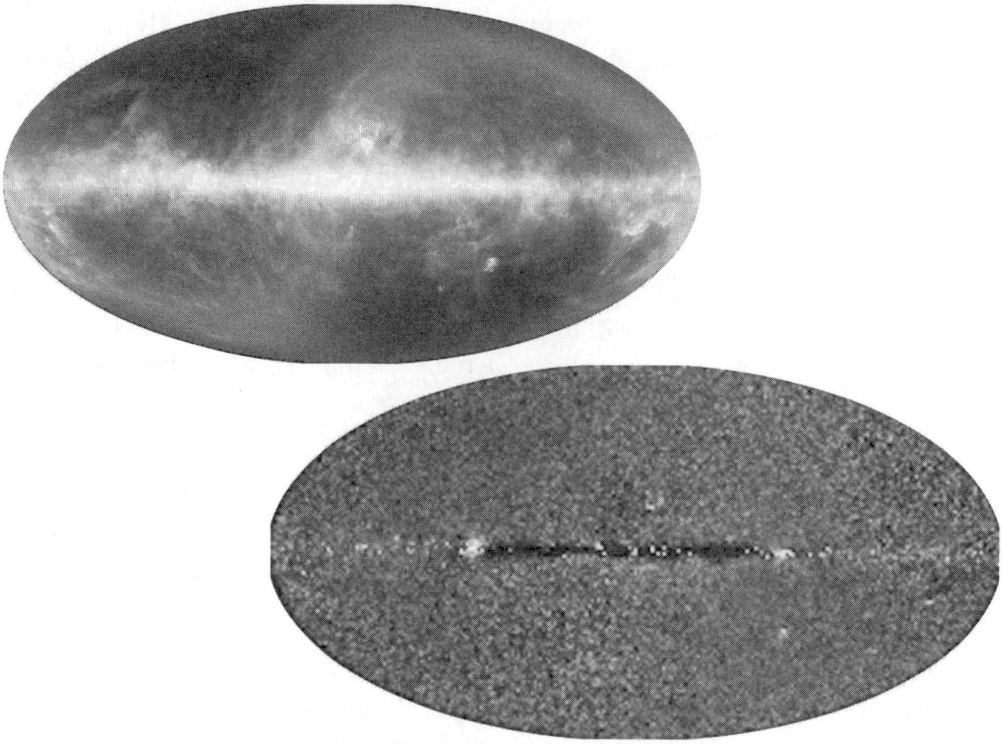

Figure 1-4. A Universe May be Shaped Líke an Egg with Two Poles

By searching for the origin of the spirit, we may comprehend the meaning of spirit. In the same way, material scientists look for the most basic structure of matter, in order to unravel the mysteries of material science.

From more than two thousand years of experience in spiritual cultivation, Daoists and Buddhists discovered the way to achieve this unification of the human spirit with the universal spirit. The first step is to recognize our spiritual body and understand it, by first understanding the energetic body, which is associated with the spirit. In the past, Qì could only be felt, but now through bioelectric research it can be tested and measured, rather than regarded as a mysterious and obscure concept.

To unify our spirit with the natural spirit, we must also open the "third eye" (Upper Dāntián or Tiānyǎn, 上丹田、天眼) at the lower center of the forehead. This opens the spiritual mind to be clear and see the true nature of reality, and to be able to access the natural spirit without obstacle. This step is called spiritual enlightenment.

To open this third eye, one first accumulates abundant Qì in the Real Lower Dāntián. Only then does one have enough energy to be led up through the spinal cord to the brain, to activate and energize it to a high level of resonance. Since spirit resides in the brain, it can likewise be raised to a higher level. When more brain cells are activated, a halo will be seen.

Years of Qì cultivation focus energy at the front of the brain, so the third eye can open. For more about this, refer to the books *Qìgōng—The Secret of Youth*, and *Qìgōng Meditation—Embryonic Breathing*.

Convert the Essence and Change It into Qì (Líànjīng Huàqì, 煉精化氣. One absorbs healthy food and air (post-birth essence) and converts it into Qì, while generating hormone (pre-birth essence) production from your glands with Qìgōng. With higher hormone levels, you can convert food essence into Qì more efficiently. Once abundant Qì is converted, you store it in the Real Lower Dāntián, which is considered the formation of the Holy Embryo (Shèngtāi, 聖胎). After this comes Ten Months Carrying the Baby (Shíyuè Huáitāi, 十月懷胎).

Nourish the Spirit with Qì (Líànqì Huàshén, 煉氣化神). Next you lead Qì up to the brain to nourish the brain cells, and raise up the spirit of vitality. You also lead Qì to the front of brain through the pituitary and pineal glands. This promotes smooth production of growth hormones and melatonin, the keys to longevity.

After many years, or many lifetimes, of meditation, you may finally open the third eye, allowing your spirit to leave your body while you are still alive. Your mind experiences gradual unification with the natural spirit, which it contacts directly. In Daoist cultivation, this is the birth of the holy baby embryo, as the spirit achieves enlightenment.

After the holy spirit baby is born, it must at first stay near your body to survive. Gradually it grows stronger. This step is called Three Years of Nursing (Sānnián Bǔrǔ, 三年哺乳).

Refine the Spirit and Return It to Nothingness (Líànshén Fǎnxū, 煉神返虛). To achieve unification with the natural spirit, you must completely free yourself from emotional bondage and remain neutral, which may take a long time. The spirit baby continues to grow stronger until it is mature and able to survive independently from you. It is said to take at least nine years of effort to do so. To keep your spiritual mind neutral, traditionally one must meditate facing the wall within a cave, which is called "nine years of facing the wall" (Jiǔnián Miànbì, 九年面壁). Then, the spirit can have independent life without needing the physical body.

The independent spirit stays peacefully in the Yīn space (Yīnjiān, 陰間) for some time without emotional disturbance. This is spiritual sleep, the state of Wújí (no extremity, 無極).

Crush the Nothingness (Fěnsuì Xūkōng, 粉碎虛空). The spirit can decide to remain in the neutral state of Wújí, but may want to reincarnate in physical form to accept the new challenge. The spirit faces a new environment to train it to a higher level. This is to "crush the emptiness" (Wújí state). After repeated cultivation, finally your spirit is united forever with the natural spirit.

This is only a brief summary of spiritual cultivation training. We will explain it in detail in later chapters, and in the next book: *Qìgōng—Grand Circulation for Spiritual Enlightenment*.

1-8. Buddhist and Daoist Qìgōng Concepts (Fójiā Yǔ Dàojiā Zhī Qìgōng Gàiniàn, 佛家與道家之氣功概念)

Because it was kept so secret, religious Qìgōng did not become as popular as other categories in China before the Qīng Dynasty (1644–1912 CE, 清朝). Only in the 20th century were the secrets gradually revealed to the public, and religious Qìgōng became popular in China. Religious Qìgōng is mostly Daoist and Buddhist, and its main purpose is to assist in the attainment of enlightenment, or what Buddhists refer to as Buddhahood.

Buddhist Qìgōng

Three main schools of Buddhist Qìgōng developed in Asia during the last two thousand years: Indian, Chinese, and Tibetan. Buddhism was created in India by an Indian prince named Gautama between 558 BCE and 478 BCE. Therefore, Indian Buddhist Qìgōng has the longest history. Buddhism was imported into China during the Eastern Hàn Dynasty (58 CE, 東漢), and Chinese Buddhists gradually learned its methods of spiritual cultivation. Their practice was influenced by traditional Chinese scholar and medical Qìgōng practices, which had been developing for about two thousand years. What resulted was a unique system of training different from its antecedents.

According to the fragmentary records available, only the philosophy and doctrines of Buddhism were passed down to the Chinese during the first few centuries following its adoption. The actual methods of cultivation and Qìgōng training were not known. There are several reasons for this:

1. Because of the difficulty of transport and communication at that time, the transfer of Buddhist documents from India to China was limited. Although a few Indian priests were invited to China to preach, problems remained.
2. Even if the documents had been transferred, because of the profound theory and philosophy of Buddhism, very few people were qualified to really translate them accurately from Sanskrit to Chinese. This problem was exacerbated by the different cultural backgrounds. Even today, different cultural backgrounds are always the main problem in translating accurately.
3. The main reason was probably that most of the actual training methods need to be taught and guided personally by an experienced master. Only a limited amount can be learned from documents. This problem was compounded by the tradition of passing information secretly from master to disciple.

The process was very slow and painful, especially with regard to the actual training methods. For several centuries it was believed that as long as you purified your mind and sincerely strove for Buddhahood, sooner or later you would succeed. This situation was not improved until Dámó wrote the *Muscle/Tendon Changing and Marrow/Brain Washing Classics* (*Yìjīnjīng, Xǐsuǐjīng*; 易筋經、洗髓經). Then at last there was a firm direction in the training to reach Buddhahood.

Before Dámó, Chinese Buddhist Qìgōng training was very similar to Chinese Scholar Qìgōng. The main difference was that while Scholar Qìgōng aimed at maintaining health, Buddhist Qìgōng aimed at becoming a Buddha. Meditation is a necessary process in training a priest to stay emotionally neutral. Buddhism believes all suffering is caused by the seven passions and six desires (Qīqíng Líùyù, 七情六慾). The seven passions are happiness (Xǐ, 喜), anger (Nù, 怒), sorrow (Āi, 哀), joy (Lè, 樂), love (Ài, 愛), hate (Hèn, 恨), and desire (Yù, 慾). The six desires are the six sensory pleasures derived from the eyes, ears, nose, tongue, body, and mind. Buddhists also cultivate within themselves a neutral state separated from the four emptinesses of earth, water, fire, and wind (Sìdà Jiēkōng, 四大皆空). They believe that this training enables them to keep the spirit independent so it can escape from the recurring cycle of reincarnation, known as "the Wheel of Life and Death" (Shēngsǐ Lúnhuí, 生死輪迴).

Tibetan Buddhism has always been kept secret and isolated from the outside world. Because of this, it is very difficult to determine precisely when Tibetan Buddhism was established. Because Tibet is near India, it is reasonable to assume that Tibetan Qìgōng training has had more influence from India than Chinese Qìgōng has. However, over thousands of years of study and research, the Tibetans established their own unique style of Qìgōng meditation. Tibetan priests are called Lamas (Lǎma, 喇嘛), and many of them also learned martial arts. Because of the different cultural background, not only are the Lamas' meditation techniques different from those of the Chinese or Indian Buddhists, but so are their martial techniques. Tibetan Qìgōng meditation and martial arts were kept secret from the outside world, and so were called Mìzōng (秘宗) which means "secret style". Because of this, and because of the different language, there are only very limited documents available in Chinese. Tibetan Qìgōng and martial arts did not spread into Chinese society until almost the Qīng Dynasty, but since then they have become popular.

Daoist Qìgōng

Líke Buddhists, Daoists believe in building up the spirit (Shén) so that it is independent and strong, to escape from the cycle of reincarnation. When a Daoist reaches this stage of enlightenment, it is said he has attained eternal life.

Daoist monks found that to enhance their spirit, they had to cultivate Qì which was converted from their Jīng (Essence). Again, the Daoist Qìgōng training process is: 1. To convert the Jīng (精, Essence) into Qì (Líànjīng Huàqì, 煉精化氣, 2. To nourish the Shén (Spirit, 神) with Qì (Líànqì Huàshén, 煉氣化神), 3. To refine the Shén and return it to nothingness (Líànshén Fǎnxū, 煉神返虛) and 4. To crush the nothingness (Fěnsuì Xūkōng, 粉碎虛空).

The first step involves firming and strengthening the Jīng (Gùjīng, 固精), converting it into Qì through meditation or other methods. This Qì is then led to the top of the head to nourish the brain and raise up the Shén. When a Daoist has reached this stage, it is called "the three flowers meet at the top" (Sānhuā Jùdǐng, 三花聚頂). The three flowers are Jīng (精), Qì (氣), and Shén (神). This stage achieves the necessary health and longevity for continued cultivation. Finally, the Daoist starts training to reach enlightenment. The biggest obstacle is one's emotions, which affect thought and upset spiritual balance. This is why Daoists retreat to the mountains, away from other people and distractions. Usually they also abstain from eating meat, feeling that it muddles thinking and intensifies the emotions, leading the spirit away from self-cultivation.

An important part of this training is Yìjīnjīng and Xǐsuǐjīng Qìgōng. Yìjīnjīng Qìgōng builds up abundant Qì in the Lower Dāntián and strengthens the body. Xǐsuǐjīng Qìgōng leads Qì to the brain to raise up the spirit, and keeps Qì circulating in the marrow so it stays clean and healthy. Your marrow produces most of your blood cells, which bring nourishment to the whole body, and removes waste products. When your blood is healthy, your whole body is well-nourished and you can resist disease effectively. When the marrow is clean and fresh, it manufactures plenty of healthy blood cells which do their job efficiently. Your whole body stays healthy, and degeneration is slowed significantly.

Although the theory is simple, the training is very difficult. One accumulates Qì at the Real Lower Dāntián and fills up your eight Qì vessels, then leads it into the bone to wash the marrow. Except for some Daoist monks, there are very few people who have lived more than 120 years, because the training is so arduous. You need a pure mind and a simple lifestyle to enable you to concentrate entirely on the training.

Many Daoist Qìgōng styles are based on the theory of cultivating both the spirit and the physical body. It is said, "Talking about human nature (spirit) and life, cultivate them both. Place the lead (Pb, Yīn) and mercury (Hg, Yáng) together. This secret is hard to comprehend. Cultivate human nature to refine self-being while cultivating life to return the essence (convert essence into Qì). Xīn is the house of the spirit while the body is the residence of the Qì. Lífe is the Qì. Those who cultivate human nature blend the body and the Xīn as a family. Jīng, Qì, and spirit must combine into one unit. Then the cultivation of life can be approached."[18] This emphasizes that to reach enlightenment, you must cultivate both body and spirit. The key is to harmonize Yīn and Yáng. Yīn is the spiritual body while Yáng is the physical body. Only when they are harmonious and the three treasures (essence, Qì, and spirit) have reached the brain, can you reach enlightenment.

In Daoism, there are generally three ways of training: Golden Elixir Large Way (Jīndān Dàdào, 金丹大道), Dual Cultivation (Shuāngxiū, 雙修), and Herb Picking Outside the Dào (Dàowài Cǎiyào, 道外採藥).

Golden Elixir Large Way teaches training Qìgōng within yourself, to find the elixir of longevity and enlightenment within your own body.

In the second approach, Dual Cultivation, a partner is used to balance one's Qì more quickly. Most people's Qì is not entirely balanced. Some are too positive, others too negative, and individual channels also are positive or negative. If you exchange Qì with a partner, you can speed your training. Dual Cultivation has two meanings: one is to cultivate Qì with a partner, and the other means cultivation of both one's human nature and physical body.

The third way, Herb Picking Outside of the Dào, uses herbs to accelerate and regulate cultivation. Herbs can be plants such as ginseng (Rénshēn, 人蔘), or animal products such as musk from the musk-deer. To many Daoists, the word "herbs" can also mean the Qì obtained from sexual practices.

According to the training methods used, Daoist Qìgōng can again be divided into two major schools: Peaceful Cultivation Style (Qīngxiūpài, 清修派), and Plant-and-Graft Style (Zāijiēpài, 栽接派). This division was especially clear after the Sòng and Yuán Dynasties (960–1368 CE, 宋、元朝). The meditation and methods of Peaceful Cultivation Style are similar to those of Buddhists. They believe the only way to reach enlightenment is Golden Elixir Large Way, in which one builds up the elixir within the body. Using a partner for cultivation is considered immoral, and causes emotional problems which may significantly affect cultivation.

However, the Plant-and-Graft Style claims that their approach of using Dual Cultivation and Herb Picking Outside of the Dào, in addition to Golden Elixir Large Way, makes the cultivation faster and more practical. For this reason, Daoist Qìgōng training is also commonly called Dāndǐng Dàogōng (丹鼎道功) which means the Dào Training in the Elixir Crucible. Daoists originally believed they could find and purify the elixir from herbs, but later realized the only real elixir is in your body. Let us discuss these two styles in more detail.

Peaceful Cultivation Style (Qīngxiūpài, 清修派). Qīng (清) means clear, pure, and peaceful. Xiū (修) means cultivation, study, and training. Pài means style or division. The basic rules of Peaceful Cultivation Daoists are to follow tradition according to the Daoist bibles. All training and study are based on the fundamental principles which Lǎozi expounded: "Objects are many, each returns to its root. When it returns to its root, it means calmness. It also means repeating life."[19] All things have their origins, and ultimately return to them. Then they are calm and peaceful. From this state, life originates again. He also said, "Concentrate Qì to attain softness, can it be soft like a baby?"[20] These two sayings of Lǎozi demonstrate the emphasis on cultivating calmness, peace, harmony, and softness. These are the basic rules of traditional Daoism, which originated from observation of natural cycles. All life originates from the roots of calmness and peace.

Peaceful Cultivation Daoists emphasize, "the method of Yīn and Yáng, harmony of the numbers (according to the *Yìjīng*), and shape follows and combines with spirit."[21] Yīn and Yáng must be in harmony and balance each other, and the appearance of the body will follow the lead of the spirit. This style believes that spiritual cultivation alone can lead them to enlightenment, so a strong physical body is not important. The body is only a temporary ladder to reach the goal of spiritual enlightenment. They emphasize sitting meditation, through which they Regulate the Body (Tiáoshēn, 調身), Regulate the Emotional Mind (Tiáoxīn, 調心), Regulate the Breathing (Tiáoxí, 調息), Condense the Spirit (Níngshén, 凝神), Tame the Qì (Fúqì, 伏氣), Absorb the Essence (Shèjīng, 攝精), and Open the Crux (Kāiqiào, 開竅). These are their seven steps of Internal Gōngfū (Nèigōng, 內功), by which they cultivate and trace back to their root, the point of calmness and peace within themselves, and finally cultivate for eternal spiritual life. Through this they endeavor to reach immortality and enlightenment.

The principles and training of Peaceful Cultivation Style are similar to those of Chán (禪) (Zen) meditation in Buddhism. Once the mind is calm and peaceful, they look for the root and meaning of life, becoming emotionally neutral as they train to reach enlightenment.

Plant-and-Graft Style (Zāijiēpài, 栽接派). Zāi (栽) means to plant, grow, or raise. Jiē (接) means to join, connect, or graft. Pài means style or division. Plant-and-Graft Style Daoists go in the opposite direction of Peaceful Cultivation Daoists. They maintain that the methods used by Peaceful Cultivation Style, such as still meditation alone, breathing, swallowing saliva, and using the Yì to lead Qì past the gates and open the vessels, are less effective and impractical. This view was expressed in the Book on Awakening to the Truth (Wùzhēnpiān, 悟真篇): "Within Yáng, the quality of Yīn essence is not tough. To cultivate one thing alone is wasteful. Working just on the shape (body) or leading (Qì) is not the Dào. To tame Qì and dine on rosy clouds is emptiness after all."[22] Meditation is the Yīn side of cultivation, and the Yīn essence in the Yáng is not strong. You also need Yáng training methods which are different from still meditation. This statement criticizes the Peaceful Cultivation Style Daoists for seeking longevity and enlightenment through meditation alone. Focusing exclusively on Yīn training, such as the taming of Qì and enjoying beautiful scenery in meditation, is empty illusion after all.

The Daoist document Maintaining Simplicity (Bàopǔzi, 抱朴子) by Gé, Hóng (葛洪) said, "The Grand Ultimate (the emperor) knows Daoist secular techniques, which he carefully keeps and respects, of thoroughly studying the ultimate emptiness, enlivening all things, then viewing its repetition, finally obtaining the Dào and entering heaven."[23] Secular techniques are those used by Plant-and-Graft Daoists. When ultimate emptiness is reached, all things start again from the beginning and come to life. When you understand the cycles which occur continually throughout nature, you comprehend the real Dào. This sentence emphasizes that even the emperor practiced Daoist secular techniques to reach enlightenment.

What then are the secular techniques of the Plant-and-Graft Division? They said: "If the tree is not rooted, the flowers are few. If the tree is old and you join it to a fresh one, peach is grafted onto willow, mulberry is connected to plum. To pass down examples to those looking for the real (Dào), this is the ancient immortal's plant-grafting method. The man who is getting old has the medicine to cure after all. Visit the famous teacher, ask for prescriptions, immediately start to study and cultivate, do not delay."[24] This says that when you are getting old, you can gain new life from mutual Qì transportation through particular sexual practices and special types of meditation.

"When clothes are torn, use cloth to patch. When the tree is senile, cultivate the soil. When man is weakening, what should be used to patch? Use Heaven and Earth to create the opportunity of variations."[25] This asks how a weakened person is to regain his energy if not from another person? The purpose of Plant-and-Graft training is "similar types working together, spiritual communication between separate bodies."[26] People training together can help each other. Spiritual communication (Shénjiāo, 神交) uses shared feeling to guide your spirit and stimulate production of hormones. Qì is exchanged in communicating with your partner. Some sexual practices stimulate hormone production while protecting and storing the Qì, which is considered the "herb" to cure aging. When done correctly, neither partner loses Qì, and both obtain the benefits of longevity.

This style of Daoism encourages a proper sex life. With this approach it is more difficult to achieve emotional neutrality and enlightenment. As a result, it mainly emphasizes a long and happy life. Han's Book of Art and Literature (Hànshū Yìwén Zhì, 漢書藝文誌) says, "The activity in the bedroom is the ultimate of personality and emotions, the ultimate of reaching the Dào. To restrain external joy, is to forbid internal emotion. Harmony between husband and wife is the scholarship of longevity."[27] Correct sexuality promotes longevity, enabling you to balance your Qì and spirit.

In addition to sexual Dual Cultivation, they also emphasize non-sexual Dual Cultivation (Shuāngxiū, 雙修). Everyone has a different level of Qì, and no one's Qì is completely balanced. In your teens, your Qì is stronger and more abundant than afterwards. Once you pass forty, your Qì supply tends to weaken and become deficient. To be healthy, your Qì should be neither excessive nor deficient. Dual Cultivation meditation helps balance each other's Qì. This can be done by two men, two women, or man and woman. It is said, "Yīn and Yáng are not necessarily male and female; the strength and weakness of Qì in the body are Yīn and Yáng."[28] "Two men can plant and graft and women can absorb and nourish."[29]

To Plant-and-Graft Daoists there are four requirements for reaching the Dào: money, partner, technique, and place. Without money you spend too much time earning a living, and you will not have time to study and cultivate. Without the right partner, you cannot find the "herb" to balance your Qì. Without correct techniques you waste time. Without the right place to train, you cannot meditate to digest the "herb".

As a Plant-and-Graft Daoist, to balance Qì with your partner, you practice techniques of retaining semen, converting it into Qì, and using the Qì to nourish your Shén (spirit). Your energized Shén directs Qì into the five Yīn organs, namely the heart, lungs, liver, kidneys, and spleen, to enhance their functions. This Qì is called Managing Qì (Yíngqì, 營氣). Your Shén also directs Qì to the skin, where it protects you against negative outside influences. This Qì is called Guardian Qì (Wèiqì, 衛氣), which may be what is known in the West as one's "aura." Your Shén also leads Qì into your bone marrow (Suǐqì, 髓氣).

Plant-and-Graft Daoists also use herbs to help Qì cultivation, believing they offer significant benefits. Peaceful Cultivation Daoists and Buddhists use herbs as well, but usually only for healing.

Daoists at this level can have long and healthy lives. But to reach even higher and attain enlightenment, one must establish a baby Shén (Shéntāi, 神胎, Shényīng, 神嬰) or spirit baby (Língtāi, 靈胎), feed it, and teach it to be independent. To reach this higher level, one slowly regulates his or her emotions. One usually needs to leave normal society and become a hermit to be able to cultivate the mind.

Even though Plant-and-Graft techniques bring quick results, many Daoists and Buddhists oppose and even despise them. Since you are human, it is easy to fall back into emotional bondage during training, preventing you from clearing your mind. Also, many who practice these techniques do not balance Qì for the mutual benefit of both partners but simply take what the partner offers, without giving anything in return. This is easy with a partner who does not know Qìgōng, and this kind of selfishness is considered immoral.

General Differences between Buddhist and Daoist Qìgōng

1. In view of training philosophy, Buddhism is conservative while Daoism is open-minded. Religious Daoism absorbed the imported Buddhist culture into their own doctrine, traditional Scholar Daoism, which is generally open-minded. Whenever they found methods or theory which could enhance their cultivation, they adopted it. This was impossible for Buddhists, who believed that any philosophy other than Buddhism is not true. In Buddhist society, new ideas on cultivation would be considered a betrayal. The sixth Chán (禪) ancestor Huìnéng (慧能), who lived during the Táng Dynasty (713–907 CE,

唐朝), changed some meditation methods and philosophy and was considered a traitor for a long time. Because of this, Chán style divided into Northern and Southern styles. This is well-known among Buddhists, and is called "sixth ancestor disrupting the passed-down method" (Líùzǔ Shuō Chuánfǎ, 六祖說傳法). Daoists have had more opportunities to learn, compare, and experience, and in many aspects have advanced faster than Buddhists. In health and longevity Qìgōng, Daoist methods are better organized and more effective than those of the Buddhists.

2. Though both Buddhists and Daoists kept their training secret for a long time, the Buddhists, especially Tibetans, were more strict than the Daoists. Before the Qīng Dynasty, although both Buddhist and Daoist Qìgōng were kept secret from lay people, at least Daoist monks could learn from their masters more easily than Buddhists. In Buddhist society, only a few trusted disciples were selected to learn the deeper aspects of Qìgōng training.
3. Daoists and Buddhists have different training attitudes. Buddhist Qìgōng emphasizes cultivating the body (Xiūshēn, 修身) and cultivating the Qì (Xiūqì, 修氣). Cultivation implies to maintain and to keep. However, Daoists focus on training the body (Líànshēn, 練身) and training the Qì (Líànqì, 練氣). Training means to improve, build up, and strengthen. Daoists look for ways to resist destiny, to avoid illness, and to extend the usual limits of longevity.
4. Buddhist Qìgōng emphasizes striving for Buddhahood, while Daoist Qìgōng focuses on longevity and enlightenment. While striving for Buddhahood, most Buddhist monks concentrate all their attention only on cultivating their spirit, regarding the body as a "smelly skin bag" (Chòupínáng, 臭皮囊). The body is used for spiritual cultivation, and is not as important as the spirit, so physical health is widely ignored in Buddhist society. By contrast, Daoists insist on a healthy physical body to achieve the final goal, emphasizing both life and natural virtue. This is called Xìngmìng Shuāngxiū (性命雙修), Dual Cultivation of human nature and life. This is why more Daoists than Buddhists have had very long lives. "If only cultivates human nature and not (physical) life, this is the first illness of cultivation."[30] "Human nature is Yīn while life is Yáng. If only cultivating Yīn Qì and not Yáng Qì, it is like the rooster carry the egg by himself, the chicken will not be complete."[31] "Human nature is at the top (head) (Níwán, 泥丸) while the life is at the navel."[32]

   Daoists found ways to strengthen the body and slow the degeneration of the organs, to achieve long life. They say, "One hundred and twenty means dying young."[4] Buddhists also do physical training, but generally only those doing martial arts, such as the Shàolín priests.

5. Buddhist spiritual cultivation has generally reached a higher level than that of the Daoists. For example, Chán meditation techniques have been highly developed, and Daoists can learn from them.
6. Almost all Buddhist monks are against such training methods as Dual Cultivation (Shuāngxiū, 雙修) or Picking the Herb from Outside the Dào (Dàowài Cǎiyào, 道外採藥) through sexual practices. Using someone else's Qì to nourish you leads to emotional involvement which may disturb your cultivation. The mind will not be pure and calm enough for spiritual cultivation. Many Daoists, however, train mainly for health and longevity instead of enlightenment, so they regard these methods as beneficial.

1-9. Importance of Qìgōng Study to the Human Race (Qìgōng Yánjiù Duì Rénlèi Zhī Zhòngyàoxìng, 氣功研究對人類之重要性)

Qìgōng is an important science which has developed through thousands of years of observation, pondering, study, and experimentation. It is the product of the study of health, longevity, and spiritual growth, based on the generally applicable Daoist theory of Yīn and Yáng.

Before the 18th century, people generally followed the Natural Way (Dào) in their lifestyles. They went to bed soon after sunset and got up at dawn. They walked a lot and had sturdy limbs. Constant labor made their torsos strong. The human body developed over millions of years of harmony with nature into their present form.

Things changed quickly with the industrial revolution in the 18th century, when machines began to replace labor through mass production. Lifestyles are now very different from the Natural Way out of which we evolved, and since the 1950s they have been changing at a breathtaking pace. The great progress of material science has left our psyche and society in tatters, and has generated many problems. We need to re-evaluate the process objectively to find a wiser, more rational path for the future.

The discovery of electricity changed lifestyles significantly. It brought great convenience, but also many problems. With artificial light came changes in our sleeping patterns. How much has this new lifestyle influenced our physical and mental structure? What Qì imbalance is caused by working a night shift? Can this account for why human sperm count continues to decline?

With the invention of aircraft, we can relocate ourselves from one side of the earth to the other within hours. How does this affect Qì circulation? Will this cause us physical or mental problems?

Because we use automobiles, we walk much less than ever before in human history. Our knees have degenerated rapidly, with knee injuries becoming very common today. Foot injuries have also increased significantly. Now, with heavily cushioned shoes, the feet are overprotected and the tendons weakened by lack of exercise. Use of the torso has seriously decreased, causing it also to weaken and degenerate. A very common problem is lower back pain and spinal injury.

Another serious problem caused by the new lifestyle is the increase in breast cancer. Only a few decades ago, a woman would usually bear about ten babies in her lifetime. Through a million years of evolution, women have developed breasts to produce milk for their babies. There is a great deal of Qì in a woman's breasts. Now, through the use of birth control, the average woman will have only one or two babies, and often will not breastfeed. The result is a great accumulation and stagnation of Qì in the breast area, which often triggers cancer. Many do not realize that human lifestyles have changed in a relatively short period, and do not know the consequences, nor their solutions.

There are many other problems caused by the rapid development of material science. Microwave ovens, fluorescent light, and high tension powerlines are recent developments, which create artificial electromagnetic waves. Our body is a living electromagnetic field which can be influenced by external fields. A human brain contains 2.5 million tiny magnetic crystals. The brain is a magnetic unit like a computer floppy disk, with the capability of thought and memory. When the brain is exposed to a varying external magnetic field, it changes our moods, our thoughts, and we can even lose our memory.[33]

From more and more discovery, we realize how much risk we have exposed ourselves to in the new electromagnetic environment created by humans. How can we protect ourselves from the energy pollution of the new electromagnetic environment, which affects our thinking, judgment, and even our health?

We have also experienced a great loss of the human spirit, caused by wide-scale ignorance and a focus on material science and material possessions. Humans are ensnared in emotional bondage, having lost their spiritual center. To recover this lost spirituality, we must learn from the past, understand it, and bring it back into daily life.

We must educate the new generation about the importance of spirit. At the age of three, a child has become familiar with the body's balance, and learned to walk and run. This is the best age to teach them to feel the mental center of their being. For example, teaching them to walk with eyes closed, they establish a stronger inner feeling and body awareness. Next, teach them to locate the residence of the spirit and to communicate with it. This develops sensitivity to the subconscious mind. This kind of inner feeling is called Nèishì Gōngfū (內視功夫), which means Gōngfū of internal vision. This kind of training is easier for children than adults, since the child's mind has not yet been contaminated by the complex emotional world, and its thinking can be simple and pure. If we teach the new generation this meditation, we can bring them to a higher level of sensitivity and understanding of the spiritual world. From this recognition of spiritual identity, children will have less confusion and their lives will be more meaningful. Those methods which lead people to blind worship should be discouraged. Blind worship can only lead us back to the past of dictatorship and spiritual abuse.

However, we cannot deny that development of material science has also improved human life significantly. For example, the average life expectancy of men increased from 47 in 1900 to 76 in 1998. We will soon be able to live to be 120 years old with the help of human growth hormone.[12-15] But we should also understand the side effects of injecting human growth hormone. If there are any cancer cells hidden in the body, growth hormone can help them spread. Hormones are catalysts in the body, enhancing its biochemical reaction (metabolism), including the metabolism of cancer cells. If blood circulation is not as abundant as it should be, growth hormone may keep the muscles and the surface of the body young, but the deep places, such as the joints, continue to age. Proper Qìgōng exercise and relaxation can minimize this problem.

From this we can summarize the importance of Qìgōng to society:

1. **Raising awareness.** When we better understand the human electromagnetic field, we can avoid exposing ourselves to harmful external electromagnetic fields.
2. **Alerting us to harmful future developments.** Many chemicals and radioactive substances are harmful and should be forbidden, and we must prevent creation of such products in the future. If we correct our path now, we may lead ourselves to a safer, more peaceful environment.
3. **Educating the next generation about spirit.** Teach them how to meditate and develop the spiritual mind. Today we have reached a good level of material science, and freed ourselves from material shortages. However, this also causes the danger of modern weapons. We face the complete destruction of the earth and human culture. If we cannot educate the next generation to be free from the emotional bondage, we will surely self-destruct. We have to wake up and enlighten our spirit, before we can expect harmony and peace on earth.
4. **Applying Qìgōng to solve today's problems.** Many illnesses which cannot be cured by modern medicine respond to traditional Qìgōng methods. Cases of cancer or arthritis have been cured by Qìgōng. Spine and lower back pain is often cured by Qìgōng, which also rebuilds the strength of the torso. The greatest benefit in practicing Qìgōng is increasing the strength of your immune system and keeping you healthy.
5. **Helping to regain our spiritual center.** Through Qìgōng practice, countless people have brought themselves back from confusion and rootlessness, to a state of self-recognition. They regain their spiritual center, understand the meaning of life, and realize their role in society. This is the path of setting us free from emotional bondage and material slavery.

6. **Developing the Yīn side of science.** From studying Qìgōng, we understand and develop the Yīn side of science, that of energy and spirit. We open the gate to understanding the spiritual side of the human being and comprehending the mission of our existence in this universe.
7. **By understanding past Qìgōng practice, we create a feasible way for future spiritual cultivation.** This will cultivate enlightenment for mankind, the unification of Heaven and Man (Tiānrén Héyī, 天人合一), of the natural spirit and the human spirit.

1-10. About This Book (Guānyú Zhèběnshū, 關於這本書)

Qìgōng is like an infinite garden which contains everything in nature, both material and spiritual, but we have never had a detailed map of it. Qìgōng masters each discovered some of the pathways to an understanding of this garden, and mysterious hidden places which manifest the beauty of nature were gradually revealed. The masters passed down their understanding through teaching students or through writing. Though each document may provide only a little information on how to reach a tiny area of the garden, it took a Qìgōng master's lifetime to obtain. Each document is a possible road sign to our goal. When the fragments are combined, we can construct a map, a theory which might take us to places of our Qìgōng garden where nobody has ever gone before. It will probably take thousands of years of effort to obtain a detailed map of nature.

So far we have only limited information about material nature, and know very little about spiritual nature. We are still confused about the meaning of life, and far from understanding the truth of nature.

We need open minds to set us free from traditional brainwashing and bondage. We should humbly face the challenge and be willing to accept the truth and the mistakes we have already committed. Only then can we realize our dream of the future. Then we will be able to think with an open mind. If nobody can prove their ideas about the universe, we should dare to postulate a theory and explanation generated by the imagination. We try to prove our assumptions, and if proven wrong, we go back to modify the theory and try again. This is the scientific method: to dare to dream, dare to accept the challenge, and dare to accept the facts and the truth.

This book offers methods to establish a firm foundation of Small Circulation, a step on the path toward the ultimate goal of spiritual enlightenment.

Many explanations here originate from my personal understanding and scientific background. I cannot guarantee the correctness of my assumptions. It is quite possible that someone with deeper understanding of this subject may step in to modify or even completely change my theory. That is the natural course of scientific study. After the assumed theory has been tested repeatedly, we will be able to confirm what is correct and what is not, and the map will become clear.

The theory and practice methods introduced in this book only originate from Chinese study. You should keep an open mind and study the same subject in other cultures. A different view of the same topic could lead you to a clearer judgment. This is especially true for spiritual cultivation, as we are still at the beginning of understanding this subject. Any past experience could offer you more information and direct you to a better path of reaching the goal. This book is not an authority on this subject, and can only offer you one cultural viewpoint.

Even though we cannot yet prove the existence of the spirit in this universe by scientific method, it does not mean it does not exist. We should continue our research to untie this knot and open the gate of spiritual science experienced by people in all different cultures.

In the second chapter of Part I, I offer a theoretic foundation of Qìgōng practice related to Small Circulation meditation. In Part II, training methods passed down from the past are introduced. From Parts I and II, you will have a clear idea of how to approach the essence of this training. Meditation methods are introduced in Part III. Many remaining questions are listed in Part IV.

In this practice, the theoretic foundation is like a map which could lead you to the goal. You should first study it and understand it clearly. If you rush into practice without comprehending the theory, you may enter the wrong path and become confused, and endanger yourself through incorrect practice.

References

1. 《莊子刻意》：〝吹呴呼吸，吐故納新，熊經鳥伸，為壽而已矣。此導引之士，養形之人，彭祖壽考者之所好也。〞

2. 李時珍《奇經八脈考》：〝蓋正經猶夫溝渠，奇經猶夫湖澤，正經之脈隆盛，則溢于奇經。〞

3. 人生七十古來稀。

4. 一百二十謂之夭。

5. 外家由外而內，從硬到軟。

6. 內家由內而外，從軟到硬。

7. 《達摩大師住世留形內真妙用訣》：〝若不知子母相守，氣雖呼吸於于內，神常勞役于外，遂使神常穢濁而神不清，神既不清，即元和之氣漸散，而不能相守也。〞

8. "Silent Sperm," Lawrence Wright, p. 42, *The New Yorker*, January 15, 1996.

9. 《黃帝內經素問・上古天真論》：〝上古之人，知其道者，法于陰陽，和于術數，食飲有節，起居有常，不妄作勞，故能形與神俱，而盡終其天年度百歲乃去。〞

10. "Complex and Hidden Brain in the Gut Makes Cramps, Butterflies and Valium," Sandra Blakeslee, Science, *The New York Times*, January 23.

11. *The Second Brain: The Scientific Basis of Gut Instinct and a Groundbreaking New Understanding of Nervous Disorders of the Stomach and Intestine*, Michael D. Gershon, New York: Harper Collins Publications, 1998.

12. "Effects of Human Growth Hormone in Men Over 60 Years Old," *New England Journal of Medicine*, Daniel Rudman, July, 1990.

13. "The Foundation of Youth," *Harvard Health Letter*, Vol. 17, Number 8, June, 1992.

14. "The Hormone That Makes Your Body 20 Years Younger," Bill Lawren, *Longevity*, Oct. 1990.

15. *Grow Young with HGH*, Dr. Ronald Klatz, Harper Collins Publishers, NY, 1997.

16. 宇宙是個大天地，人身是個小天地。

17. "Measuring Stardust's Glow," Earl Lane, *Newsday*, January 10, 1998.

18. 《性天風月通玄記・師徒傳道》：〝論性命，要雙修，將鉛汞，兩下投，這消息，難參透，修性即煉己，修命即還丹。心是神之舍，身是氣之宅。命即氣也，修性之人，把身心混作一家，精氣神打成一片。修命之能事備矣。〞

19. 老子云：夫物芸芸，各復歸其根，歸根曰靜，是謂復命。

20. 專氣致柔，能嬰兒乎。

21. 法於陰陽，和於術數，形與神俱。

22. 悟真篇云：陽裡陰精質不剛，獨修一物轉羸尪。勞形按引皆非道，服氣餐霞總是狂。

23. 抱朴子云：太上知玄素之術，守敬篤，致虛極，萬物並作，以觀其復而得道飛昇。

24. 無根樹，花正微，樹老將新接嫩枝，桃寄柳，桑接梅，傳於修真作樣兒，自古神仙栽接法，人老原來有藥醫。訪名師，問方兒，下手速修莫太遲。

25. 衣破用布補，樹衰以土培，人損將何補，乾坤造化機。

26. 同類施工，隔體神交。

27. 漢書藝文誌云：房中者，性情之極，至道之極，制外藥，禁內情，和夫婦，及壽考之學也。

28. 陰陽不必分男女，體氣強弱即陰陽。

29. 兩個男人可栽接，一對女人能採補。

30. 只知修性不修命，此是修行第一病。

31. 《道鄉集》："性為陰，命為陽，只修陰氣，不修陽氣，即‵牝雞自卵，其雛不全。′"

32. 性在泥丸，命在臍。〔性潛于頂，命歸于臍。〕

33. "Pulsing Magnets Offer New Method of Mapping Brain," Sandra Blakeslee, *The New York Times*, May 21, 1996.

Chapter 2

Theoretical Foundations

2-1. Introduction (Jièshào, 介紹)

The Chinese concept of Dào (道) is commonly translated as the Natural Way. The *Yìjīng* (*Book of Changes,* 易經, 1122–1115 BCE) says, "One Yīn and One Yáng is called Dào."[1] The fundamental concept of Dào is the coexistence of Yīn and Yáng aspects of nature. This concept was later refined by Lǎozi (老子) (604–531 BCE). In his book *Dào Dé Jīng* (道德經), Chapter 24, he said, "Dao begets one, one produces two, two generate three, and three derive into millions of objects."[2] Dào is the natural causative force which creates the first single object from emptiness, and later this one (Wújí state of no extremity) divides into two aspects, and continues to derive into millions of objects and lives.

Chapter 25 of *Dào Dé Jīng* says, "There is an undiscriminated thing formed before the heaven and the earth (Yīn and Yáng). Extremely quiet, existing alone and without change, repeating cyclically without end, the mother of heaven and earth. I do not know its name and so call it Dào."[3] Dào exists since the very beginning, before heaven and earth, quietly, alone, and unchanging in its original virtue. When the Dào makes Wújí (no extremity) derive into Yīn and Yáng, it sets in motion the patterns of opposing forces and natural cycles. This derivation from Wújí to Yīn and Yáng is the origin of millions of things and therefore the mother of life.

Lǎozi believed Dào is responsible for all of creation and life. "Dào is the most mysterious of the mysterious, the door (origin) of all marvelousness."[4] "When Dào is born, the natural virtues are raised, objects are formed, and the natural state will be complete."[5] Millions of variations of nature derive from the Dào. Once this natural pattern is complete, the natural cycles are established and repeated. For us to fit into this nature, Lǎozi explained, "Man copies the earth, the earth follows heaven, heaven models itself after the Dào, the Dào follows nature."[6] It does not matter how big, such as heaven, or how small, such as a microbe, all follow the same energy patterns and the same Dào of nature.

Dào creates a single object from nothing, and from this single object, it divides into Yīn and Yáng. When Yīn and Yáng interact with each other harmoniously, millions of lives are created and derived. It is said in Huáinánzi (淮南子), "Dào begins from one, one does not beget, therefore dividing into Yīn and Yáng. When Yīn and Yáng harmonize with each other, millions of objects are born."[7]

Lǎozi pointed out the derivation from Wújí (無極) to Yīn and Yáng can proceed either way. Wújí can derive into Yīn and Yáng and Yīn and Yáng can be united to become Wújí. He said in Chapter 1, "Nothing, is the beginning of the pre-heaven (Wújí) state, the mother of millions of objects. Always nothing, wish to see its marvelousness, always existing, wish to see it expand."[8] Dào changes from nothing to something, and from something back to nothing, always changing from one to the other.

In order to understand the theoretical foundation of Chinese Qìgōng meditation, you must first study its history, tracing back the philosophic origins of Chinese culture. Qìgōng is an integral part of Chinese culture. If you separate them, you lose the root and essence of the art.

The oldest Chinese philosophy relates to the development of nature, especially human nature. The *Yìjīng* (*Book of Changes*, 1122 BCE) is the first book to offer a detailed clear discussion. Under its influence, the Dào (natural way) was followed by the Chinese people.

Yìjīng, *Great Biography* (*Yì Dàzhuàn*, 易大傳) said,

> *The ancestor named Bāoxī became king of heaven and earth. He looked up to see the phenomenal changes of the heavens, looked down to observe the natural rules of the earth, watched the instinctive behavior of birds and animals and how they interacted with the earth. He adapted to the changes of things he saw around him, he adopted the recurring cycles of objects, he then created the Eight Trigrams. This was used to understand the virtue of the divine and the behavior of millions of lives.*
>
> 易大傳曰："古者包羲氏之王天下也。仰則觀象於天，俯則觀法於地。觀鳥獸之文，與地之宜。近取諸身，遠取諸物。於是始作八卦，以通神明之德，以類萬物之情。"

Bāoxī (包羲) (2852–2737 BCE) was the ruler of China. The heaven and the earth means the kingdom. After he carefully observed the patterns of natural cycles and the behavior of plants and animals, he created the Eight Trigrams (Bāguà, 八卦), which are used to interpret and trace the patterns of nature. The theory of trigrams has significantly influenced Chinese culture.

Yìjīng (易經) also said,

> *Therefore, Yì (Change) has Tàijí (Grand Ultimate), and begets two poles (Yīn and Yáng). Two poles produce four phases. Four phases give rise to Bāguà (Eight Trigrams). Bāguà determines good or bad fortune, from good or bad fortune, the great career is created.*
>
> 是故易有太極，是生兩儀，兩儀生四象，四象生八卦，八卦定吉凶，吉凶生大業。

Only because there is Tàijí, is there change. From Tàijí, the Two Poles (Yīn and Yáng) are created from Wújí (no extremity or nothingness) and the two poles again derive into four phases. These four phases produce the Eight Trigrams. From the Eight Trigrams, the patterns of natural cycles can be understood, and good or bad fortune predicted. To be prosperous in business, follow the good luck patterns and avoid the bad luck patterns of nature. All derivations originate from Tàijí. Tàijí is the Dào or natural force which makes division and unification take place.

A Daoist classic, *Jìnsīlù* (近思錄) said,

> *Wújí begets Tàijí. When Tàijí moves, the Yáng is born. When movement reaches its extremity, again calm, generating the Yīn. When calmness reaches its extremity, again moving. One moves and one is calm, mutually as the root. Yīn and Yáng are discriminated and the two poles completed.*
>
> 無極生太極，太極動而生陽，動極復靜；靜而生陰，靜極復動。一動一靜，互為其根，分陰分陽，兩儀至焉。

Through this recurring cycle of Yīn and Yáng, millions of lives are begotten. The causative force is called Tàijí. The ancient Daoist classic, *Glossary Talking by Zhūzi* (Zhūzi Yǔlèi, 朱子語類) said, "What is called Tàijí, is the root of millions of things in heaven and earth."[9]

Wáng, Zōng-Yuè (王宗岳, 1750 CE) described Tàijí,

> *What is Tàijí? It is generated from Wújí and is a pivotal function of movement and stillness. It is the mother of Yīn and Yáng. When it moves, it divides. At rest it reunites.*
>
> 太極者，無極而生，動靜之機，陰陽之母也。動之則分，靜之則合。

Tàijí is neither Wújí nor Yīn and Yáng, but the natural force or Dào which makes the divisions and unifications happen. It is the cause and origin of life and death, the way of the natural cycle.

Chinese culture is based on the theory of Tàijí, and of Yīn and Yáng. When the theory is applied to Qìgōng, the first important goal of practice is the harmony and balance of Yīn and Yáng (Yīnyáng Xiétiáo, 陰陽諧調). To reach this harmonious state of balance, you adjust Yīn and Yáng, through the methods of Kǎn (Water, 坎) and Lí (Fire, 離).

When this theory is applied to human health, the physical body is considered Yáng, while the mental and the spiritual bodies are considered Yīn. To have a long, healthy life, you must also consider your spiritual condition. Mind and spirit are the foundation of life, and although they cannot be seen, they are nevertheless the origins and the causes of physical manifestation. When this foundation is firm and strong, the manifestation of life can be strong. To achieve health and longevity, cultivate both mental and physical bodies. This is called Dual Cultivation of human nature and life (Xìngmìng Shuāngxiū, 性命雙修). Human nature means the inner nature, the original spirit carried with us since birth. Lífe here means the limited physical life.

When you adjust yourself into harmony internally and externally, it is called "balance the body and mind" (Shēnxīn Pínghéng, 身心平衡). This allows you to live longer, enabling spiritual cultivation to reach enlightenment or Buddhahood, the final goal of cultivation.

Fortunately material science is highly developed, allowing us to verify things which were inexplicable in the past. Nevertheless, many mysteries remain that are waiting to be investigated from a scientific point of view. We live in a very exciting and challenging era, in which ancient mysteries and experiences can be comprehended using today's science. The documents passed down by thousands of Qìgōng experts provide us with clues, some more useful than others.

I am like a puzzle player. In front of me are thousands of pieces of the puzzle of Qìgōng practice. I try to choose those which are useful and valuable, discarding those which mislead. Through my efforts I have compiled a map of Qìgōng, not as detailed as I would like, but nevertheless a clear guide to prevent confusion and the fear of getting lost.

A clear and detailed map is necessary, but I cannot accomplish this mammoth task by myself in a single lifetime.

1. Thousands of ancient documents remain to be translated, interpreted and explained. This requires qualified scholars familiar with Qìgōng practice who are also masters of ancient Chinese writing, to understand the special terminology used.

2. We need experienced Qìgōng practitioners to translate these ancient documents into other languages correctly. This is no easy task since a Chinese word can have many different meanings, depending on where, how, and when it is used.
3. We need open-minded scientists and medical experts to offer opinions on the merits of these ancient practices. They need to challenge and attempt to verify the ancient experience in a scientific context.
4. We need a foundation with strong financial support to bring the various experts together to discuss every aspect of Qìgōng practice. From these conferences, information would be compiled, studied, researched, experimented with, and finally published. Without government support, or the interest of various scientific groups, it will be hard to accomplish this task.

In this chapter, I try to explain many mysteries in Qìgōng practice based on my personal limited scientific background. These possible explanations remain to be verified, but until then they remain the most probable hypothesis.

We first review the Chinese medical concept of the Qì channels and vessels. With this foundation, we use the scientific view to discuss the concept of Chinese Qìgōng in section 3. In section 4, the meaning and the purpose of Qìgōng meditation is discussed.

The training theory of Muscle/Tendon Changing and Marrow/Brain Washing Qìgōng is summarized in section 5, followed by Small Circulation, Grand Circulation, and Enlightenment Meditation in sections 6, 7, and 8 respectively.

2-2. Qì Vessels and Channels (Qìmài Yǔ Jīngluò, 氣脈與經絡)

We have two bodies: the physical body and the Qì (bioenergetic) body. The physical body can be seen, but Qì must be felt. The Qì body is the foundation of the physical body, of living cells, and of our lives. The Qì body is not only related to our cells, but also to our thinking and spirit, since it is the main energy source which maintains the brain's functioning. Therefore, Qì imbalance or stagnation are the root of any physical sickness or mental disorder.

Western medical science has long studied the physical body, while for the most part ignoring the Qì body. This has begun to change in the last two decades, but scientific understanding of the Qì body, and how it affects health and longevity, is still in its infancy. Under these circumstances, we may still accept the ancient Chinese understanding of our body's Qì network.

Twelve Primary Qì Channels and the Eight Vessels

From the viewpoint of Chinese medicine, the Qì circulatory system in the body has Eight Vessels (Bāmài, 八脈), Twelve Primary Qì Channels (Shíèrjīng, 十二經), and thousands of secondary channels branching out from the primary channels (Luò, 絡).

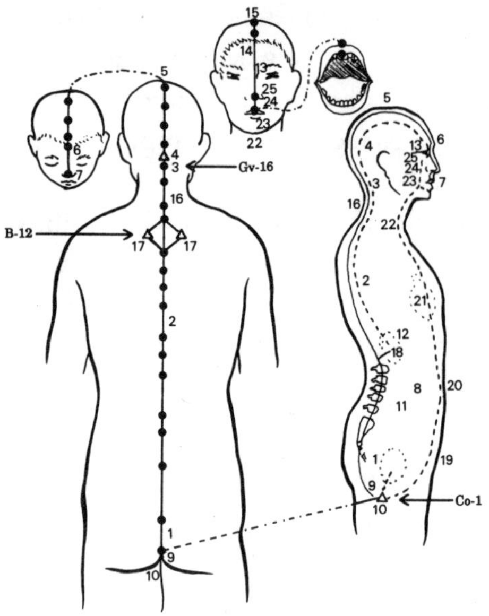

Figure 2-1. The Governing Vessel (Dūmài)

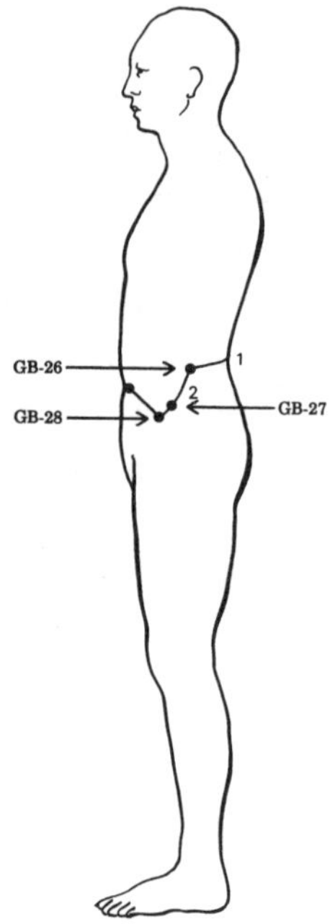

Figure 2-2. The Girdle (Belt) Vessel (Dàimài)

On two of the vessels (Governing and Conception Vessels) and the twelve primary Qì channels, there are more than seven hundred acupuncture cavities through which Qì can be adjusted. In this way, Qì circulation in the body, especially in the internal organs, can be regulated into a harmonious state, sickness cured, and health maintained. Here, we briefly review these three circulatory networks. For more about this Qì network, refer to Chinese acupuncture books or my books, *The Root of Chinese Qìgōng* and *Qìgōng Massage*.

Eight Vessels (Bāmài, 八脈)

a. The eight vessels include four Yáng vessels and four Yīn vessels, which balance each other.

b. The Four Yáng Vessels are:

Governing Vessel (Dūmài, 督脈) (Figure 2-1)
Girdle (or Belt) Vessel (Dàimài, 帶脈) (Figure 2-2)
Yáng Heel Vessel (Yángqiāomài, 陽蹺脈) (Figure 2-3)
Yáng Línking Vessel (Yángwéimài, 陽維脈) (Figure 2-4)

The Four Yīn Vessels are:

Conception Vessel (Rènmài, 任脈) (Figure 2-5)
Thrusting Vessel (Chōngmài, 衝脈) (Figure 2-6)

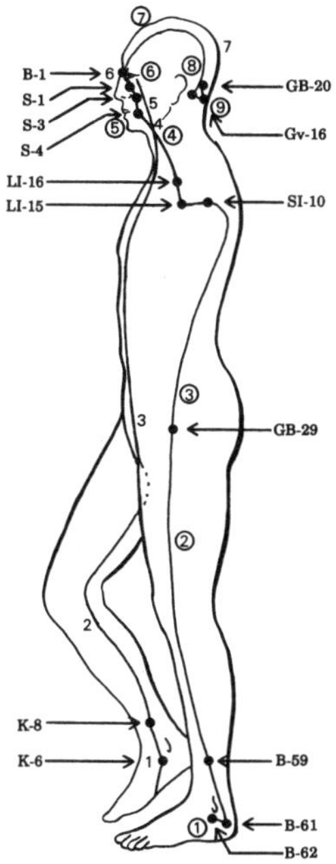

Figure 2-3. The Yáng Heel Vessel (Yángqiāomài) and the Yīn Heel Vessel (Yīnqiāomài)

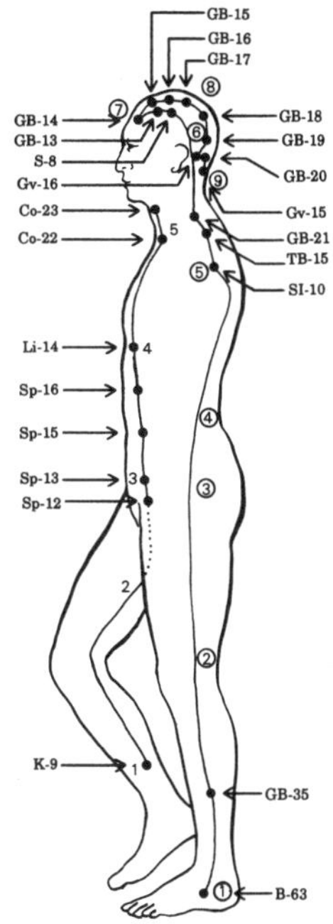

Figure 2-4. The Yáng Línking Vessel (Yángwéimài) and the Yīn Línking Vessel (Yīnwéimài)

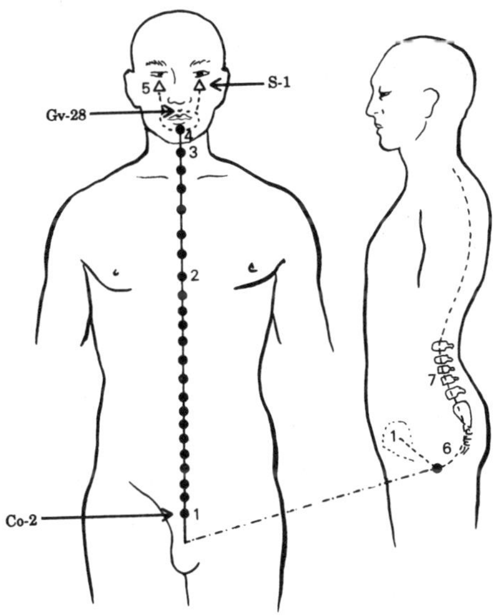

Figure 2-5. The Conception Vessel (Rènmài)

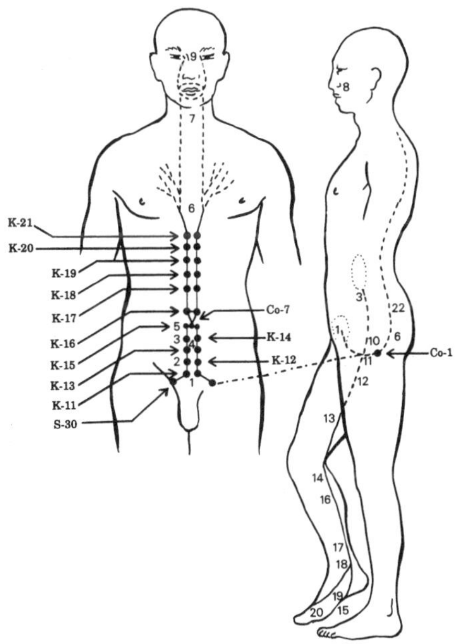

Figure 2-6. The Thrusting Vessel (Chōngmài)

Yīn Heel Vessel (Yīnqiāomài, 陰蹻脈) (Figure 2-3)
Yīn Línking Vessel (Yīnwéimài, 陰維脈) (Figure 2-4).

c. According to Chinese medicine, vessels function as reservoirs, connected to the twelve primary Qì channels and regulating Qì circulating in these channels. When the Qì level in some specific channel is too high, one or more of the reservoirs absorbs the excess, and if the Qì is too low, the shortfall will be supplied from these vessels. In this way, harmony is maintained.

d. Two Yáng vessels, Governing and Girdle Vessels, and two Yīn vessels, Conception and Thrusting Vessels, are in the torso. The other four vessels are in pairs, located in the legs. There are no vessels in the arms.

e. Among the eight vessels, the Governing and Conception Vessels are the most important, since they regulate the twelve primary Qì channels. The Governing Vessel regulates Qì in the six primary Yáng channels, while the Conception Vessel regulates Qì in the six primary Yīn channels. There are acupuncture cavities on these two vessels, but none on the other six. However, there are many cavities on the six vessels which belong to the twelve primary Qì channels, considered to be gates where Qì passes between the vessels and channels.

f. The methods for filling the vessels with Qì are very important. When their Qì is abundant, the regulating potential of the primary Qì channels is high. The Governing and Conception Vessels are the most important, since they regulate the twelve primary Qì channels. Qì circulates in them, and is distributed to the twelve primary Qì channels throughout the day.

g. In Religious Qìgōng meditation for enlightenment, the Thrusting Vessel (Spinal Cord) is very important. It connects the brain and the perineum, and Qì is abundant in this vessel around midnight. During these hours we sleep, and the body is very relaxed. The body does not need much Qì to support its activities, and Qì circulates abundantly in the spinal cord to nourish the brain and sexual organs. Hormone production increases at night. When the brain is nourished, the spirit is raised and enlightenment can be achieved. Again, for more detail, refer to my book, *Qìgōng—The Secret of Youth*.

h. The Governing Vessel, up the middle of the back, is the main vessel supplying Qì to the nervous system branching out from the spinal cord. The nervous system consists of physical cells which need to be nourished with Qì to function and stay alive. To maintain abundant Qì circulation in this vessel, your physical health is very important. Injury or damage along the course of this vessel will cause the Qì supply to the nervous system to be stagnant and irregular. To have abundant Qì circulating in this vessel, increase the storage of Qì in the Lower Real Dāntián (Zhēn Xiàdāntián, 真下丹田), which is the main

Qì reservoir or bioelectric battery in our body. We discuss this subject in more detail in Chapter 6.

i. The Yáng Girdle Vessel is very important, and is the only vessel in which Qì circulates horizontally. It is from this vessel that we feel our balance. Qì in this vessel is Yáng and expands outwards. As with a tight-rope walker, the longer the balancing pole, the easier it is to keep balance. Qìgōng practitioners and martial artists train this vessel to improve balance and stability of body and mind. Then you can find your center and be rooted, so your spirit can be raised.

j. Lǐ, Shí-Zhēn (李時珍) (1518–1593 CE) said in his book, The Study of Strange Meridians and Eight Vessels (Qíjīng Bāmài Kǎo, 奇經八脈考), "The Yáng Línking Vessel dominates the Qì of the surface (Guardian Qì) while the Yīn Línking Vessel dominates the Qì of the inner body. The Yáng Heel Vessel dominates the Yáng of the body's left and right sides, while the Yīn Heel Vessel dominates the Yīn of the body's left and right sides. The Governing Vessel dominates the Yáng at the back of the body, while the Conception and Thrusting Vessels dominate the Yīn in front. The Girdle Vessel regulates all vessels horizontally."[10]

The Twelve Primary Qì Channels and Their Branches (Shíèrjīng Luò, 十二經絡)

a. The six Yáng channels and six Yīn channels balance each other.

b. The six Yáng channels are:

Arm Yáng Brightness Large Intestine Channel (Shǒu Yángmíng Dàchángjīng, 手陽明大腸經) (Figure 2-7)

Leg Yáng Brightness Stomach Channel (Zú Yángmíng Wèijīng, 足陽明胃經) (Figure 2-8)

Arm Greater Yáng Small Intestine Channel (Shǒu Tàiyáng Xiǎochángjīng, 手太陽小腸經) (Figure 2-9)

Leg Greater Yáng Bladder Channel (Zú Tàiyáng Pángguāngjīng, 足太陽膀胱經) (Figure 2-10)

Arm Lesser Yáng Triple Burner Channel (Shǒu Shàoyáng Sānjiāojīng, 手少陽三焦經) (Figure 2-11)

Leg Lesser Yáng Gall Bladder Channel (Zú Shàoyáng Dǎnjīng, 足少陽膽經) (Figure 2-12)

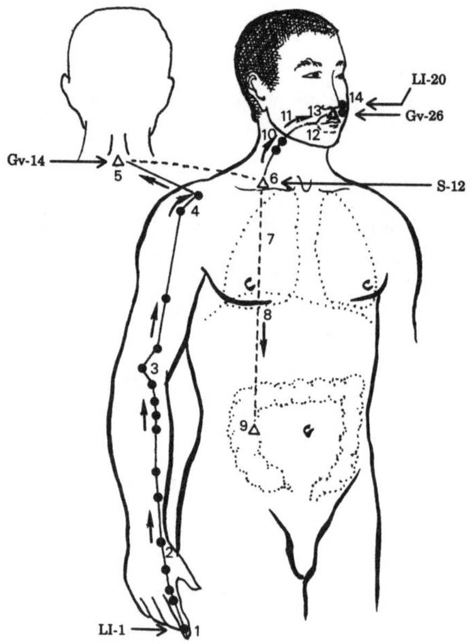

Figure 2-7. The Large Intestine Channel of the Hand-Yáng Brightness

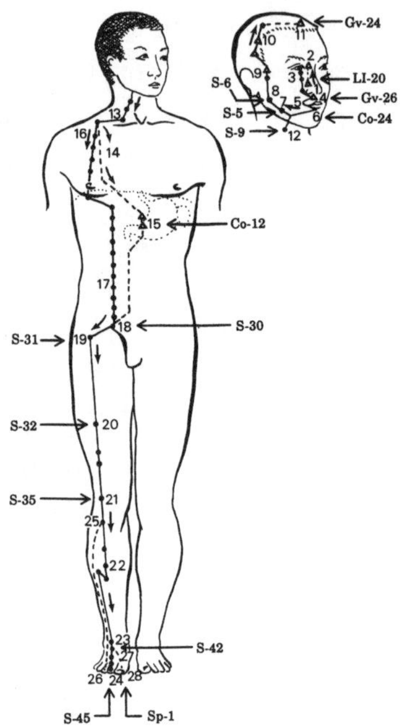

Figure 2-8. The Stomach Channel of the Foot-Yáng Brightness

The Six Yīn channels are:

Arm Greater Yīn Lung Channel (Shǒu Tàiyīn Fèijīng, 手太陰肺經) (Figure 2-13)

Leg Greater Yīn Spleen Channel (Zú Tàiyīn Píjīng, 足太陰脾經) (Figure 2-14)

Arm Lesser Yīn Heart Channel (Shǒu Shàoyīn Xīnjīng, 手少陰心經) (Figure 2-15)

Leg Lesser Yīn Kidney Channel (Zú Shàoyīn Shènjīng, 足少陰腎經) (Figure 2-16)

Arm Absolute Yīn Pericardium Channel (Shǒu Juéyīn Xīnbāoluòjīng, 手厥陰心包絡經) (Figure 2-17)

Leg Absolute Yīn Líver Channel (Zú Juéyīn Gānjīng, 足厥陰肝經) (Figure 2-18)

c. One end of each channel connects to an extremity, and the other end to an internal organ. Each channel has many acupuncture cavities through which its Qì can be regulated. This is the basic theory of acupuncture.

d. Thousands of secondary channels (Luò, 絡) branch out from each primary one. These lead Qì to the surface of the skin and to the bone marrow. This

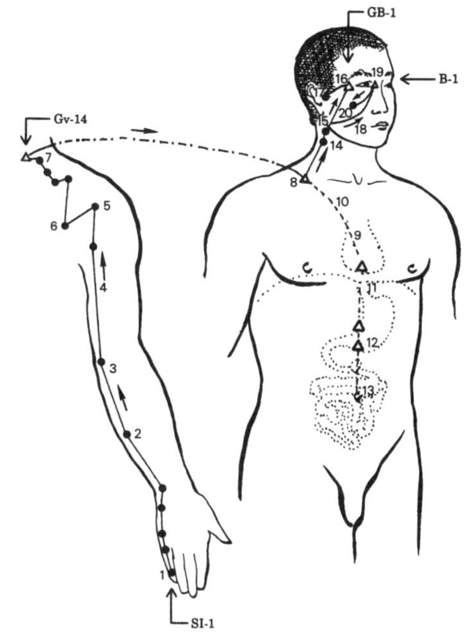

Figure 2-9. The Small Intestine Channel of the Hand-Greater Yáng

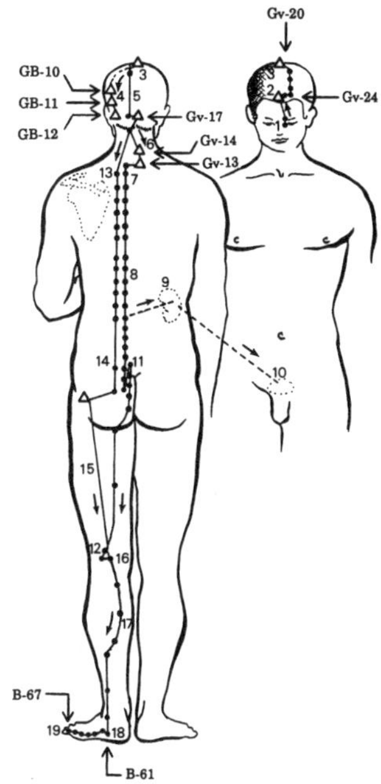

Figure 2-10. The Urinary Bladder Channel of the Foot-Greater Yáng

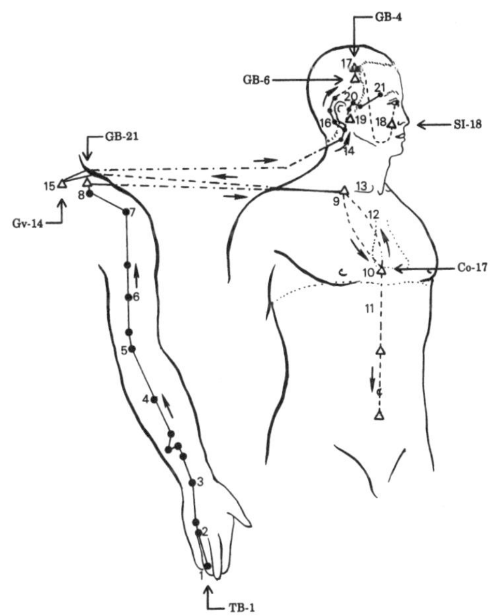

Figure 2-11. The Triple Burner Channel of the Hand-Lesser Yáng

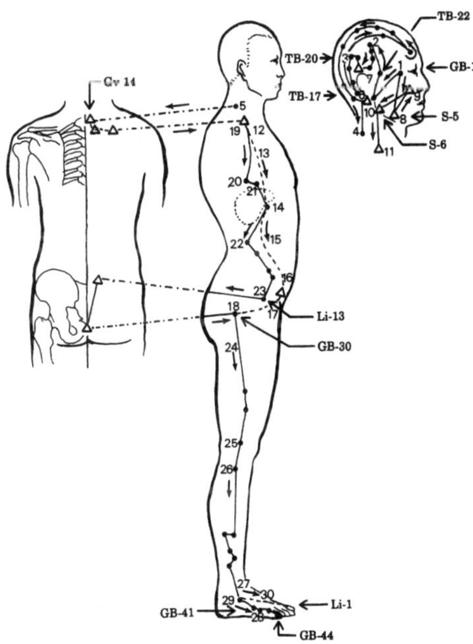

Figure 2-12. The Gall Bladder Channel of the Foot-Lesser Yáng

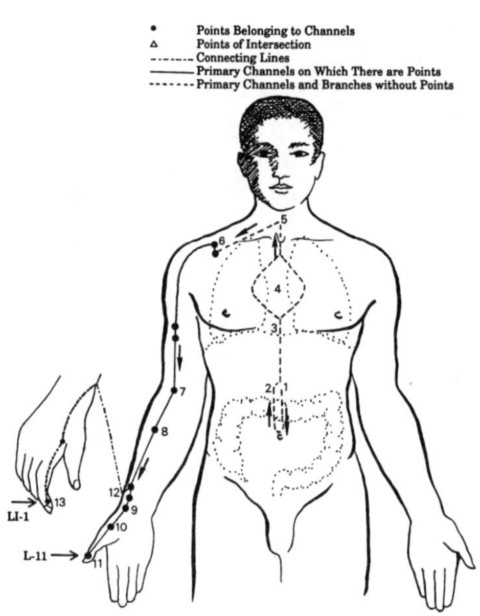

Figure 2-13. The Lung Channel of the Hand-Greater Yīn

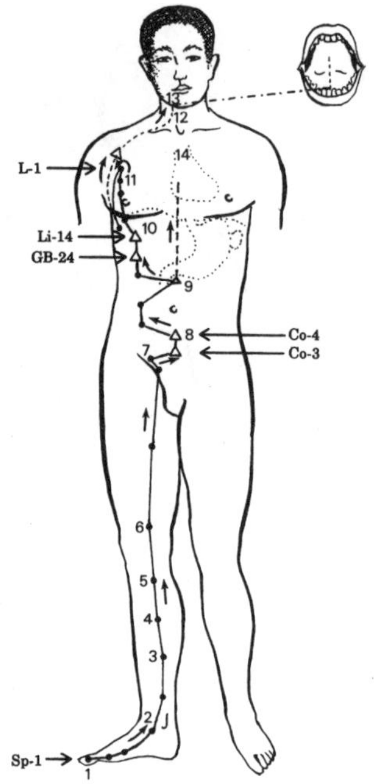

Figure 2-14. The Spleen Channel of the Foot-Greater Yīn

is very similar to the artery and capillary system except that, instead of blood, Qì is distributed.

2-3. Human Qìgōng Science (Rénlèi Zhī Qìgōng Kēxué, 人類之氣功科學)

Modern science has started to accept Qìgōng concepts, but has far to go to reach profound understanding. The observations in this section are from my personal understanding, and from information already published. For a satisfactory explanation, many assumptions are needed, so use logic and a scientific mind to judge. Question all assumptions and explanations. Only once we have verified the theory can we trust it fully.

In this section, a human bioelectric network is postulated and compared to ancient Chinese medical concepts. We define the human biobattery, both in the traditional Chinese concept and also from the viewpoint of modern Western science.

A Modern Definition of Qì (Qì Zhī Jìndài Dìngyì, 氣之近代定義)

In ancient China, people had no knowledge of electricity. They only knew from acupuncture that when needles were inserted into acupuncture cavities, some kind of energy other than heat was produced, which often caused shock or a tickling sensation. When the Chinese became acquainted with electromagnetism, they realized that this energy

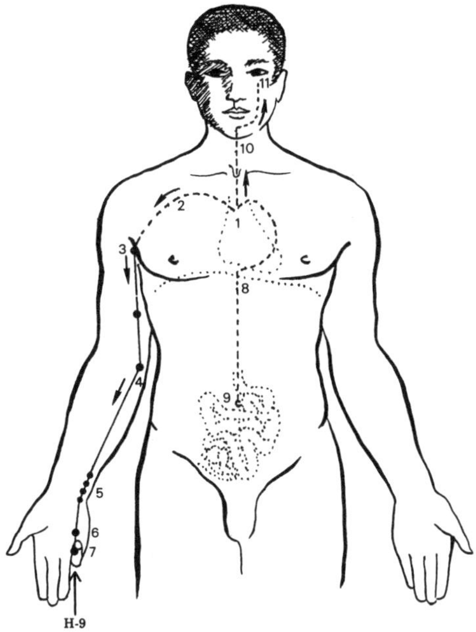

Figure 2-15. The Heart Channel of the Hand-Lesser Yīn

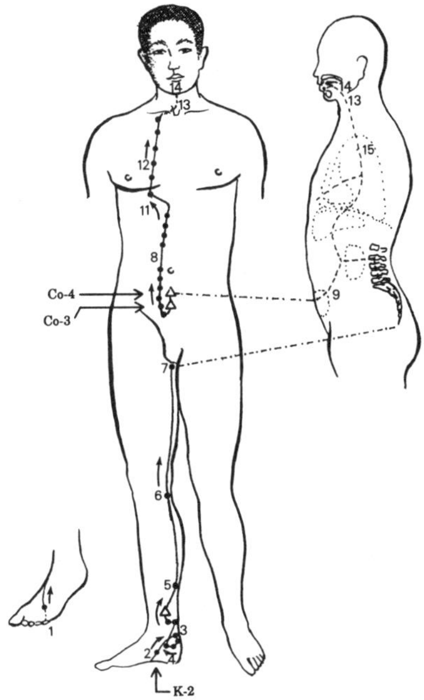

Figure 2-16. The Kidney Channel of the Foot-Lesser Yīn

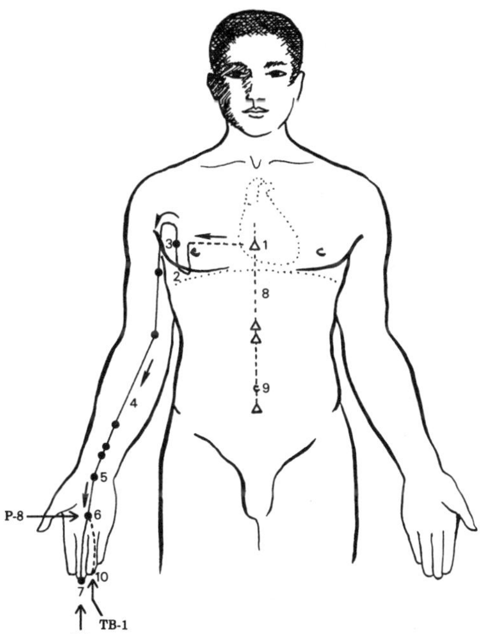

Figure 2-17. The Pericardium Channel of the Hand-Absolute Yīn

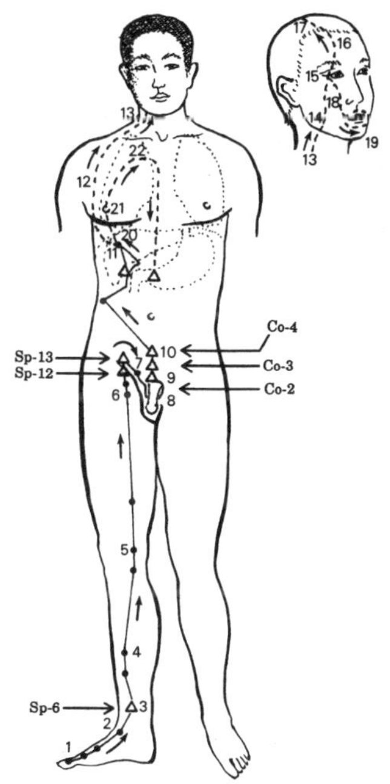

Figure 2-18. The Líver Channel of the Foot-Absolute Yīn

circulating in the body, which they called Qì, might be the same thing as what today's science calls bioelectricity.

The human body is constructed of many different electrically conductive materials, and forms a living electromagnetic circuit. Electromagnetic energy is continuously generated in the body through biochemical reaction, which assimilates food and air, and circulates electromotive force (EMF) within the body.

It is constantly affected by external electromagnetic fields such as that of the earth or electrical fields generated by clouds. When you practice Qìgōng, you need to be aware of these external factors and take them into account.

Countless experiments have been conducted in China and Japan to study how external electromagnetic fields affect the body's Qì field. Many acupuncturists use magnets and electricity in their treatment. They attach a magnet to the skin over a cavity and leave it there for a period of time, where its magnetic field gradually affects Qì circulation in that channel. Alternatively, they insert needles into cavities and then run an electric current through the needle to reach the Qì channels directly. Although researchers claim success in their experiments, they have not been able to explain the theory behind them. Conclusive proof remains elusive, and many unanswered questions remain. Of course, this theory is new, and will take more research before it is verified and understood. At present, many conservative acupuncturists are skeptical.

To unravel this knot, we look at what modern Western science has discovered about bioelectromagnetic energy. Many reports on bioelectricity research have been published, and frequently the results closely relate to what is experienced in Qìgōng training and Chinese medicine. During the electrophysiological research of the 1960s, investigators discovered that bones are piezoelectric. In other words, when they are stressed, mechanical energy is converted to electrical energy in the form of electric current.[11] This might explain one of the practices of Marrow Washing Qìgōng in which stress on the bones is increased to increase Qì circulation.

Dr. Robert O. Becker has done important work in this field. In his book, *The Body Electric*, he reports on much of the research concerning the body's electric field.[12] It is presently believed that food and air are the fuels which generate electricity in the body through biochemical reaction. This electricity is circulated throughout the body by means of electrically conductive tissue, one of the main energy sources keeping cells alive.

When you are injured or sick, your body's electrical circulation is affected. If this circulation of electricity stops, you die. Bioelectric energy not only maintains life, it also repairs damage. Researchers seek ways of using external electromagnetic fields to speed up recovery from injury. Richard Leviton reports, "Researchers at Loma Línda University's School of Medicine in California have found, following studies in sixteen countries with over 1,000 patients, that low-frequency, low-intensity magnetic energy has been successful in treating chronic pain related to tissue ischemia, and has also worked well in clearing up slow-healing ulcers. In 90 percent of patients tested, it increased blood flow significantly."[13]

He reports that every cell functions like an electric battery, able to store electric charge. "Other biomagnetic investigators take an even closer look to find out what is happening, right down to the level of the blood, the organs, and the individual cell, which they regard as a small electric battery."[13] This convinces me that our entire body is essentially a big battery assembled from millions of small ones. All of them together activate the human electromagnetic field.

Much research relates to acupuncture. Dr. Becker reports that the conductivity of the skin is much higher at acupuncture cavities, and it is now possible to locate them precisely by measuring the skin's conductivity (Figure 2-19).[12] Many reports show a scientific basis for the acupuncture which has been practiced in China for thousands of years.

Some researchers use the theory of bioelectricity to explain ancient miracles attributed to the practice of Qìgōng. Albert Huebner reports, "These demonstrations of body electricity in human beings may also offer a new explanation of an ancient healing practice. If weak external fields can produce powerful physiological effects, it may be that fields from human tissues in one person are capable of producing clinical improvements in another. In short, the method of healing known as the laying on of hands could be an especially subtle form of electrical stimulation."[11]

Another phenomenon reported is the halo seen around the head of a Qìgōng practitioner who reaches a high level during meditation. This is commonly shown in paintings of Jesus Christ, Buddha, Orthodox and Catholic saints, and various Oriental immortals. Frequently the light is pictured as surrounding the whole body. This phenomenon may be explained by the body electric theory. When one cultivates Qì to a high level, it may accumulate in the head. It may interact with the oxygen molecules in the air, ionize them and cause them to glow.

Although the link between the theory of the body electric and the Chinese theory of Qì is becoming more accepted, there are still many questions to be answered. For example, how does the mind actually generate EMF to circulate the electricity in the body? How is the human electromagnetic field affected by the multitude of other electric fields which surround us, such as radio or electrical appliances? How can we readjust our electromagnetic field and survive in outer space or on other planets where the magnetic fields are completely different from that on earth? The future of Qìgōng and bioelectric science is challenging and exciting. We need to use modern technology to understand the inner energy world which, for the most part, has been ignored by Western society.

A Modern Definition of Qìgōng (Qìgōng Zhī Jìndài Dìngyì, 氣功之近代定義)

If we accept that the internal energy (Qì) circulating in our bodies is bioelectricity, we can formulate a definition of Qìgōng based on the principles of physics.

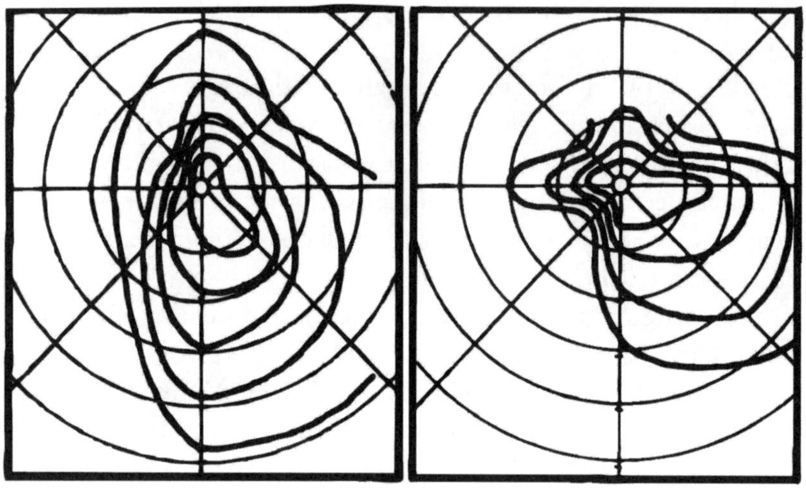

Figure 2-19. Electrical Conductivity Maps of the Skin Surface over Acupuncture Points

Let us assume that the circuit shown in Figure 2-20 is similar to that in our bodies. Although we now have some understanding of this circuit from acupuncture, we still do not know in detail exactly what the body's circuits looks like. We know there are Twelve Primary Qì Channels (Qì rivers) and Eight Vessels (Qì reservoirs). There are also thousands of small Qì channels (Luò, 絡) which allow Qì to reach the skin and bone marrow. In this circuit, the twelve internal organs are connected and mutually related through these channels. There is also a Dāntián (丹田, elixir field) biobattery which stores the Qì.

In the illustration, you see that:

1. The Qì channels are like wires which carry electric current.
2. The internal organs are like electrical components such as resistors and solenoids.
3. The Qì vessels are like capacitors, which regulate the current in the circuit.
4. The Dāntián is like a battery, which stores charge and provides EMF.

How do you keep this electrical circuit functioning efficiently? Your first concern is the resistance of the wires which carry current. In a machine, we use a wire with high conductivity and low resistance, otherwise the current may melt it. It should be of a material like copper or even gold. In your body, you keep current flowing smoothly, removing anything which causes stagnation. Fat has low conductivity, so use diet and exercise to remove excess from your body. Relaxation to open the Qì channels is the first practice in Tàijíquán and many Qìgōng exercises.

How do you maintain the electrical components, your internal organs? Your organs burn out from too much current (Yáng) or too little (Yīn). To avoid these problems in a machine, you use a capacitor to regulate the current. When there is too much current, the capacitor absorbs and stores the excess, and when it is weak, the capacitor supplies

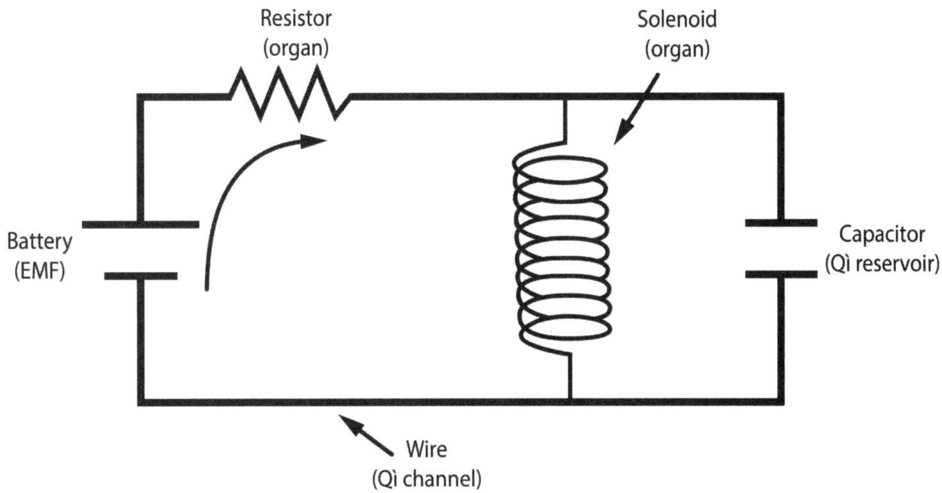

Figure 2-20. The Human Bioelectric Circuit is Similar to an Electric Circuit

current to the circuit. The eight Qì vessels are your body's capacitors. Qìgōng increases their level of Qì to supply current when needed, and keep the internal organs functioning smoothly. This is especially important as you get older, when your Qì level is generally lower.

For a healthy circuit, you address the components themselves. If they are weak or of poor quality, the circuit suffers. Qìgōng maintains and rebuilds the internal organs. There is an important difference between the circuit in the diagram, and the Qì circuit in our bodies. The body is alive, and with proper Qì nourishment, all of the cells can be regrown and the state of health improved. For example, if you jog three miles today, and keep jogging regularly, you can gradually increase the distance to five miles, as your body rebuilds and adjusts to the circumstances.

If we increase Qì flow through our internal organs, they become stronger and healthier. The increase must be slow and gradual so they can adjust to it. To increase Qì flow, you work with EMF. Imagine two containers filled with water and connected by a tube. If both have the same water level, water will not flow. However, if one side is higher than the other, the water will flow from that container to the lower. In electricity, this potential difference is called electromotive force. The higher the EMF, the stronger the current will be.

The key to effective Qìgōng practice is reducing resistance in the Qì channels, and increasing the EMF in your body. There are six sources of EMF in the body which can increase the flow of bioelectricity.

1. **Natural energy.** Your body is made of conductive material, so its electromagnetic field is affected by the sun, moon, clouds, gravity, and other energies around you. The sun, moon, and the earth's gravity affect Qì circulation significantly. We are now also affected by energy pollution by modern technology, such as radio, TV, microwave ovens, computers, and mobile telephone networks.
2. **Food and air.** To maintain life, we absorb food and air through our mouths and noses. These are converted into Qì through the biochemical reaction in the chest and digestive system (called the Triple Burner in Chinese medicine). EMF is generated which circulates Qì through the body. A major part of Qìgōng is devoted to getting proper food and fresh air.
3. **Thinking.** The mind is the most important source of bioelectric EMF. Any time you move to do something, you first generate an idea (Yì, 意). This idea generates EMF and leads Qì through the nervous system, to energize and move the appropriate muscles. The more you concentrate, the stronger the EMF, and the stronger the flow of Qì you lead to the muscles to energize them. The mind is the most important factor in Qìgōng training.
4. **Exercise.** Exercise converts stored food essence (fat) into Qì, building up EMF. Many Qìgōng styles utilize movement for this purpose.
5. **Converting Pre-Birth Essence into Qì.** The hormones produced by our endocrine glands are called Pre-Birth Essence in Chinese medicine. They are converted into Qì to stimulate the function of the body, increasing vitality. Balancing hormone production when you are young, and increasing its production when you are old, are important subjects in Chinese Qìgōng.
6. **Medical Methods.** In Chinese medicine, methods such as acupuncture, moxibustion and massage generate EMF to regulate irregular Qì in the body. These have become important methods of treatment in Chinese medicine.

The human body has an electrical circuit. To circulate bioelectricity requires a battery or power supply. There are three places which store Qì, called Dāntiáns (elixir field). One is called the Lower Dāntián, located one or two inches below the navel (Xià Dāntián, 下丹田). The second is at the lower sternum, called the Middle Dāntián (Zhōng Dāntián, 中丹田). The third is the lower central forehead, or third eye, called the Upper Dāntián (Shàng Dāntián, 上丹田).

The Lower Dāntián is the residence of Water Qì, called Original Qì (Yuánqì, 元氣), generated from Original Essence (Yuánjīng, 元精). In this area is a cavity called Qìhǎi (Co-6, 氣海, Qì ocean). This produces Qì elixir, abundant as the sea.

To accumulate Qì in the Lower Dāntián, you move your abdomen (Lower Dāntián) through abdominal breathing. This exercise is called Qǐhuǒ (起火), which means

Starting the Fire, and is also called Back to Childhood Breathing (Fǎntóng Hūxī, 返童呼吸). After exercising the Lower Dāntián for about ten minutes, you feel warmth in the lower abdomen, as Qì accumulates there. Daoists call the abdominal area Dānlú (丹爐), which means "elixir furnace."

What happens when the abdomen moves? It has about six layers of muscle and fat sandwiched between layers of fascia (Figure 2-21). When your mind moves the abdominal muscles, there is muscular contraction and relaxation, turning fat into bioelectricity. When bioelectricity encounters resistance from the fasciae, it turns into heat. Fat and fasciae are poor electrical conductors, while muscles are relatively good conductors.[11,12,13] When these materials are sandwiched together, they act like a battery. Through abdominal movement, energy is stored and manifests as warmth.

Real Lower Dāntián. The front of the abdomen is not the real Dāntián, but in fact a False Dāntián (Jiǎ Dāntián, 假丹田). It generates Qì to a high level, but does not store it for long. It is located on the path of the Conception Vessel, so whatever Qì builds up, circulates in the Conception and Governing Vessels. It cannot be a battery as we understand the term, as a real battery should store the Qì. Where, then, is the Real Lower Dāntián (Zhēn Xiàdāntián, 真下丹田)?

Daoists teach that the Real Lower Dāntián is at the center inside the abdomen, at the physical center of gravity in the large and small intestines (Figure 2-22).

Life begins with sperm from the father entering an egg from the mother, forming the original human cell (Figure 2-23).[14] This cell divides into two cells, then four, and so on. When this group of cells adheres to the internal wall of the uterus, the umbilical cord starts

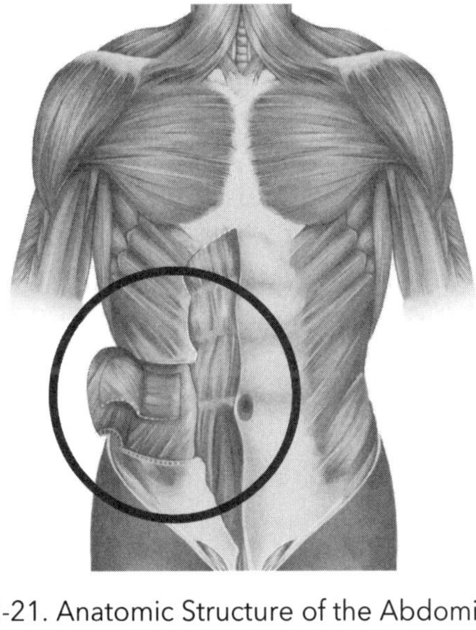

Figure 2-21. Anatomic Structure of the Abdominal Area

to develop. Nutrition and energy for further cell multiplication is absorbed from the mother through this cord. The baby's abdomen moves up and down, pumping nutrition and energy into its body. Immediately after birth, air and nutrition are taken in through the nose and mouth, through the mouth's sucking action and the lungs' breathing. The child slowly forgets the natural movement of the abdomen. This is why Abdominal Breathing is called "Back to Childhood Breathing."

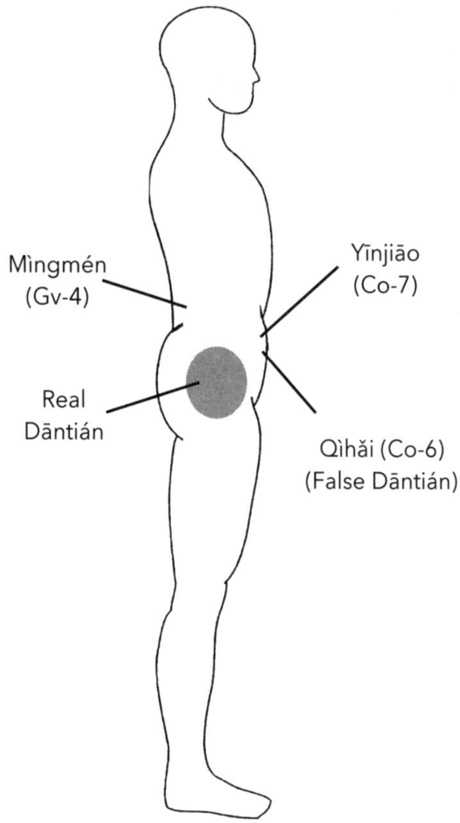

Figure 2-22. The Real Lower Dāntián and the False Lower Dāntián

If your first human cell were still alive, where would it be? Most likely it died long ago—approximately one trillion cells die in the body each day.[15] But if this first cell were still alive, it would be located at our center of gravity. From this center, the cells multiply evenly outwards until the body is fully constructed. To maintain this process, Qì must be centered here and radiate outward. In the embryonic state, this is the center of gravity and Qì. As we grow after birth, this center remains.

The physical center of gravity is occupied by the Large and Small intestines (Figure 2-24). There are three kinds of muscle in our bodies, classified according to our ability to control them. The first is the heart muscle, in which electrical conductivity is the highest. The heart beats all the time, regardless of our attention, and through practice and discipline we can only regulate its beating, not start or stop it. The second category of muscles are those which contract automatically, but over which we can exert significant control if we make the effort. The diaphragm which controls breathing, our eyelids, and certain sexual responses are examples of this muscle type, and their electrical conductivity is lower than the first type. The third kind of muscle is directly controlled by our conscious mind. Their electric conductivity is the lowest of the three groups.

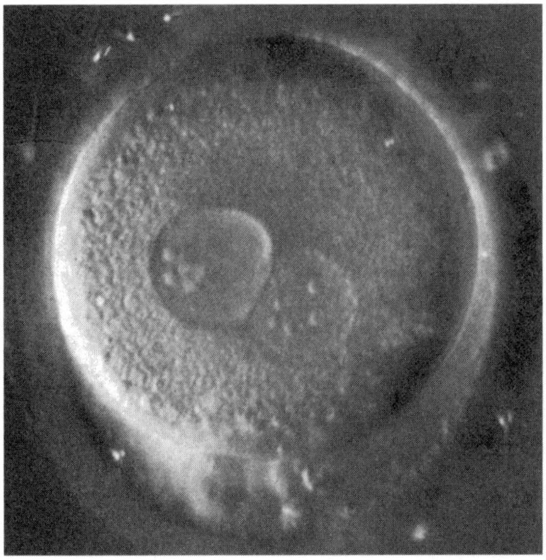

Figure 2-23. Original First Human Cell

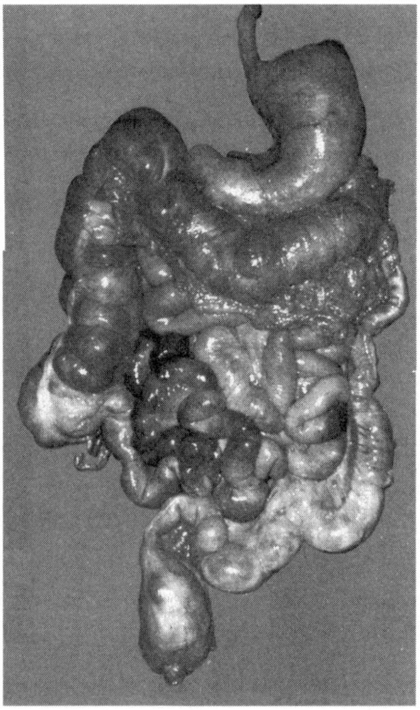

Figure 2-24. Anatomic Structure of the Real Dāntián–Large and Small Intestines

The total length of your Large and Small Intestines is approximately six times your body's height (Figure 2-25). With such long electrically conductive tissue sandwiched between the linings, which it is reasonable to believe are poor conductors, it acts like a huge battery in our body (Figure 2-26).[16] So the center of gravity, rather than the False Dāntián, is the real battery in our body.

Second Brain. According to a 1996 report in The New York Times, the human body has two brains: one in the head, and the other in the digestive system, which is known as the Enteric Nervous System.[17,18] Though these two brains are separated physically, they function as one through the connection of the spinal cord, which is highly conductive tissue (Figure 2-27).

The article explained that the upper brain thinks and remembers, storing data, and uses electrochemical charges. The lower brain has memory but not the capacity for thought. This discovery confirms the Chinese belief that the Real Lower Dāntián, in the large and small intestines, stores Qì, while the Upper Dāntián governs thinking and directs the Qì. The upper brain thinks, so it should be able to generate EMF, while the lower brain should have a large capacity for storing this charge. In other words, the lower brain is the human battery in which the life force resides. Once the upper brain generates an idea (EMF), the charge is directed from the lower brain, through the spinal cord and nervous system, to activate the appropriate part of the body.[18]

According to Ohm's Law in physics,

$$\Delta V = i\,R$$

where ΔV is potential difference or EMF, i is current, and R is resistance.[19]

If R is constant, then the higher the potential or EMF, the stronger the current generated. If we assume the resistance of our body remains constant, then the more we concentrate the EMF, the stronger the Qì flow will be. This parallels the Qìgōng concept that the more you concentrate, the higher your energy level. Qìgōng trains higher levels of concentration through still meditation. If EMF is constant, that means the mind's concentration remains the same. Then, the lower the R, the higher the current flow will be. According to Qìgōng theory, the more you relax, the more Qì can flow.

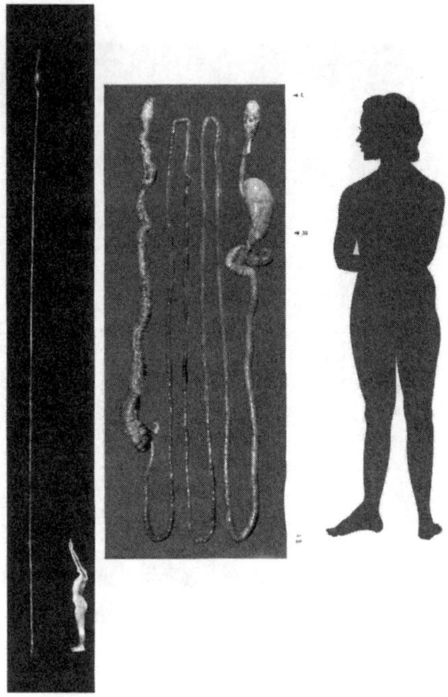

Figure 2-25. The Large and Small Intestines are About Six Times Your Height

We also examine the formula for manifestation of physical power:

$$\text{Power} = \Delta V \times i = i^2 R$$

The power generated depends on the current and the resistance. When one manifests physical strength, one tenses the body. This increases the body's resistance, energy (current) is trapped in the muscles and power manifested. It is the same in external hard martial arts styles, such as Tiger and Eagle, which focus on building the muscles and tendons to manifest power to its highest level.

The approach of the soft internal martial styles and Internal Elixir Qìgōng is quite different. Current is the energy manifested, and its influence on power is much more significant, since current is squared in the formula. Therefore, practitioners pay more attention to cultivating a stronger Qì flow. Meditation is vital for this, since it generates EMF to move the current. Smooth Qì circulation requires physical resistance or tension to be at a minimum, so relaxation is the key to the internal styles.

The most focused manifestation of power which can be generated should come from both energy and muscle, both the current and the resistance. Sacrifice either one, and power is reduced. Soft-hard martial styles of Qìgōng, such as White Crane, Xíngyìquán,

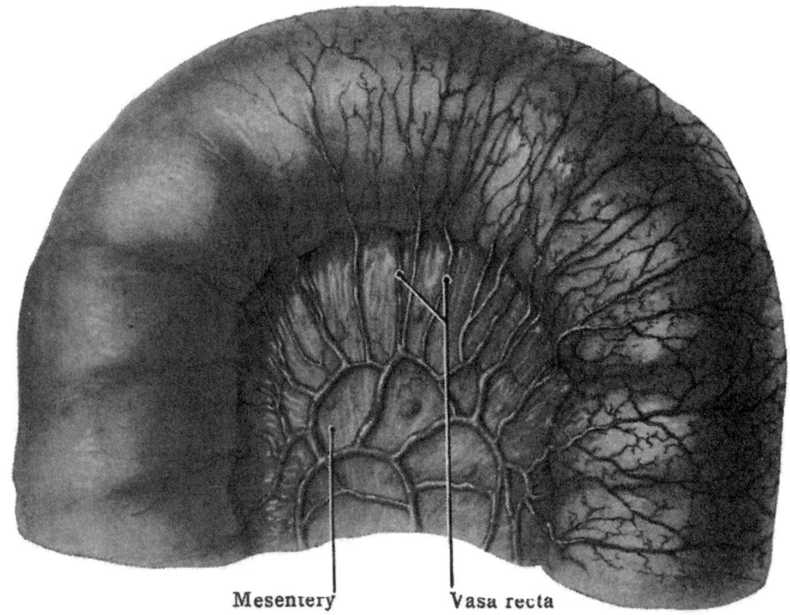

Figure 2-26. Low Electrically Conductive Materials Such as Mesentery, Outer Casing, and Water in and Around the Intestines Makes the Entire Area Act Líke a Battery
(Used with permission: James E. Anderson, M.D., Grant's Atlas of Anatomy, 7th ed., ©Williams and Wilkins)

and Dámó's Yìjīnjīng, emphasize both Qì (current) and tension (resistance). They do so by keeping the body as relaxed as possible, while using the concentrated mind to lead Qì to the body. Once Qì is led from the Lower Dāntián to the limbs, right before impact, they suddenly tense the body. These are called soft-hard styles, emphasizing both internal and external manifestation of power.

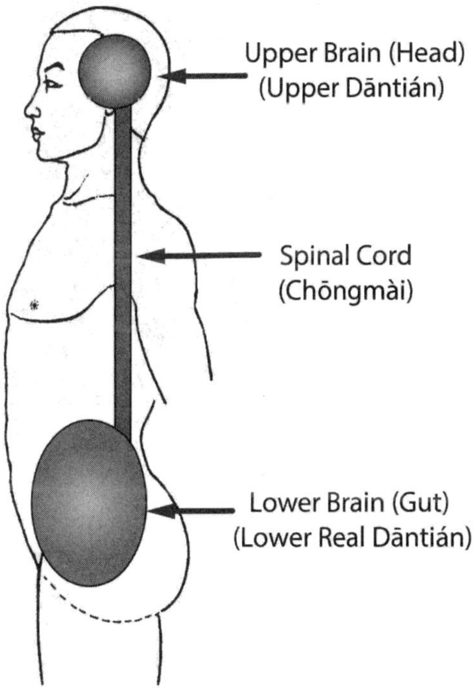

Figure 2-27. Two Polarities (Brains) of a Human Body

Middle Dāntián. The Middle Dāntián is located at the diaphragm, which is a membranous muscular partition separating the abdominal and thoracic cavities (Figure 2-28). It functions in respiration and is a highly electrically conductive material. Above and below it are fasciae, which isolate the internal organs from the diaphragm. Here again is a good electrical conductor isolated by poor electrical conductors, thus able to store electricity or Qì. Since it is between the lungs and the stomach, which assimilate Post-Birth Essence (namely air and food) into energy, the Qì accumulated in the Middle Dāntián is classified as Fire Qì (Huǒqì, 火氣). Naturally, this Fire Qì can also agitate your Emotional Mind.

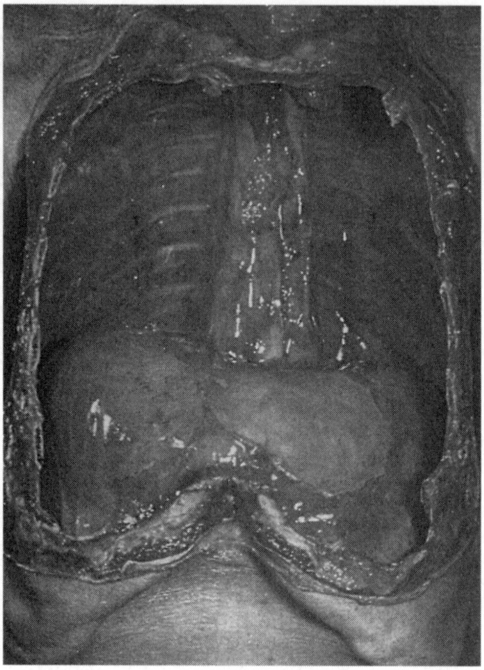

Figure 2-28. The Middle Dāntián is Connected to the Diaphragm

Upper Dāntián. The brain is the Upper Dāntián. The brain and the spinal cord constitute the central nervous system, having the highest electrical conductivity in the body. The brain is segregated into separate portions by the arachnoid mater, a delicate membrane of the spinal cord and brain, lying between the pia mater and dura mater (Figure 2-29). It is reasonable to assume that these tissues are poor electrical conductors. This is another giant energy center which consumes a great amount of Qì, although it does not produce any itself.

In this way we can compare ancient experience with modern scientific understanding. Let us also look at Qìgōng from another scientific point of view, this time chemical.

Cell Replacement. When we breathe, we inhale oxygen and exhale a lot of carbon in the form of carbon dioxide (Figure 2-30). Where does this carbon come from, and how much is actually processed out through breathing? The first source of carbon is from the food (glucose) we eat. Food is converted into energy, yielding carbon dioxide.[20]

$$\text{glucose} + 6O_2 \longrightarrow 6CO_2 + 6H_2O$$

$$\Delta G^{o\prime} = -686 \text{ Kcal (energy content)}$$

The second source of carbon is from dead cells. The body is constructed mainly from carbon, hydrogen, oxygen and nitrogen, while other elements such as calcium (Ca), potassium (P), chlorine (Cl), sulfur (S), potassium (K), sodium (Na), magnesium (Mg), iodine (I), and iron (Fe) comprise much less of our body weight.

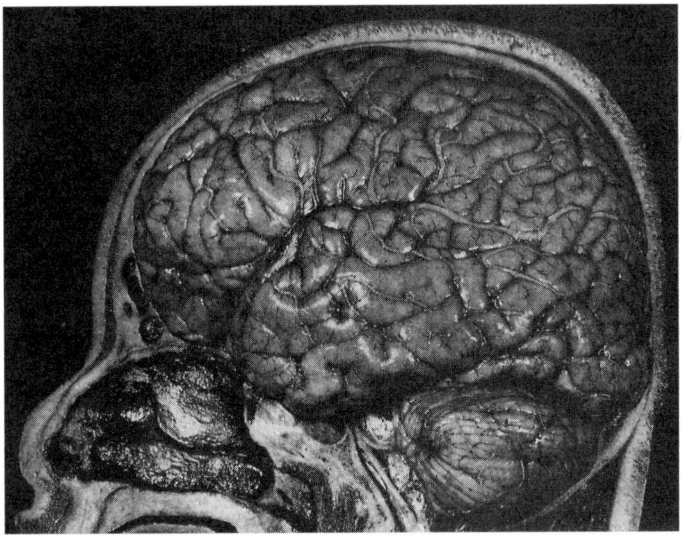

Figure 2-29. The Upper Dāntián—The Human Brain

As many as a trillion cells die in the body every 24 hours.[15] The average lifespan of a skin cell is 28 days. Different cells, such as those of bone, marrow, or liver, each have their own individual lifespans. We rely on our respiration to expel the carbon from the dead cells and to supply living cells with fresh oxygen. Carbon and other minerals are replenished from the food we eat. This process is vital to the formation of new cells and the continuation of life.

The cell replacement process is ongoing and continuous. Health during our lifetime depends on how smoothly and quickly it is carried out. If there are more new healthy cells to replace the old cells, you live and grow. If the cells replaced are as healthy as the original cells, you remain young. If fewer cells are produced or if the new ones are not as healthy as the original ones, then you age.

To produce healthy cells requires hydrogen, oxygen, carbon, and other minerals which we absorb from air or food. Air quality, water purity, and the choice of food become critical factors when considering your health and longevity.

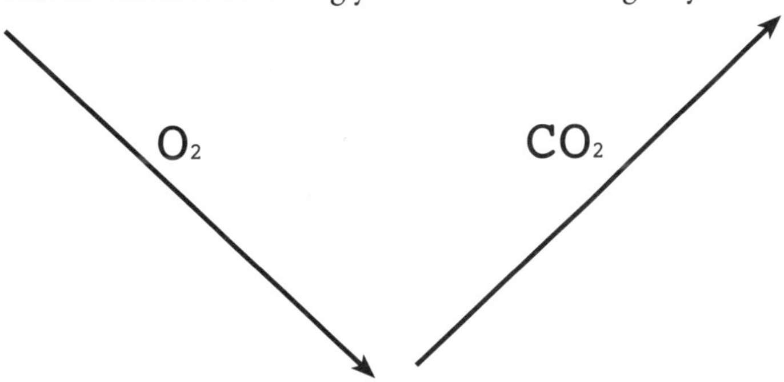

Figure 2-30. We Inhale to Absorb Oxygen and Exhale to Expel Carbon Dioxide

Air and water are being contaminated by pollution, especially in cities and industrial areas. The quality of food we eat depends on their source and processing methods. It is not easy to find the same pristine environment as in ancient times. However, we must adapt to our new environment and choose our way of life wisely.

Since carbon comprises such a major part of our body, absorbing good quality carbon is an important issue in modern health. You may obtain it from animal products or from plants. Carbon from plants is generally more pure than that taken from animals.

Red meat is more contaminated then white meat, so is more likely to disturb and overstimulate your Emotional Mind and confuse your thinking. Fish is another good source of carbon, but of course some fish are better than others. Shrimp is high in cholesterol, which can increase the risk of high blood pressure.

Due to the high level of impurities in most animal products, Qìgōng practitioners have spent a lot of time and effort searching for ways to efficiently absorb the protein they needed from plants, such as peas and beans. Soy beans are one of the best of these sources. They are inexpensive and easy to grow, but for a non-vegetarian it can be difficult for the body to produce the enzymes required to digest an all-vegetable diet. Humans evolved as omnivores, and the craving for meat can be strong. Even today, we still have canine teeth, used to tear off raw meat in ancient times. The natural enzymes in the body are more tailored to digesting meat. If we placed meat and corn in human digestive enzymes, the meat would dissolve in a matter of minutes, while the corn could take hours. So it is generally easier for the body to absorb the carbon it needs from meat than from plants.

This does not mean that we are unable to absorb plant protein efficiently. The key is that if an enzyme is present to begin with, then its production can be increased within your body, but it will take time. If you wish to become a vegetarian, you must reduce the intake of meat products slowly and allow your body to adjust to it, otherwise you may experience protein deficiency.

We must consume a variety of foods instead of concentrating only on those that are high in protein, to ensure we absorb all the various vitamins and trace minerals the body requires. Although they comprise only a minor proportion of our bodies, they are still essential in order for it to run smoothly. Calcium is important for bone development, and iron is crucial for healthy blood.

Nutrition is only one side of the coin. When a person ages quickly it may be due to poor Qì storage and circulation as opposed to malnourishment. Without an abundant supply, Qì circulation will not be regulated efficiently and your physical body will begin to degenerate. Qìgōng builds up the Qì in your Eight Vessels and helps you circulate it in your body. This Qìgōng training includes Wàidān (External Elixir) and Nèidān (Internal Elixir) practice, which we discuss in the next section.

While nutrition and Qì circulation are very important, the efficiency of the whole cell replacement process depends on the blood cells, which carry water, oxygen, and nutrients everywhere in the body through the blood circulatory network. From arteries and capillaries, the components for new cells are brought to even the most remote places in the body. The old cells absorb everything required from the bloodstream and divide to produce new cells. The remaining material from the dead cells is brought back through the veins to the lungs. Through respiration, the dead cells are expelled as carbon dioxide. Qì is vital for the process of cell division. Every blood cell is actually a dipole or small battery, storing bioelectricity and releasing it.[11] In Chinese medicine, it is understood that blood and Qì are always together. Where there is blood, there is Qì, and vice versa. The term Qì-Xuě (Qì-Blood, 氣-血) is often used in Chinese medicine.

The arteries are located deep beneath the muscles, while the veins are near the skin surface. The color of the blood in the arteries is red, because of the presence of oxygen. In the veins it looks blue, due to the absence of oxygen and the presence of carbon. Cell replacement starts inside the body, moving outward. If we tense more, blood circulation will be stagnant and the cell replacement process slower. Most cell replacement occurs at night, as we relax during sleep. So the importance of sleep in promoting health and longevity is obvious.

We must consider the means of ensuring steady production of healthy blood cells to maintain health and prevent premature aging. Without sufficient blood cells, the cell replacement process stagnates, and you degenerate swiftly.

Blood cells have a certain lifespan. When old ones die, new ones must be produced from the bone marrow to replace them. Bone marrow is the major blood factory of the body. When a person turns thirty, the marrow near the end of the bone cavities begins to turn yellow, as fat accumulates there. Red blood cells are no longer produced in the yellow area (Figure 2-31).[21] Qìgōng practitioners believe the degeneration of the bone marrow is due to insufficient Qì supply, and so Bone Marrow Washing Qìgōng was developed.

Hormone production also affects cell replacement. Hormones act as catalysts in the body. When hormone levels are high, we are more energized, and cell replacement proceeds faster and more smoothly. When hormone production is low, cell replacement will be slow and we age quickly. By increasing hormone levels, we extend life significantly.[22]

Maintaining healthy hormone production is a major concern in Qìgōng practice. Glands which produce hormones were recognized since ancient times, but hormones themselves were not well understood. They understood that the essence of life was stored in the kidneys. Today, we know this essence is actually the hormones produced by the adrenal glands on the top of the kidneys. They believed that through stimulation of the testicles and ovaries, the life force could be increased. From still meditation practice, they learned to lead Qì to the brain to raise up the spirit of vitality. It is led to the pituitary gland to stimulate growth hormone production. These practices are effective paths to longevity. Hormone levels decline significantly once our bones are complete, around the age of 30. Once the body has finished constructing itself, it triggers the reduction of hormone levels.

To prevent illness, we also consider our immune system. When Qì storage is abundant, you get sick less. Every white blood cell is like a fighting soldier who needs food to maintain his strength. When Qì is strong, the immune system is strong. Skin breathing was developed to lead Qì to the surface of the skin and strengthen the Guardian Qì (Wèiqì, 衛氣), the energetic component of the immune system near the skin surface.

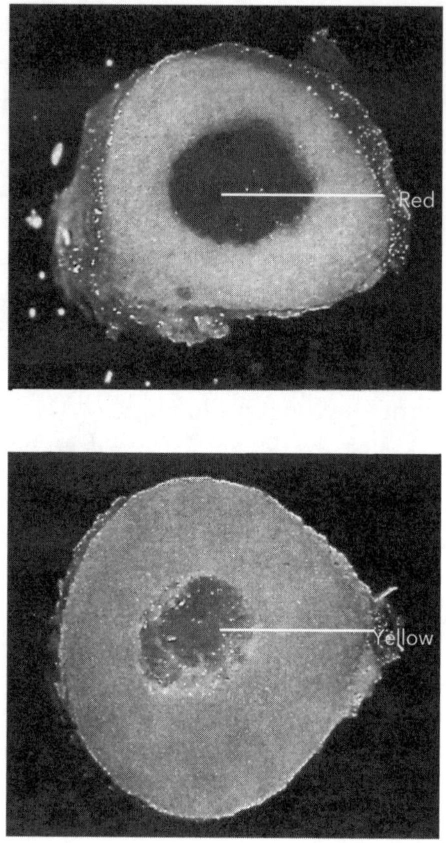

Figure 2-31. Structure of a Long Bone. Red Bone Marrow and Yellow Bone Marrow

2-4. Meaning and Purpose of Meditation (Jìngzuò Zhī Yìyì Yǔ Mùdì, 靜坐之意義與目的)

Many different schools of meditation have developed to serve a wide range of purposes. Meditation has existed in some form in almost every culture around the world, especially in religious societies. In some of these societies religious meditation has reached a very high level.

In China, different schools of meditation exist in almost all levels of society. In medical and scholar society, meditation is called Jìngzuò (靜坐), which means to sit quietly. It is used to bring the mind to a neutral, harmonious, and calm state. Many illnesses and mental problems are caused by emotional disturbances, so if we neutralize these emotional imbalances, we remove the causes of illness and emotional pain. This meditation is considered suitable for lay society, and was designed for regulating the mind and not aggressively pursuing regulation of the spirit.

Chinese martial society also uses meditation to seek the meaning of life and to raise the spirit. When the meaning of life is comprehended during meditation, a peaceful mind is attained, namely Yīn calmness. Then, Qì is led effectively to the body for Yáng power manifestation. Balancing this Yīn and Yáng, a martial artist reaches a level of deep martial skill and profound understanding of harmony and peace. Most well-known Chinese martial styles such as Shàolín (少林), Tàijí (太極), Wǔdāng (武當), Éméi (峨嵋), Tiānshān (天山), Qīngchéng (青城), and Kūnlún (崑崙) were developed in the monasteries. Their meditation methods were influenced strongly by religious meditation and in many ways cannot be separated.

Religious meditation is called Zuòchán (坐禪) in Buddhism, meaning "sit for Chán," and Dǎzuò (打坐) in Daoism, meaning "to sit." "Chán" means to cultivate, refine or pursue the state of Buddhahood. In the Buddhist *A Han Classic* it says (*Āhánjīng*, 阿含經), "Sit for Chán and ponder the origin, do not be neglectful and lazy."[23] Through Chán meditation, you search for the source of spiritual life.

The final goal of religious meditation is enlightenment (Daoist) or Buddhahood (Buddhism). Religious meditation is the highest level of meditation in Chinese society. Aspirants strive not only to achieve peace and harmony by neutralizing the Emotional Mind, but also for unification with the natural spirit (Tiānrén Héyī, 天人合一). To achieve this, abundant Qì storage in the Lower Real Dāntián must strengthen the physical body and nourish the brain to an enlightened state. When the body is strong, life will be long, allowing more time for spiritual cultivation. When the brain is nourished sufficiently, the third eye can be opened. Then the spirit is reunited with the natural spirit, and the purpose of life attained.

First, establish the goal of your mediation training. Are you cultivating a peaceful mind, or martial skill, or enlightenment? Then determine the path to reach your goal. How do you find the correct way? How committed are you? Do you have enough patience, perseverance, and a strong enough will to actively pursue your goals? Without a clear idea of where you are going and how to get there you will soon lose your way and give up.

The Small Circulation Meditation introduced in this book originates from Chinese religious society. Its first goal is to store abundant Qì at the Lower Real Dāntián. The second goal is leading Qì to circulate in the two major Qì vessels, the Conception and Governing Vessels (Rènmài, Dūmài, 任脈・督脈). When the Qì is strong and circulating smoothly in these two vessels, the Qì circulating in the Twelve Primary Qì Channels is strong, and the body strong and healthy.

In the next section, we summarize the purposes of general meditation. Small Circulation, Grand Circulation, and Enlightenment meditation will be discussed later in this chapter.

Purposes of General Meditation

The search for a peaceful mind. The most common purpose of meditation is to train the mind to be relaxed, calm and harmonious. Without meditation, the mind is generally emotionally agitated by surrounding circumstances, being scattered, confused, and excited. Through meditation with deep breathing, we can calm and clear the mind.

Using an EEG (Electroencephalogram), four separate groups of brainwaves (oscillating electrical currents) have been classified according to their frequency bands, with different activities related to each band.

These four categories are: (Figure 2-32)[24]

1. Beta activity (above 13 Hz): Occurs in bursts in the anterior part of the brain and is associated with mental activity.
2. Alpha activity (8-13 Hz): Relaxation, daydreaming.
3. Theta activity (4 to less than 8 Hz): Drowsy or asleep.
4. Delta activity (below 4 Hz): Deep sleep and coma.

When we are awake and thinking deeply (Beta), there is a lot of activity, but its amplitude is low. On average, 13 or more thoughts pass through our brain per second. By contrast, in the Alpha state of relaxation, although the signals are still almost as weak, the number of oscillations is significantly reduced. This implies that a calm mind has more clarity and focus. In the Theta state of drowsiness or sleep, the number of oscillations is also reduced, but the thoughts are more irregular. In deep, sound sleep (Delta), the number of oscillations is reduced substantially, while the amplitude is significantly increased. In scientific terms, the power of oscillation is as follows:[25]

$$P \propto \text{Frequency}^2 \times \text{Amplitude}^2$$

"Power is directly proportional to Frequency squared times Amplitude squared."

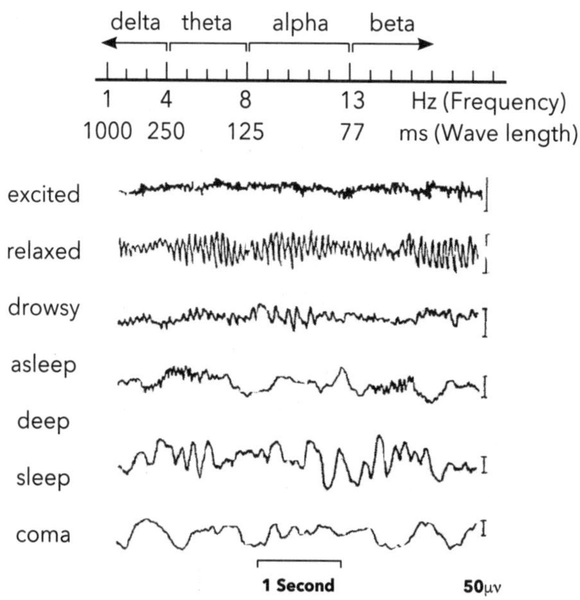

Figure 2-32. Typical Brain Wave Patterns from a State of Excitement to One of Deep Coma

In deep sleep, although your conscious mind is not deeply involved in thought (frequency reduced), the brain cells obtain a large supply of nutrition, oxygen, and Qì nourishment. In this calm state, there is less disturbance in the brain. Under these extremely calm and relaxed conditions, if you can control your consciousness without falling asleep, you can build up a better sensitivity for energy correspondence with the outside world. This is one of the desired states in meditation practice.

In meditation, you try to reach the stage at which the brainwaves are between Theta and Delta. It seems you are sleeping, yet your conscious mind is still governing the being. In this semi-sleeping or self-hypnotic state, the brain's sensitivity or energy correspondence with other brainwaves or natural vibrations reaches a peak. It is in this state that a meditator seeks the connection between his spiritual being and the spirit of nature.

Improving health and healing. When the mind is relaxed and calm, the body will be too. The more profound meditative state the mind reaches, the deeper the body can relax. When both mind and body relax, the Qì circulates smoothly and naturally. In this way, irregular Qì circulation due to illness or any other reason can be regulated to a healthy state of harmony. This is the main method used in Chinese medicine for healing and maintaining health. During deep meditation and relaxation, mind-body communication is efficient, Qì circulation is stronger, and the healing process faster.

During deep meditation, the breathing will be deep, soft and slender, which enables you to absorb oxygen and expel carbon dioxide more efficiently. Each brain cell consumes about twelve times as much oxygen as other cells, so a steady oxygen supply is crucial to keep the brain healthy. Deep exhalation of carbon dioxide disposes of waste from remote parts of the body. This is important for replacement of cells in the body.

To find the center of self-being. When you calm down, your mind becomes clearer and your thought process more logical. You must prevent your mind from wandering to memories or into fantasy, called "entering the devil" (Rùmó, 入魔). The best is to pay attention to the breathing, and keep the mind honest and truthful.

There are four steps to reach the final goal of spiritual freedom. The first is self-recognition (Zìshì, 自識), where the mask you wear starts to drop off, allowing you to recognize your spiritual being more clearly. Mistakes you have made and lies you have told are buried in your subconscious and will gradually arise in your conscious awareness. Your subconscious mind is always truthful and associated with the spiritual being. Once you discard the mask you have been wearing, you must face the real you. You encounter the past and analyze it. Not only that, to attain deep emotional balance, you search for ways to release feelings of guilt hidden deep inside. This process makes you humble, helps you understand yourself better, and finally helps you find the center of your being.

The next step is self-awareness (Zìjué, 自覺). By paying attention, you become aware of your spiritual being and the problems existing within yourself. You become more aware of your thinking and behavior, as well as that of others. You analyze your existence, your problems, and the role you should play in society. Through this self-awareness meditation process, you establish a calm and peaceful mind which harmonizes you with others and with nature.

To search for and understand the meaning of our lives. The third stage of cultivation is called self-awakening (Zìxǐng, Zìwù, 自醒・自悟). Through this stage you pay attention, collect information, and understand yourself and your environment. Many people, after this awakening process, see how ugly human nature is and decide to separate from lay society and become hermits or monks. Others build up their self-confidence and make their lives more meaningful.

The search for spiritual freedom. Realizing that we are being abused by political and spiritual leaders, the search begins for freedom from spiritual bondage (Jiětuō, 解脫), known as spiritual independence. When you reach this stage, your spiritual being can be independent and does not need to rely on others.

To comprehend the meaning of the universe. Many non-religious people try through meditation to comprehend the meaning, root, or origin of nature, searching for the truth of the Dào. The first step is to search for the root of our lives (Shēngmìng Zhīběn, 生命之本). Since our lives are a part of nature, from understanding the root of our lives, we comprehend the meaning of nature. To keep and cherish this root is called embracing the origin (Bàoyuán, Bàoyī, 抱元・抱一).

The three origins of our lives are Original Essence (Yuánjīng, 元精), Original Qì (Yuánqì, 元氣), and Original Spirit (Yuánshén, 元神). Original spirit is the origin of the others, since it exists before physical life begins. Searching for the spiritual root is the most important cultivation in Chinese society. Daoists say, "Cultivate the Xīn (Emotional Mind) to cultivate the natural being. Keep the center and embrace the origin."[26] Scholarly society says, "Pay attention to the Xīn to cultivate the natural being. Maintain the center to fully comprehend the origin."[27]

By contrast, the Buddhist family says: "Understand the Xīn clearly to grasp human nature. Millions of methods return to one."[28] The medical family says: "Void Xīn (humble mind) to stabilize the human natural being, cherish the origin and keep it."[29] The "one" is explained in a classic entitled the Classic of Great Peace (Tàipíngjīng, 太平經). It says, "Ponder to keep one, why? What is one? The beginning of the counting numbers. What is one? The Dào of begetting. What is one? The beginning of the raising of the Qì? What is one? The root principle of the universe."[30] The "one" means the very origin of all matter and energy. According to the *Book of Changes* (*Yìjīng*, 易經), this "one" means the state of Wújí (無極), of no extremity. The Daoist book, *The Complete Book of Principal Contents of Life and Human Nature* (*Xìngmìng Guīzhǐ Quánshū*, 性命圭旨全書) says, "What the scholar means by the one, is to use the original body to understand human nature."[31] It is also said in Daoist family that, "Dào, use the one to understand thoroughly."[32]

Even in secular meditation practice, the goals of meditation can be divided into levels ranging from beginner to profound. All of these spiritual regulation processes are also pursued by other Qìgōng groups such as martial artists.

2-5. Muscle/Tendon Changing and Marrow/Brain Washing Qìgōng (Yìjīnjīng Yǔ Xǐsuǐjīng, 易筋經與洗髓經)

We should be familiar with the Qìgōng practice of Muscle/Tendon Changing (Yìjīnjīng, 易筋經) and Marrow/Brain Washing (Xǐsuǐjīng, 洗髓經). Small Circulation meditation plays a major role in this practice.

Our two bodies are the physical (Yáng) body and the energy (Yīn) body. The physical body consists of skin, muscle, tendon, ligament, bone, and marrow. The energy body refers to the structure supplying Qì to the physical body and the brain.

Many Qìgōng practitioners consider the Yīn (Qì) body to be some kind of mental or spiritual body. Qì is neutral, supplying energy to the physical body for movement, and to the brain to support thought and behavior. But since thought and mental behavior are so closely related to spiritual cultivation, Chinese religious society considers the spiritual body to be the same as the Yīn body. The physical body is called Mìng (命) which means life, while the spiritual body is called Xìng (性), which means human nature, namely the natural spirit we are born with.

Muscle/Tendon Changing and Marrow/Brain Washing Qìgōng are religious Qìgōng training methods, created and passed down by an Indian monk, Dámó, in a Chinese Buddhist monastery called the Shàolín Temple (少林寺) (Figures 2-33 and 2-34). In Dámó's classic, he emphasizes that to achieve spiritual enlightenment, we need a long and healthy life, which will allow us more time for spiritual cultivation. Muscle/Tendon Changing Qìgōng describes how to condition the body, while Marrow/Brain Washing Qìgōng teaches how to build up an abundant supply of Qì with which to nourish the brain and promote its function to a higher level. Then, the final goal of spiritual enlightenment can be reached:

> *The Xǐsuǐjīng says a man's body is touched by love and desire, and formed with shape, contaminated by sediment and dirtiness. If you wish to cultivate the real meaning of Buddhism, (Spirit) moving and stopping at will, then the five viscera and six bowels, four limbs and hundreds of bones must be completely washed clean individually. (When you are) pure and can see calmness and peace, (you) can cultivate and enter the domain of Buddhahood. If you do not cultivate this way, (your cultivation) will not have foundation and origin. Read till here, then know that believers thought that "acquiring the marrow" was not just a comparison.*
>
> 洗髓經者，謂人之生，感於愛慾，一落有形，悉皆滓穢；欲修佛諦，動障真如，五臟六腑，四肢百骸，必先一一洗滌淨盡，純見清虛，方可進修，入佛智地，不由此經進修，無基無有是處；讀至此，然後知向者所謂得髓者，非譬喻也。

The Yìjīnjīng says that outside of the bone and marrow, under the skin and meat (muscles), there is nothing but the tendons and vessels which connect the body and transport the blood and Qì. All these are post-birth body, and must be promoted (trained). Borrow them to cultivate the real (Dào). If you do not promote them, you see weakening and withering immediately. If you see this just as ordinary training, how could you reach the final goal? If you give up and do not train them, there is no strength for cultivation, and nothing can be achieved. (When I) read till here, then I know that what were called skin, meat, and bones are also not a comparison and not a casual comment.

易筋者，謂髓骨之外，皮肉之內，莫非筋聯絡周身，通行血氣，凡屬後天，皆其提挈，借假修真，非所贊勷，立見頹靡，視作泛常，曷臻極至？舍是不為，進修不力，無有是處；讀至此，然後知所謂皮肉骨者，非譬喻，亦非漫語也。

From these two paragraphs, you can see that Muscle/Tendon Changing is for developing the body, while Marrow/Brain Washing is for spiritual advancement. This concept was very important to religious Qìgōng meditators. The ultimate goal of both Buddhist and Daoist study is to reach Buddhahood or enlightenment. They believe it normally takes hundreds of lifetimes to cultivate the spirit, and that gradually, lifetime after lifetime, you progress toward the final destination. If each lifetime is long, you have more time for spiritual cultivation. The physical conditioning is critical, especially as the most effective period for spiritual cultivation is after the age of forty. Normally, before then, the spirit of your new life is still maturing to be able to make contact with your pre-birth spirit. If you live a long and healthy life, you have enough time to develop your spirit to a higher level. The longer your life, the higher the level of cultivation, of maturity and wisdom your spirit can reach.

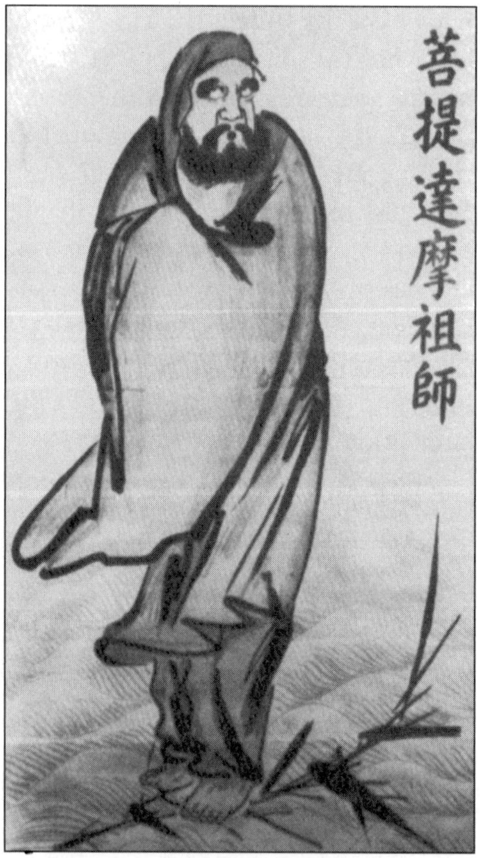

Figure 2-33. Dámó

The importance of longevity to spiritual cultivation was well understood by Daoists but was somewhat neglected by Buddhists. Daoists believe that the physical body and spiritual body are of equal importance and should be cultivated together. It is called "dual cultivation of spiritual virtues and physical life" (Xìngmìng Shuāngxiū, 性命雙修) in Daoist society. This was not the case in Buddhist society. Buddhists believe our physical body is only a temporary residence for the spirit, and spending time to build up physical strength is wasting precious time that could be spent on spiritual cultivation. Let us summarize the differences of approach to Muscle/Tendon Changing and Marrow/Brain Washing training in Buddhist and Daoist societies.

1. Although Buddhists developed these two training classics, they kept them strictly secret, without much opportunity to develop and evolve. Once Daoists learned them, they continued to research and develop them, and it seems the Daoist methods and theory are more complete and systematic than those of the Buddhists.
2. The Daoists have revealed more of their training to the public than the Buddhists have. Daoist training can produce health and longevity faster than the Buddhist training can, and can be practiced by seculars who do not wish to give up their normal existence for a life of seclusion. For this reason, more Daoist training documents have been found than Buddhist. However, the original theory, principles, and training methods were recorded in the Buddhist bibles.
3. Due to this constant research and development, many training techniques developed by the Daoists are more effective and efficient than the Buddhist

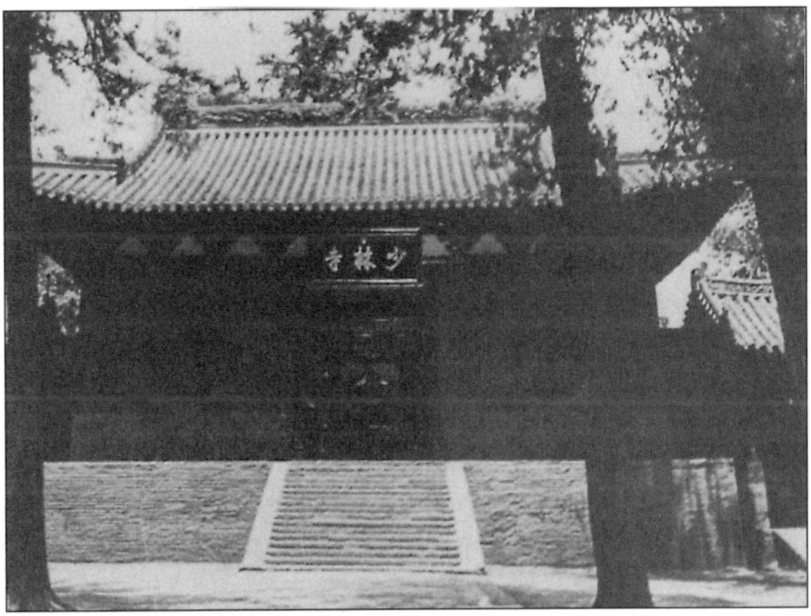

Figure 2-34. Shàolín Temple

alternatives, to improve health and increase longevity. However, when the training reaches the higher levels of spiritual cultivation found in the *Xǐsuǐjīng*, it seems the Buddhist methods of training are more effective. The Buddhists focus on training for the future instead of the present, while the Daoists to a certain extent pay more attention to the present.

4. Daoists have developed many techniques such as dual cultivation or Picking the Herb from Outside of the Dào to assist the Xǐsuǐjīng training. Some Daoists encourage gaining Qì balance through dual meditation or sexual practices. Sexual Qìgōng has always been forbidden in the Buddhist monasteries. This is probably the most significant difference between the two schools of training.
5. Daoist Xǐsuǐjīng training comprises both physical and spiritual practices, while the Buddhist approach is mainly spiritual. Daoist training begins with many physical exercises, such as massaging the testicles. The physical stimulation generates semen, which is converted into Qì either physically or mentally. The Daoist documents discuss many physical training techniques, while the Buddhist training emphasizes meditation.
6. Daoists have researched the use of herbs to assist Qìgōng training, while the Buddhists have never paid much attention to this. The Daoist documents have more herbal prescriptions than the Buddhist documents.

Kǎn and Lí in Yìjīnjīng and Xǐsuǐjīng (Yìjīnjīng Yǔ Xǐsuǐjīng De Kǎn-Lí, 易筋經與洗髓經的坎離)

In any style of Qìgōng, you balance Yīn and Yáng by controlling Kǎn (坎, Water) and Lí (離, Fire). Tàijíquán trains slow meditative physical movements which are examples of Lí, and may make your body too Yáng. You balance this with still meditation, which is Kǎn and neutralizes excess Yáng. In moving Tàijí forms, there is also Kǎn and Lí adjustment. While the movement is Lí, which causes Yáng, the calm mind is Kǎn, which neutralizes the Yáng. In still meditation, while the stillness of the physical body is Kǎn and causes Yīn, the Qì must be actively led to circulate in the body, which is Lí and results in Yáng, which balances the Yīn. In all Qìgōng practices, if there is Yīn, there must be Yáng to balance it, and vice versa.

It is the same with the Yìjīnjīng and Xǐsuǐjīng training. They are based on this Yīn and Yáng concept. The Yìjīnjīng is Lí because it generates Qì and causes Yáng, while the Xǐsuǐjīng is Kǎn, utilizing and storing Qì, and causing Yīn. The Yìjīnjīng deals with the muscles, tendons, and skin, which are visible externally, while the Xǐsuǐjīng deals with the marrow and brain, which must be felt internally. While the Yìjīnjīng training emphasizes the physical body, the Xǐsuǐjīng training focuses on the spiritual. Thus Yīn and Yáng are balanced and coexist harmoniously.

In the Yìjīnjīng, the physical stimulation and exercises are considered Lí, and cause the body to become Yáng, while the still meditation for the Small Circulation is Kǎn, calming Lí and makes the body more Yīn. In the physical stimulation Lí training, external strength is Lí, while internal mental strength is Kǎn. In still meditation, the physical body is still and Kǎn, while the Qì led by the mind and moving internally is Lí.

The same theory prevails in Xǐsuǐjīng training. The physical stimulation to increase the Original Essence production is Lí, while the techniques of internal cultivation, which are used to lead Qì to the marrow and brain, are Kǎn.

The key to successful Qìgōng training is Yīn and Yáng balance, and the means to achieve this is adjustment of Kǎn and Lí. This fundamental theory is the foundation of Qìgōng practice.

The Role of Small Circulation in Yìjīnjīng and Xǐsuǐjīng (Xiǎozhōutiān Zài Yìjīnjīng Yǔ Xǐsuǐjīng Zhōng De Jiǎosè, 小周天在易筋經與洗髓經中的角色)

1. **To store and enhance Qì in the Real Lower Dāntián to an abundant level.** To recondition the body from weak to strong, and to flood the brain with Qì for brain washing, you require abundant Qì, without which you cannot progress. The way to build up the Qì and store it in the Real Lower Dāntián is through Embryonic Breathing (Tāixí, 胎息) techniques, which are discussed later.
2. **To raise the level of Qì circulation in the Conception and Governing Vessels.** Once Qì is abundant in the Real Lower Dāntián, the second goal of Small Circulation training is to lead it to the Conception and Governing Vessels (Rènmài, Dūmài; 任脈・督脈). It circulates smoothly in these two vessels, which act as Qì reservoirs, and in the twelve channels, which function as rivers. With abundant Qì in the reservoirs, the Qì in the rivers can be regulated efficiently. The Conception Vessel regulates the Qì level of the six primary Yīn channels, while the Governing Vessel regulates the six primary Yáng channels. These twelve channels connect the Qì from the limbs to that of the internal organs. Once Qì is abundant and circulating smoothly in these twelve channels, your physical body will be stronger and healthier.

Small Circulation is actually a Muscle/Tendon Changing practice to recondition the body, while Embryonic Breathing helps establish the Qì storage necessary for the Marrow/Brain Washing practice.

2-6. What Is Small Circulation? (Héwèi Xiǎozhōutiān? 何謂小周天？)

In this section, we discuss the three common Qì paths in Qìgōng meditation practice (Figure 2-35). From this we may define Small Circulation. Each of these three paths has its own training theory, purposes, and methods. Generally speaking, the Fire Path described below is recognized as Small Circulation.

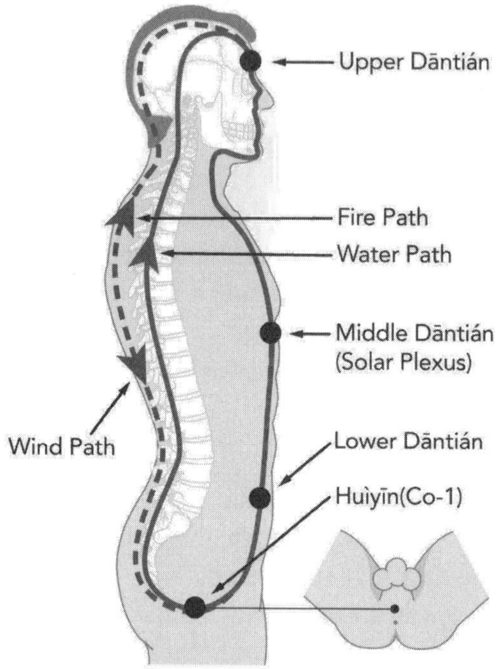

Figure 2-35. The Fire, Water and Wind Paths of Qì Circulation

Three Paths

Fire Path (Small Circulation Meditation) (Huǒlù, 火路). In Fire Path circulation, having built up abundant Qì in the Real Lower Dāntián (Zhēn Xiàdāntián, 真下丹田) through Embryonic Breathing, you then use your mind to lead Qì to the Conception and Governing Vessels (Rènmài, Dūmài; 任脈・督脈). You enhance the Qì in these two Qì reservoirs and then circulate it up the Governing Vessel and down the Conception Vessel, thereby regulating Qì circulation in the Twelve Primary Qì Channels, linking the internal organs and the limbs. This strengthens and energizes the physical body and enhances the Guardian Qì (Wèiqì, 衛氣), making your body Yáng. Thus the Fire Path meditation is Lí (Fire, 離) and generates fire in the body.

There are a few documents relating to the practice of Fire Path circulation. The book *Great Attainment of Acupuncture and Moxibustion* (*Zhēnjiǔ Dàchéng*, 針灸大成) says, "Slowly swallow a mouthful of air and lead Qì into the Dāntián. The impulse begins at the Mìngmén (命門, navel or Qìhǎi), lead it in the Governing Vessel, pass the Tailbone (Wěilǘ, 尾閭), ascend up to the Níwán (泥丸, crown), to chase and move (initiate or awaken) the origin of human nature. Then lead it down the Conception Vessel, pass the Multi-Towers (Chónglóu, 重樓, throat) and down to return to Qìhǎi (Co-6, 氣海). Two vessels revolving up and down. The front descends and the rear ascends, continuously and without stopping... After practicing for a long time, the tricky gates open automatically. The Qì circulates smoothly in hundreds of meridians and hundreds of sicknesses will not be initiated."[33] In the book *Antithetic Writing of Regulating the Path* (*Lǐyuè Piánwén*, 理瀹駢文), it says, "Close the eyes and sit quietly. The nose inhales clean air. Expand the abdomen to enable internal Qì to descend to the Lower Dāntián under the navel. Transport Qì past the perineum, along the Governing Vessel and past the Tailbone (Wěilǘ, 尾閭), Squeezing Spine (Jiájí, 夾脊, between the shoulder blades) and Jade Pillow (Yùzhěn, 玉枕), the three gates. Reach Bǎihuì (Gv-20, 百會) cavity on top of the head, follow the face to the tongue and connect with the Conception Vessel, descend down along the front of the chest, to finally reach the Dāntián and again circulate in the original path. Where there is Qì stagnation or pain, inhale and think of the place, and exhale to lead the Qì back to the Dāntián. This can strengthen the body and repel sickness. It is also called Sānmèiyìn (Samadhi, 三昧印)."[34]

From these two ancient documents, we may assume that Small Circulation meditation is the same as Fire Path meditation.

Water Path (Enlightenment Meditation) (Shuǐlù, 水路). The Water Path is the hardest but most effective method of using Kǎn (Water, 坎) to neutralize the body's Yáng. It is trained in Marrow/Brain Washing (Xǐsuǐjīng, 洗髓經). The mind directs Qì from the Real Lower Dāntián via the Huìyīn (Co-1, 會陰) up through the Thrusting Vessel (Chōngmài, 衝脈, spinal cord) to nourish the brain. When the brain is well nourished, the spirit can be raised for enlightenment. Water Path training calms the mind, but also helps lead Qì into the center of the body for marrow washing. Since bone marrow is where your body produces white and red blood cells, abundant Qì there promotes their production. Red blood cells carry oxygen and other nutrients required for cell replacement, slowing degeneration of your body. When white blood cells are abundant and healthy, the immune system is strong, preventing illness. Water Path Qìgōng meditation is for enlightenment or Buddhahood. We will discuss this in detail in future publications on the topics of Grand Circulation and Enlightenment Meditation.

Wind Path (Kǎn Lí Meditation) (Fēnglù, 風路). The Wind Path is considered to be a reversed Small Circulation. In the Wind Path, the Water Qì accumulated in the Real Lower Dāntián is led by the mind to circulate in the path which exactly reverses the path of the Fire Path Qì circulation. There are many reasons for this Wind Path Qì circulation. First, through reversing the natural Qì circulation, it is possible to cool down your overexcited mental and physical body. This is because when you practice the Wind Path Qì circulation, you are slowing down the natural Qì circulation. Second, through it you can lead the Water Qì from the Real Lower Dāntián upward to cool down the Fire Qì accumulated in the Middle Dāntián (Zhōng Dāntián, 中丹田) (diaphragm). In this way, the mental and physical body can also be cooled down. This process is commonly called "Kǎn-Lí." However, to Enlightenment Meditation practitioners, the Wind Path is crucial to conceive a Spiritual Embryo (Língtāi, 靈胎) at the Huángtíng (黃庭) cavity located between the Middle Dāntián and Real Lower Dāntián. In this practice, as mentioned earlier, the Water Qì is led upward to meet the Fire Qì which is led downward from the Middle Dāntián and they meet each other at the Huángtíng. This process is also called "Kǎn-Lí" (坎-離) which causes the interaction of the Yīn and Yáng. From this Yīn-Yáng interaction, with the focused attention of the Shén, a new Spiritual Embryo can be produced.

Small Circulation meditation is generally practiced as Fire Path Qìgōng meditation. Its two main purposes are to enhance the Qì (Chōngqì, 充氣) in the Real Lower Dāntián (Zhēn Xiàdāntián, 真下丹田) and to lead the Qì (Yǐnqì, 引氣) to circulate smoothly in the Conception and Governing Vessels.

In Daoist society, the name for Small Circulation is Yīn-Yáng Circulation Small Heavenly Cycle (Yīn-Yáng Xúnhuán Yī Xiǎozhōutiān, 陰陽循環一小周天). In Buddhist society it is called Sānmèiyìn (三昧印) or Sānmódì (三摩地), adopted from the Sanskrit word Samhadi. Since both societies have very different names for the same practice it indicates that Small Circulation has been practiced intensely by both Daoist and Buddhist societies.

In *Anthology of Daoist Village* (Dàoxiāngjí, 道鄉集), it says, "The Cycling Heaven (Small Circulation) of the Daoist family is the same as Turning the Wheel of Law (Zhuǎnfǎlún, 轉法輪) of the Buddhist family. The principles are the same though the approaches are different. It was the descendant people themselves that separated them."[35] Small Circulation is called Xiǎozhōutiān (小周天) which means Small Heavenly Cycle. Since humans are an integral part of nature, Qì circulation in the human body should resemble and be influenced by the Qì circulation between heaven and earth. Therefore, the head is referred to as Tiānlínggài (天靈蓋), which means Heavenly Spiritual Cover, while the perinium is called Hǎidǐ (海底) which means sea bottom. The Qì circulation between Heaven and Earth is called Dàzhōutiān (大周天), or Grand Heavenly Cycle. Qì circulating within the human body between the head and the perinium is called Xiǎozhōutiān (小周天), or Small Heavenly Cycle. Qì circulation through the Conception and Governing Vessels is closely related to and influenced by that of Heaven and Earth in 24-hour cycles.

Buddhist society also referred to Small Circulation meditation as Zhuǎnfǎlún (轉法論) which means Turning the Wheel of Natural Law. Fǎlún (法論) was translated from the Indian word Dharmachakra which is a common name for Buddhism.[36] In the book, *The Complete Book of Principal Contents of Life and Human Nature* (*Xìngmìng Guīzhǐ Quánshū*, 性命圭旨全書) says, "The Buddhist family call it Ruling Wheel (Fǎlún, 法輪), the Daoist family call it Heavenly Cycle (Zhōutiān, 周天), and Confucians call it Circulating the Heavenly Court (Xíngtíng, 行庭). But all have the same basis."[37] This document also describes the methods of practice in turning the Ruling Wheels. The interaction of Yīn and Yáng governs nature, and comprises the natural Ruling Wheels which influence the variations of the Qì circulation in Heaven and Earth.

Lǐ, Shí-Zhēn (李時珍) (1518-1593 CE) wrote in his book *The Study of Strange Meridians and Eight Vessels* (*Qíjīng Bāmài Kǎo*, 奇經八脈考), "The Conception and Governing Vessels are the body's Zǐ (midnight) and Wǔ (noon). It is the Dào (Natural Way) of increasing the Yáng fire and decreasing the Yīn water. It is also the place where Kǎn and Lí interact."[38] When one circulates Qì smoothly in these two vessels, it flows smoothly throughout the rest of the body, without stagnation. This is the basis for longevity.

There were a few points in particular that he emphasized.

1. The flow of Qì in the Conception and Governing Vessels is closely related to the time of day.
2. We adjust Yīn and Yáng through constant practice of Kǎn and Lí.
3. Kǎn and Lí interact on the path of the Conception and Governing Vessels.
4. The smooth flow of Qì in these two vessels affects the flow in the twelve primary channels (rivers, Jīng, 經) and countless secondary Qì channels (streams, Luò, 絡).
5. Smooth Qì flow in these two vessels is the foundation of longevity.

Summary

1. The are many different schools of meditation practice. Normally, Small Circulation refers to the circulation of Qì in the Conception and Governing Vessels.
2. Small Circulation likens the Qì flow in the Yīn Conception and Yáng Governing Vessels with the Qì flow between Heaven and Earth, in nature as a whole.
3. Small Circulation is to some extent a process which occurs naturally. The meditation practice just uses the mind to enhance the process.
4. The natural flow of the Conception and Governing Qì follows the time of day, which will be discussed in more detail later.
5. The full name of Small Circulation is Yīn-Yáng Circulation Small Heavenly Cycle (Yīn-Yáng Xúnhuán Yī Xiǎozhōutiān, 陰陽循環一小周天) in Daoist society. In Buddhist society it is called Sānmèiyìn (三昧印) or Sānmódì (三摩地), from the Sanskrit Samadhi, meaning steadiness. Buddhists also refer to it as Zhuǎnfǎlún (轉法論), or Turning the Wheel of Natural Law.

2-7. What Is Grand Circulation? (Héwèi Dàzhōutiān? 何謂大周天？)

Internal Grand Circulation Meditation (Zìwǒ Dàzhōutiān Jìngzuò, 自我大周天靜坐)

Through Internal Grand Circulation meditation, your mind leads Qì to any part of the body. You first develop the sensitivity to feel each part of your body internally, from the skin to the bone marrow. The deeper your mind reaches in meditation, the more profound and effective this practice will be.

With practice, you lead the Qì to the remotest places within the body for healing. If your Qì is strong, you may also use it to heal and nourish other people, commonly referred to as Qì Massage (Qìànmó, 氣按摩) or External Qì Healing (Wàiqì Líáofǎ, 外氣療法). Martial artists use Grand Circulation to energize the body.

Primary Qì Channel Circulation Meditation (Shíèrjīng Dàzhōutiān Jìngzuò, 十二經大周天靜坐). The main purpose of this meditation is to enhance circulation in the Twelve Primary Qì Channels, so the internal organs grow strong and healthy. Qì distribution to the arms and legs also improves, which strengthens the physical body.

There is a specific natural order of Qì circulation from one channel to another, with certain times of day in which a channel's Qì is strongest. This cycle is called Zǐwǔ Líúzhù (子午流注), or midnight to noon major Qì flow. If you understand this natural Qì flow timing, you can adopt the correct path and timing for your practice.

Joint Grand Circulation Meditation (Guānjié Dàzhōutiān Jìngzuò, 關節大周天靜坐). The purpose here is to circulate Qì in the bone marrow and within the joints, as well as in the primary channels. This is especially important for Qì healers, enabling them to project Qì outside the body.

Four Gates Breathing Circulation (Sìxīn Hūxī Dàzhōutiān Jìngzuò, 四心呼吸大周天靜坐). The purpose of Four Gates Breathing is to lead Qì from the Real Lower Dāntián to the four gates. Two of these gates called Láogōng (P-8, 勞宮), meaning Labor Palace, belong to the Pericardium Channel and are located at the center of the palms (Figure 2-36). The other two gates are called Yǒngquán (K-1, 湧泉), which means Gushing Spring. They belong to the Kidney Channel and are located at the front center of the soles (Figure 2-37).

These four cavities are the main gates which regulate the Qì level of the heart and kidneys. When Qì flows smoothly to them, the body is healthy, and great power is generated in the limbs. Four Gates Meditation is emphasized in Chinese martial arts, especially in the internal arts. It has been discussed at length in the YMAA books *The Essence of Tàijí Qìgōng* and *The Essence of Shàolín White Crane*.

Skin/Marrow Breathing Circulation (Fūsuǐxī Dàzhōutiān Jìngzuò, 膚髓息大周天靜坐). Again, this leads Qì to the skin surface to enhance your Guardian Qì (Wèiqì, 衛氣), and stores Qì in the bone marrow as Marrow Qì (Suǐqì, 髓氣). When Guardian Qì is

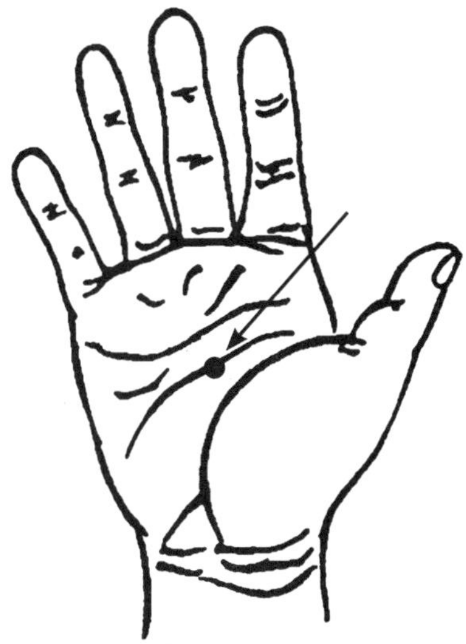

Figure 2-36. The Láogōng (P-8) Cavity

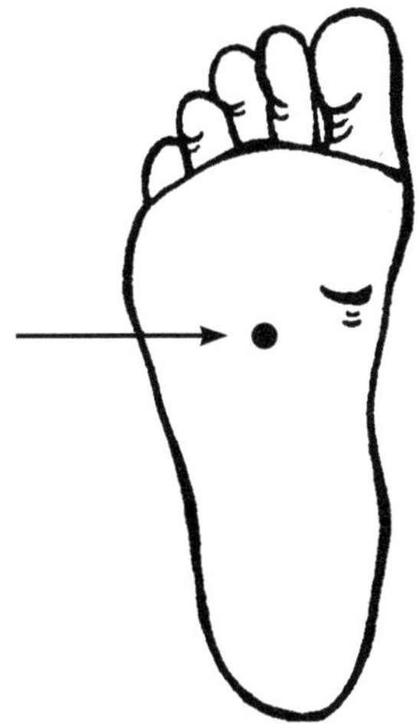

Figure 2-37. The Yǒngquán (K-1) Cavity

strong, your immune system functions efficiently. When Marrow Qì is strong, the bone marrow produces a regular supply of healthy blood cells.

Grand Circulation Meditation with a Partner (Shuāngxiū Dàzhōutiān Jìngzuò, 雙修大周天靜坐)

Once abundant Qì is stored in your Real Lower Dāntián and you can circulate it smoothly throughout your body, you can heal and nourish other people. Dual Cultivation (Shuāngxiū, 雙修), as it is called, is the foundation of Qì healing. It is the most effective method for Qìgōng healers to train to exchange Qì with other people. Through this practice, two healthy people can nourish one another and elevate their training spirit significantly. Dual Cultivation is one of the most effective ways of accelerating spiritual enlightenment. We will discuss this subject in the book *Qìgōng Grand Circulation for Spiritual Enlightenment*.

Grand Circulation Meditation with Great Nature (Tiānrén Héyī Dàzhōutiān Jìngzuò, 天人合一大周天靜坐)

Grand Circulation Meditation with the Earth (Dìrén Dàzhōutiān Jìngzuò, 地人大周天靜坐). In this meditation you project your Qì beyond the body and exchange it with your environment, such as with the earth, trees, animals, and the air, all of which have their own Qì fields. It is possible to absorb Qì from around you, enhancing your own Qì level. In China, trees are regularly used for Qì regulation purposes. The difference between this Qì exchange and that involving a human partner is that these objects do not have a mind that we are able to recognize, so they cannot use their mind to lead their Qì as they exchange it with you.

Grand Circulation Meditation with Heaven (Tiānrén Dàzhōutiān Jìngzuò, 天人大周天靜坐). Grand Circulation Meditation with Heaven is also called Fifth Gate Meditation. Its purpose is to achieve spiritual unification with the universe, Tiānrén Héyī (天人合一). You lead Qì up through the Thrusting Vessel (Chōngmài, 衝脈) to the brain, nourish and energize it to a high energy state. The spirit grows and the third eye gradually opens. This is called enlightenment (Wùzhēn, 悟真). Having opened the third eye, there are no obstacles to communication between you and the surrounding environment, and you comprehend many things which cannot be understood by others. You communicate with others without speaking, as your telepathic capabilities develop. You comprehend the meaning of life and of nature.

2-8. What is Enlightenment Meditation? (Héwèi Xiāndào Jìngzuò?, 何謂仙道靜坐？)

To grasp the meaning of the universe, we combine our Qì with that of nature. Animals still have this spiritual connection, but humans lost it long ago. Due to the development of the human intellect and emotions, our spirit separated from that of nature, and our thoughts are contaminated by emotions and desires. Animals have not developed as we have, so they are still connected with nature, and their behavior is in line with the natural way of life. At birth we have a similar connection with the natural Qì and spirit. But as we grow, our minds are molded by the masked environment created by human minds. To survive in society we mask our faces, suppressing our natural spiritual instincts. Many people retire to the mountains for spiritual cultivation, to free themselves from this emotional bondage, attain a neutral state of mind, and sense the natural spirit more clearly.

To achieve unification with the natural spirit, one must open the third eye (Upper Dāntián, Shàng Dāntián, 上丹田) by concentrating Qì inside it. First build up Qì in the Real Lower Dāntián (Zhēn Xiàdāntián, 真下丹田), then lead it up to nourish the brain. Build up Qì there, using Embryonic Breathing (Tāixí, 胎息). Only when the Qì stored in the Real Lower Dāntián has reached an abundant level will there be enough Qì to open the third eye.

To reach enlightenment, Daoists and Buddhists say you pass through four stages. The first is Self-Recognition, in which you remove the mask you wear. You see yourself clearly, recognizing and understanding your thought processes, and acknowledging what kind of person you really are. The second stage is Self-Awareness, in which you analyze past events and become aware of your interaction with your environment. The third stage, Self-Awakening, involves searching for freedom from emotional bondage. Finally, you attain the stage of Freedom from Spiritual Bondage, in which your ego and desires disappear. Your spirit establishes contact with the natural spirit, and you gain the Truth of Nature, or the Dào.

Daoists further classify these four stages of cultivation into sixteen steps, described in the document *The Golden Elixir Methods of Regulating the Inner Mind—Procedures of Training Internal Elixir* (*Jīndān Xīnfǎ·Liàn Nèidān Bùzhòu*, 金丹心法・練內丹步驟).[39]

1. **A strong will** (Lìzhì, 立志). The first step towards enlightenment is to establish a strong will, without which you will not finish the training.
2. **Maintain good morality** (Duānpǐn, 端品), including both the mental and the physical. Although you know right from wrong, you might ignore it and wander the path of sin. When wrong thought manifests, you harm yourself and others. Thoughts and behavior which cause harm to others is considered immoral in Buddhist and Daoist societies.
3. **Confession** (Huǐguò, 悔過). Once you have corrected your lines of thought and action, you contemplate bad deeds you committed in the past. Buddhists and Daoists believe past transgressions leave a stain on your conscience. Unless you recognize and admit your past mistakes, you continue to repeat them. At this stage you discard the mask you have been wearing.
4. **Transform into goodness** (Qiānshàn, 遷善). You now recognize your good and bad personality traits, as you accentuate the positive and discard the negative ones. Once your mind is ready, you open your third eye. If you still have things to hide, you will be unable to open it, lest you let other people see into your mind.
5. **Build a firm spiritual foundation** (Zhújī, 築基), where your Wisdom Mind (Yì) gains ascendancy over your Emotional Mind (Xīn). Your judgment becomes clear, guided by wisdom instead of by emotion.
6. **Cultivate yourself** (Líànjǐ, 煉己). The next stage is to refine your thinking, as you comprehend the meaning of your spiritual life, and your spiritual body develops rapidly. Your thinking diverges from mainstream society, and you may decide to separate from secular society to avoid distractions. When you meditate, it is as though your physical body disappears, and you feel transparent and light. This is called "getting rid of the view of the body" in Buddhism.
7. **Establish the furnace** (Ānlú, 安爐), and strengthen your spirit to survive separation from your physical body. Otherwise, once your body dies, your spirit must find a replacement in which to reincarnate, to prevent it gradually deteriorating and ceasing to exist. Buddhists and Daoists seek to develop their spiritual bodies to have independent eternal life without returning to the path of reincarnation.
8. **Picking the herb** (Cǎiyào, 采藥) involves conversion of essence, both Original Essence (Yuánjīng, 元精) and Post-Birth Essence, into Qì. Original Essence is comprised of genetically determined hormones. Post-Birth Essence is derived from our air and food. To enhance the conversion process, practice methods of increasing hormone production in the body, take herbs which can easily be converted into Qì, and ensure that you are consuming good quality food and fresh air.

9. **Starting the fire** (Qǐhuǒ, 起火) involves building up Qì in the Lower Dāntián through abdominal breathing. There are two alternative methods of abdominal breathing. The first is called Normal Abdominal Breathing (Zhèng Fùhūxī, 正腹呼吸) or Buddhist Breathing (Fójiā Hūxī, 佛家呼吸). The second is called Reverse Abdominal Breathing (Fǎn Fùhūxī or Nì Fùhūxī, 反腹呼吸・逆腹呼吸), or Daoist Breathing (Dàojiā Hūxī, 道家呼吸).
10. **Ceasing the fire** (Xíhuǒ, 熄火) involves storing the Qì you have built up, instead of manifesting it in the physical body. Only then will you be able to control the body's Qì and maintain its Yīn-Yáng balance. You store the Qì in the Real Dāntián (Zhēn Xiàdāntián, 真下丹田), the human biobattery, through Embryonic Breathing (Tāixí, 胎息).
11. **Generate the Embryo** (Jiétāi, 結胎). Original Essence is called Original Qì (Yuánqì, 元氣), or Water Qì (Shuǐqì, 水氣). It is pure and calming. However, Qì at the Middle Dāntián, or sternum, originates from Post-Birth Essence, namely air and food. It is called Post-Heaven Qì (Hòutiānqì, 後天氣) and considered to be Fire Qì (Huǒqì, 火氣), which is contaminated and liable to disturb and excite your Emotional Mind. So the Water Qì, or Kǎn (坎), can make you more Yīn, while the Fire Qì, or Lí (離), can make you more Yáng. To generate new life in the form of a Spiritual Embryo (Shéntāi, 神胎), Yīn and Yáng must interact through the method of Kǎn and Lí (坎離). Lead the Water Qì up from the Lower Dāntián or Real Lower Dāntián, and the Fire Qì down from the sternum, to meet at the Huángtíng (黃庭) cavity between sternum and navel. With continued practice, a Spiritual Embryo is generated. This converts Qì into spirit, and is called Ten Months of Pregnancy (Shíyuè Huáitāi, 十月懷胎).
12. **Nursing the baby** (Yǎngyīng, 養嬰). After ten months of pregnancy, the Spiritual Embryo is born, meaning the third eye has opened, and the spirit can leave the body and return to it at will. This is known as Refining Spirit and Returning it to Nothingness (Líànshén Fǎnxū, 煉神返虛), or Three Years of Nursing (Sānnián Bǔrǔ, 三年哺乳).
13. **Accumulation of good deeds** (Jīxíng, 積行). You now train your spirit in the finer differences between good and evil. By this stage, you have promoted your spirit to a very high level.

14. **Train Gōng** (Xínggōng, 行功) to establish a connection between your new spirit and the natural spirit. By training your spirit to separate from the physical body for longer intervals and traveling greater distances, it will gradually become independent.
15. **Facing the wall** (Miànbì, 面壁). This is called Crushing the Nothingness (Fěnsuì Xūkōng, 粉碎虛空), or Nine Years of Facing the Wall (Jiǔnián Miànbì, 九年面壁). You prepare to separate your spiritual body from your physical body permanently. You face the wall and ponder your life once more, to ensure you really wish to free yourself from all human bondage.
16. **Flying to ascend** (Fēishēng, 飛升). Now that you are ready to separate your spiritual and physical bodies, you choose the day to separate them permanently. This is the final stage of cultivation, Unification of Heaven and Man (Tiānrén Héyī, 天人合一).

It should now be easier to understand the first few steps of spiritual cultivation, although the training methods and the meaning of cultivation may remain hidden until one reaches a more profound stage. It is similar to how our perspective of the world changes as we mature.

Summary of Spiritual Enlightenment Cultivation

1. The first step is Small Circulation Meditation, the foundation of Internal Elixir (Nèidān, 內丹) Qìgōng practice. By training it, you build up Qì and store it in the Real Lower Dāntián, the human bioelectric battery. You also use the mind's ability to generate EMF to circulate Qì in the two main vessels which supply Qì to the Twelve Primary Qì Channels. This leads to an abundant Qì supply for the physical body and is the key to strengthening the body for health and longevity.
2. After Small Circulation, you train Grand Circulation Meditation, with methods of improving Qì circulation throughout the entire body, and exchanging Qì with others and with your environment. From this Qì communication, you start to understand the natural spirit, which is the initial step in understanding nature for the purpose of unification with the spirit of heaven.
   You use the mind's EMF, leading Qì to the surface of the skin to strengthen Guardian Qì, including the immune system. You also lead Qì to the marrow to maintain its health and proper function, which is vital to longevity.
   You lead Qì to the four gates: two Láogōngs and two Yǒngquáns. These are four of the five gates used to establish a connection with the environment. The fifth gate is your third eye which is related to the practice of enlightenment.

Finally, you exchange Qì with other people, animals, or natural objects. You may adjust other people's Qì into a more harmonious and balanced state, which is the key to Qìgōng healing.

3. The final goal of meditation is spiritual enlightenment, achieved by opening the third eye. The spirit can leave and enter the body at will, and survive without the support of the physical body. Finally, the physical body is left behind and the practitioner gains eternal spiritual life.

References

1. 《易》曰：〝一陰一陽之謂道。〞

2. 《道德經・四十二章》：〝道生一，一生二，二生三，三生萬物。〞

3. 《道德經・二十五章》：〝有物混成，先天地生。寂兮寥兮，獨立而不改，周行而不殆，可以為天下母。吾不知其名，強字之曰道。〞

4. 《道德經・一章》：〝玄之又玄，眾妙之門。〞

5. 《道德經・五十一章》：〝道生之，德畜之，物形之，勢成之。〞指萬物變化。

6. 《道德經・二十五章》：〝人法地，地法天，天法道，道法自然。〞指以自然為法。

7. 《淮南子・天文訓》：〝道始于一，一而不生，故分為陰陽，陰陽和合而萬物生。〞

8. 《道德經・一章》：〝無，名先天之始；有，名萬物之母。常無，欲以觀其妙；常有，欲以觀其徼。〞指事物正在變化之中。

9. 《朱子語類》：〝謂之太極者，所以指天地萬物之根。〞

10. 李時珍《奇經八脈考》：〝陽維主一身之表，陰維主一身之里，陽蹻主一身左右之陽，陰蹻主一身左右之陰，督主身後之陽，任、沖主身前之陰，帶脈橫束諸脈以總約之。〞

11. "Lífe's Invisible Current," by Albert L. Huebner, *East West Journal*, June 1986.

12. *The Body Electric*, by Robert O. Becker, M.D. and Gary Selden, Quill, William Morrow, New York, 1985.

13. "Healing with Nature's Energy," by Richard Leviton, *East West Journal*, June 1986.

14. *A Child Is Born,* by Lennart Nilsson, A DTP/Seymour Lawrence Book, 1990.

15. 解剖生理學 (*A Study of Anatomic Physiology*) 李文森編著。華杏出版股份有限公司, Lǐ, Wén-Sēn, Táipéi, 1986.

16. *Grant's Atlas of Anatomy*, James E. Anderson, 7th Edition, Williams & Wilkins Co., 9-92, 1978.

17. "Complex and Hidden Brain in the Gut Makes Stomachaches and Butterflies," by Sandra Blakeslee, *The New York Times*, Science, January 23, 1996.

18. *The Second Brain: The Scientific Basis of Gut Instinct and a Groundbreaking New Understanding of Nervous Disorders of the Stomach and Intestine*, Michael D. Gershon, New York: Harper Collins Publications, 1998.

19. *Fundamentals of Physics*, Holliday and Resnick, pp. 512-514. John Wiley & Sons, Inc., 1972.

20. *Bioenergetics*, by Albert L. Lehninger, pp. 5-6, W. A, Benjamin, Inc. Menlo Park, California, 1971.

21. *Photographic Anatomy of the Human Body*, by J. W. Rohen, 邯鄲出版社, Táipéi, Táiwān, 1984.

22. "Restoring Ebbing Hormones May Slow Aging," by Jane E. Brody, *The New York Times*, July 18, 1995.

23. 《阿含經》：〝坐禪思惟，莫有懈怠。〞

24. *The New Encyclopedia Brittanica*, Vol. 4, Encyclopedia Brittanica Inc., 1993.

25. *Fundamentals of Physics*, David Holliday and Robert Resnick, p. 308, John Wiley & Sons, Inc. New York, NY, 1970.

26. 道家：修心養性，守中抱一。

27. 儒家：存心養性，執中貫一。

28. 佛家：明心見性，萬法歸一。

29. 醫家：虛心定性，抱元守一。

30. 《太平經》：〝以思守一，何也？一者，數之始也；一者，生之道也；一者，元氣所起也；一者，天地之綱紀也。〞

31. 《性命圭旨全書・大道說》：〝儒之一貫者，以此本體之一而貫之也。〞

32. 道，一以貫之。

33. 《針灸大成》：〝徐徐咽氣一口，緩緩納入丹田，沖起命門，引督脈過尾閭，而上升泥丸；追動性元，引任脈降重樓，而下返氣海。兩脈上下，旋轉如圓，前降後升，絡繹不絕。‧‧‧‧‧久而行之，關竅自開，脈絡流通，百病不作。〞

34. 《理瀹駢文》：〝閉目靜坐，鼻吸清氣，鼓腹使內氣下降臍下丹田，運氣過肛門，沿督脈尾閭、夾脊、玉枕三關，到頭頂百會穴，順面部至舌與任脈接，沿前胸而下，至丹田復順原徑路循行。患在何處，收氣即存想其處，放氣則歸于丹田。可強身卻病。又名三昧印。〞

35. 《道鄉集》：〝仙家之周天，即佛家轉法輪，理同各異，而後人便自分開。〞

36. 法輪，原是佛教用語，為梵文 Dharmachakra 的意譯，是對佛教的喻稱。

37. 《性命圭旨》：〝釋家謂之法輪，道家謂之周天，儒家謂之行庭，都是同一內容。〞

38. 李時珍《奇經八脈考》：〝任督兩脈，乃身之子午也，乃丹家陽火陰符升降之道，坎水離火交媾之鄉。〞人能通此兩脈，則百脈皆通，自然周身流轉無有停壅之患，而長生久視之道斷在此矣。

39. 金丹心法‧練內丹步驟：〝立志、端品、悔過、遷善、築基、煉己、安爐、采藥、起火、熄火、結胎、養嬰、積行、行功、面壁、飛升。〞

Part II

Meditation Training Procedures

CHAPTER 3

Four Refinements

3-1. INTRODUCTION (JIÈSHÀO, 介紹)

First we will compare the concepts of Jīng (essence, 精), Qì (bioelectricity, 氣), and Shén (spirit, 神). A clear understanding of Jīng, Qì, and Shén is critical for effective Qìgōng training. They are the root of your life and your Qìgōng practice. Jīng, Qì, and Shén are called Sānbǎo (三寶, Three Treasures), Sānyuán (三元, Three Origins), or Sānběn (三本, Three Foundations). A Qìgōng practitioner firms his Jīng (Gùjīng, 固精; Gù means to firm, solidify, retain, and conserve), and then converts it into Qì. This is Liànjīng Huàqì (煉精化氣), which means to refine the Jīng and convert it into Qì. He leads Qì to the head to nourish Shén. This is Liànqì Huàshén (煉氣化神), which means to refine the Qì and convert it into Shén. Finally, he uses his energized Shén to end (govern) his temperament. This is Liànshén Liǎoxìng (煉神了性), namely to refine the Shén to end human nature.

This conversion process enables you to gain health and longevity. During the course of your training you must pay a great deal of attention to these three elements. If you keep these three elements strong and healthy, you will live a long and healthy life. If you neglect or abuse them, you will be sick frequently and age rapidly. Each one of these three elements or treasures has its own root, which you must strengthen and protect.

Jīng (精). The Chinese word Jīng (精) can mean various things depending on context. It can be used as a verb, adjective, or noun. As a verb, it means to refine. For example, to refine or purify a liquid to a high quality is called Jīngliàn (精煉). As an adjective, it denotes something refined, polished, and pure without mixture. People say Jīngxì (精細) for a work of art, which means delicate and painstaking. Jīngliáng (精良) means of excellent quality. When Jīng describes wisdom or personality, it means keen and sharp, e.g., Jīngmíng (精明), which means keen and clever. Jīng can describe a plan or idea as profound, astute, and carefully considered.

Used as a noun, Jīng means the essence. It can mean spirit or ghost. Chinese believe semen is a man's refined essence, so Jīng also means sperm or semen.

Jīng, as essence, exists in everything, as the primal substance or original source from which anything is made and which exhibits the true nature of that thing. In animals or humans, it means the very original and essential source of life and growth. This Jīng is the origin of the Shén (Spirit), which makes an animal different from a tree. In humans, Jīng is passed down from the parents. Sperm is called Jīngzǐ (精子), which means the sons of essence. When this essence is mixed with the mother's Jīng (egg), a new life is generated which is, in certain fundamental respects, an intertwinement of the Jīngs of both parents. The child is formed, the Qì circulates, and the Shén grows. The Jīng which has been carried over from the parents is called Yuánjīng (元精), or Original Essence.

Original Essence is the fountainhead and root of your life. As you absorb the Jīng of food and air, you convert their Jīngs into Qì to supply your body's needs. In Qìgōng society, Jīng usually refers to Yuánjīng (元精). Yuánjīng differs in quantity and quality from person to person and is affected significantly by your parents' health and living habits while they conceived you. Generally speaking, it does not matter how much Yuánjīng you have carried over from your parents, if you know how to conserve it, you will have more than enough for your lifetime. Although you probably cannot increase the quantity of your Jīng, it is possible to improve its quality through Qìgōng training.

Conserving and firming your Yuánjīng is of primary importance. To conserve means to refrain from abuse and excess sexual activity, through which you would lose Yuánjīng faster and your body would degenerate more rapidly. To firm your Jīng means to store and maintain it, and keep your kidneys strong. Kidneys are the residence of Yuánjīng, and when they are strong, Yuánjīng will be firm and not lost without reason. The firming of Yuánjīng is called Gùjīng (固精). This is the first step in training before you can improve its quality. To conserve and firm your Jīng, you must first know its root, where it resides, and how to convert it into Qì.

Before birth, your Yuánjīng is rooted in your parents. After birth, it resides in the kidneys, which now become its root. When you keep this root strong, you will have plenty of Yuánjīng to supply to your body. The meaning of "kidneys" encompasses both Internal Kidneys (Nèishèn, 內腎) and External Kidneys (Wàishèn, 外腎): the kidneys themselves, along with the adrenal glands, are the Internal Kidneys, while the gonads are the External Kidneys. Internal and external kidneys are closely connected and interrelated, and weak Qì in one will weaken the other.

You were created from the union of one egg and one sperm, which managed to reach and penetrate the egg before any of the other millions of sperm. From this, one human cell formed which started to divide, from one to two, from two to four, and so on, to form the embryo. Its health is determined by the original sperm and egg generated from the parents' Jīng. It remains immersed in liquid, receiving all its nutrition and oxygen from the mother through the umbilical cord, which connects at the navel, close to the Lower Dāntián and to the body's center of gravity. The umbilical cord is long, and the baby draws nutrients in with a pumping motion of its abdomen.

Once you are born, you breathe in oxygen through your nose and receive food through your mouth. You no longer need the abdominal motion to pump in nutrients through the umbilical cord, so it gradually stops, and you forget to use it. The Lower Dāntián (Xià Dāntián, 下丹田), or abdomen, is the source of Original Qì converted continuously from the Yuánjīng. The Lower Dāntián is located on the Conception Vessel, one of the eight Qì reservoirs in the body which regulate the Qì flow in the other Qì channels. Qì in the Lower Dāntián is Water Qì (Shuǐqì, 水氣), able to cool down the Fire Qì (Huǒqì, 火氣) generated from the Jīng of food and air, which resides at the Middle Dāntián, or sternum.

To be strong and healthy, conserve your Yuánjīng. This is like the principal in your savings account, an original investment which will continue to return interest as long as it is conserved. Jīng produces Qì, and by preserving it, you will continue to have Jīng and Qì. An unhealthy lifestyle may damage and reduce your Yuánjīng.

To conserve Yuánjīng, control your sexual activity. The gonads are called External Kidneys (Wàishèn, 外腎), as sperm is a product of Yuánjīng and the Jīng from food and air. Ejaculations exhaust your Yuánjīng and shorten your life. You need not stop sexual activity altogether. The proper amount of sexual activity is encouraged, to energize and activate the Jīng, and convert Jīng to Qì more efficiently. Jīng is like fuel, and Qì is like energy generated from this fuel. The more efficiently you convert fuel into energy, the more energy you have.

Appropriate sexual activity energizes the Qì to nourish the Shén, balance your mind, and enhance your courage and morale. The proper amount depends on one's age and state of health. The Jīng in the External Kidneys is the main source of Qì in the four major Yīn Qì vessels in the legs (Yīn Heel and Yīn Línking Vessels on each leg). These four Qì reservoirs keep the legs strong and healthy. If your legs are weakened by sexual activity, you are losing too much Jīng.

Qì (氣). Qìgōng describes the close relationship between Qì and blood circulation. Where Qì goes, blood follows. This is called Qì-Xuě (Qì Blood, 氣血). Qì provides the energy the blood cells need for life and movement. Blood stores Qì, and helps to transport air Qì to every cell of the body.

The cells and tissues are like machines, each with its own unique function, and without current they die. The routes of the blood circulatory system, the nervous system, and the lymphatic system correspond with the course of the Qì channels, because Qì is the energy they need to function. The organs process raw materials into the finished product. Some raw materials are brought in for the energy with which other raw materials are converted into finished goods. The raw materials for your body are food and air, and the finished product is life.

The Qì in your body is like the electric current which the factory obtains from coal or oil. The factory has many wires connecting the power plant to the machines, and other wires connecting telephones, intercoms, and computers. There are also many conveyer belts, elevators, wagons, and trucks to move material from one place to another. It is no different in your body, where there are systems of intestines, blood vessels, complex networks of nerves, and Qì channels to distribute blood, sensory information, and energy. Unlike the digestive, circulatory, and central nervous systems, all of whose supportive vessels can be observed as material structures in the body, Qì channels cannot be observed as physical objects. These systems all have similar configurations throughout the body.

In a factory, different machines require different levels of current. It is the same for your organs, which require different levels of Qì. If a machine is supplied with an improper level of power, it will not function normally and may even be damaged. In the same way, when the Qì level is either too positive or too negative in your organs, they will be damaged and will degenerate more rapidly. In order for a factory to function smoothly and productively, it not only needs high quality machines, but also a reliable power supply. The same goes for your body. The quality of your organs is largely dependent upon what you inherited from your parents. To maintain them in a healthy state and to insure that they function well for a long time, you must have an appropriate Qì supply.

Qì is affected by the quality of air you inhale, the food you eat, your lifestyle, and also your emotions and personality. Food and air are the fuel source, your lifestyle is how you run the machines, and your personality is the management of the factory.

This clarifies the role Qì plays in your body. However, the metaphor used is an oversimplification. The behavior and function of Qì is much more complex than the power supply in a factory. You are neither a factory nor a robot, but a human being with feelings and emotions, which influence your Qì circulation. For example, when you pinch yourself, the Qì in that area is disturbed. This is sensed through the nervous system and interpreted by your brain as pain. No machine can do this. Moreover, after you have felt pain, unlike a machine, you react either through instinct or conscious thought. Human feelings and thought affect Qì circulation in the body, whereas a machine cannot influence its power supply. To understand and control your Qì, you must feel its flow, rather than just use the intellect.

The body has two general types of Qì. The first is called Pre-birth Qì, Original Qì (Yuánqì, 元氣), or Xiāntiānqì (Pre-Heavenly Qì, 先天氣). It is converted from Yuánjīng, which you received at conception, which is why Original Qì is also called Pre-birth Qì.

The second type is Post-birth Qì or Hòutiānqì (Post-heaven Qì, 後天氣). This is drawn from the Jīng (essence) of the food and air we take in. Its residence is the Middle Dāntián, the diaphragm. It circulates and mixes with the Pre-birth Original Qì. Together, they circulate through the Governing Vessel (Dūmài, 督脈) and Conception Vessel (Rènmài, 任脈), from where they are distributed to the entire body.

Pre-birth Qì is Water Qì (Shuǐqì, 水氣) because it can cool down the Post-birth Qì, which is Fire Qì (Huǒqì, 火氣). Fire Qì brings the body to a positive Yáng state, which stimulates the emotions, scattering and confusing the mind. Water Qì cools your body down, and helps the mind become clear, neutral, and centered. Fire Qì supports the emotional body, while Water Qì supports the wisdom part.

As Fire and Water Qì mix, they not only circulate to the Governing Vessel and Conception Vessel, but also to the Thrusting Vessel (Chōngmài, 衝脈), leading Qì directly up through the spinal cord to nourish the brain and energize the Shén and soul. These are very important in Qìgōng practice.

Qì is divided into two major categories, according to its function. The first is Yíngqì (Managing Qì, 營氣), because it manages and controls body functions. This includes the functions of the brain and organs, and also body movement. Yíngqì is also divided into two types. The first circulates in the channels and is responsible for organ function. The circulation of Qì to the organs and the extremities continues automatically as long as you have enough Qì in your reservoirs and you maintain your body in good condition. The second type of Yíngqì is linked to your Yì (mind, intention). When your Yì decides to do something, for example to lift a box, this type of Yíngqì automatically flows to the muscles needed to do the job. This Qì is directed by your thoughts, and closely related to your feelings and emotions.

The second major category of Qì is Wèiqì (Guardian Qì, 衛氣). This forms a shield on the surface of the body to protect you from negative external influences. It is also involved in the growth of hair, the repair of skin injuries, and many other functions of the skin. It is led through millions of tiny channels to the surface of the skin, and can even reach beyond the body. When your body is Yáng, Wèiqì is strong and your pores open. When your body is Yīn, Wèiqì is weak and your pores close to prevent Qì from being lost.

In summertime, your body is Yáng and your Qì is strong, so your Qì shield may extend well beyond your physical body, with the pores wide open. In wintertime, your body is relatively Yīn, and you conserve Qì to stay warm and keep pathogens out. The Qì shield shrinks to be close to the skin surface.

Wèiqì functions automatically in response to environmental changes, but is also influenced significantly by your feelings and emotions. For example, when you feel happy or angry, the Qì shield will be more open than when you are sad or scared. To maintain health, Yíngqì must function smoothly, while strong Wèiqì protects you from negative outside influences such as cold.

The key is training and raising the Shén (spirit), which directs and controls the Qì. When ill or facing death, those with strong Shén, indicative of a strong will to live, often survive. Those who are apathetic or depressed generally do not last long. A strong will to live raises the Shén, energizing Qì and keeping you alive and healthy. To raise Shén, first energize your brain with Qì, to concentrate more effectively. Your mind will be steady, your will strong, and your Shén raised.

It is important to generate Water Qì and learn to use it effectively. It can cool down Fire Qì, slowing the degeneration of the body. It also helps to calm the mind and keep it centered, allowing you to judge things objectively. Qìgōng practice will help you sense and direct it effectively. Water Qì comes from conversion of Yuánjīng, and they both have the kidneys as their root. Once generated, it resides in the Lower Dāntián below the navel. To conserve it, keep your kidneys firm and strong.

Shén (神). It is very difficult to find an English word to precisely express Shén. As in so many other cases, the context determines the translation. Shén can be translated as spirit, god, immortal, soul, mind, divine, and supernatural.

When you are alive, Shén is the spirit which is directed by your mind. When your mind is not steady, it is said Xīnshén Bùníng (心神不寧), which means the Emotional Mind and spirit are not at peace. The Emotional Mind (Xīn) can energize and stimulate one's Shén to a higher state, but at the same time one must restrain the Emotional Mind with the Wisdom Mind (Yì). If the Yì can control the Xīn, the mind as a whole will be concentrated, and the Yì will be able to govern the Shén. When one's Shén is excited, however, it is not being controlled by the Yì, so we say Shénzhì Bùqīng (神志不清), which means the spirit and the will (generated from Yì) are not clear. In Qìgōng it is very important for you to train your wisdom Yì to control your emotional Xīn effectively. To achieve this, Buddhists and Daoists train themselves to be free of emotions and attachments, as only in this way can they build a strong Shén completely under their control.

When healthy, you use your Yì to protect your Shén and keep it at its residence, the Upper Dāntián. Even when energized, it is still controlled by your Yi. However, when you are very sick or near death, your Yì weakens, and your Shén leaves its residence to wander around. When you are dead, your Shén separates completely from the physical body. It is then called a Hún (魂) or soul. Often the term Shénhún (神魂) is used, since the Hún originated with the Shén. Sometimes Shénhún also refers to the spirit of a dying person, since his spirit is between Shén and Hun.

When your Shén is stronger and reaches a higher state, you can sense more sharply, and your mind is more clever and inspired. The world of living human beings is usually considered a Yáng world (Yángjiān, 陽間), and the spirit world after death is considered a Yīn world (Yīnjiān, 陰間). When your Shén reaches this higher, more sensitive state, your mind transcends its normal capacity. Ideas beyond your usual grasp can be understood and controlled, and you may develop the ability to sense or even communicate with the Yīn world. This supernatural Shén is called Líng (靈), describing one who is sharp, clever, nimble, and able to quickly empathize with people and things. When you die, this supernatural Shén (Língshén, 靈神) does not die with your body right away, but still holds your energy together as a ghost (Guǐ, 鬼). Therefore, a ghost is also called Língguǐ (靈鬼), meaning spiritual ghost, or Línghún (靈魂), meaning spiritual soul.

Líng is the supernatural part of the spirit. If strong enough, it lives long after physical death and has plenty of opportunity to reincarnate. However, once one reaches the stage of enlightenment or Buddhahood when alive, after death the spirit leaves the cycle of reincarnation to live forever. These spirits are called Shénmíng (神明), which means spiritually enlightened beings, or simply Shén (神), which here implies this spirit has become divine. Normally, if you die and your supernatural spirit is not strong, it has only a short time to search for a new residence in which to be reborn before its energy disperses. In this case, the spirit is called Guǐ (鬼, ghost).

Your Jīng and Qì may nourish Shén (Yǎngshén, 養神) and strengthen Líng. When this Língshén (靈神) is strong enough, you may separate from the physical body at will. Having reached this stage, your body may live for hundreds of years. People who can do this are called Xiān (仙), which means god, or immortal fairy. Since Xiān originated with the Shén, it is sometimes called Shénxían (神仙), or immortal spirit. The Xiān is a living person whose Shén has reached enlightenment or Buddhahood. After death, his spirit is called Shénmíng (神明).

The foundation of Qìgōng training is to firm your Shén, nourish, and grow it until it is mature enough to separate from your physical body. To do this, you must know where the Shén resides, and how to keep, protect, nourish and train it. It is also essential to know the root or origin of your Shén.

Your Shén resides in the Upper Dāntián, namely the brain. When you concentrate on the third eye, the Shén can be firmed. Firm here means to keep and to protect. When someone's mind is scattered and confused, his Shén wanders. This is called Shénbù Shǒushè (神不守舍), which means the spirit is not kept at its residence.

According to Qìgōng theory, though your Xīn (Emotional Mind, 心) can raise up the spirit, it can also confuse your Shén, so that it leaves its residence. Your Yì (Wisdom Mind) must constantly restrain and control Shén at its residence.

When Shén is highly energized, it conducts the Qì effectively. It is the force which keeps you alive, and the control tower for Qì. When it is strong, your Qì is strong and you can lead it efficiently. When it is weak, your Qì is weak and the body degenerates rapidly. Líkewise, Qì supports the Shén, energizing it and keeping it sharp, clear, and strong.

You must understand the root of your Shén and how to nourish its growth. Original Essence (Yuánjīng, 元精) is the essential life inherited from your parents, your most important source of energy. Your Original Qì (Yuánqì, 元氣) is created from Original Essence, and it mixes with Qì from food and the air to supply energy for growth and activity. This mixed Qì nourishes Shén as well. While Fire Qì energizes your Shén, Water Qì strengthens the Wisdom Mind to control the energized Shén. The Shén kept in its residence by Yì and nourished by Original Qì, is called Original Shén (Yuánshén, 元神). So the root of your Original Shén is your Original Essence. When your Shén is energized but restrained by your Yì, it is called Jīngshén (精神), which means Essence Shén, or spirit of vitality.

Original Shén is the center of your being, making you calm, clearing your mind, and firming your will. When you concentrate on doing something, it is called Jùjīng Huìshén (聚精會神, gathering Jīng to meet Shén). Use Original Essence to raise up Original Shén. Since this Shén is nourished by Original Qì, which is Water Qì, it is considered Water Shén.

At a higher level of practice, cultivating Shén becomes most important. The final goal is to generate a Holy Embryo (Xiāntāi, 仙胎), nourishing it until it is born and becomes independent. For the average practitioner, however, the final goal of cultivating Shén is to raise it up through Qì nourishment, while maintaining control with the Yi. This raised Shén directs and governs Qì efficiently and helps achieve health and longevity.

Shén and the brain cannot be separated. Shén is the spiritual aspect of your being, generated and controlled by your mind. The mind generates the will which keeps the Shén firm. The Chinese commonly use Shén (Spirit) and Zhì (Will) together as Shénzhì (神志) because they are so closely related. When Shén is raised and firm, this raised spirit strengthens the will. They are mutually related and assist each other. Thus, the material foundation of your spirit is your brain. "Nourish your Shén" means to nourish your brain. The original source of nourishment is your Jīng, which is converted into Qì, and led to the brain to nourish and energize it. In Qìgōng practice, this process is called Fǎnjīng Bǔnǎo (返精補腦), meaning to return the Jīng to nourish the brain.

Now with a clear understanding of Jīng, Qì, and Shén, you may grasp the interplay of these three treasures in Qìgōng practice, and how to use them to reach spiritual enlightenment. There are four necessary steps in training:

- **Refining the Essence and Converting It into Qì** (Liànjīng Huàqì, 煉精化氣)
  - One Hundred Days Building the Foundation (Bǎirì Zhújī, 百日築基)
- **Purifying Qì and Converting It into Spirit** (Líànqì Huàshén, 煉氣化神)
  - Ten Months of Pregnancy (Shíyuè Huáitāi, 十月懷胎)
- **Refining Spirit and Returning It to Nothingness** (Líànshén Fǎnxū, 煉神返虛)
  - Three Years of Nursing (Sānnián Bǔrǔ, 三年哺乳)
- **Crushing the Nothingness** (Fěnsuì Xūkōng, 粉碎虛空)
  - Nine Years Facing the Wall (Jiǔnián Miànbì, 九年面壁)

The Dào of reaching enlightenment, or becoming a Buddha, requires years of training. "One hundred days of building the foundation" refers to the formation of the embryo of a spirit baby, commonly called Shèngtāi (Holy Embryo, 聖胎) or Língtāi (Spiritual Embryo, 靈胎). This is followed by ten months of nourishing and growing, three years of nursing, and finally educating this spirit as it grows stronger and becomes independent. This builds up an independent spiritual body. After physical death, this spiritual body lives on, not needing to return to the path of reincarnation.

After this Xǐsuǐjīng training secret was revealed to seculars, a change took place in the training. Because the final goal of enlightenment or Buddhahood was not their main reason to practice and is so hard to attain, many secular practitioners looking only for longevity trained only the first three steps of training and ignored the fourth, so there are very few documents describing this final step.

3-2. Refining the Essence and Converting It into Qì (Liànjīng Huàqì, 煉精化氣)

One Hundred Days of Building the Foundation (Bǎirì Zhújī, 百日築基) is the first step in forming a Spiritual Embryo (Língtāi, 靈胎), or Holy Embryo (Shèngtāi, 聖胎). Many secular practitioners looking only for longevity consider this spiritual baby as an elixir of longevity. Healthy, harmonious interaction of Yīn and Yáng Qì is necessary to form it. Yīn is the mother, while Yáng is the father. Yīn and Yáng Qì must be abundant, each strong enough to balance the other. To build abundant Yīn and Yáng Qì in your body, you must practice the correct methods. For Yīn and Yáng to interact harmoniously, you must also adjust Kǎn and Lí (坎離) (Figure 3-1). You lead Yīn and Yáng Qì to the Huángtíng (yellow yard, 黃庭) to interact harmoniously.

What is the Holy Embryo, or Spiritual Embryo? "Baby Embryo, means golden elixir. To produce the golden elixir is to carry the baby embryo."[1] Elixir is the Qì which extends your life. Since it is as precious as gold, it is commonly called golden elixir. To establish an Spiritual Embryo means to build up and to store Qì at the Huángtíng cavity. The Daoist Xuē, Dào-Guāng (薛道光) wrote, "What is the baby? It is the elixir. The elixir is unique and is the real sole Qì. It is the mother's Qì of heaven and earth. Mother swallows air, belonging to the five internal organs, yielding the baby's Qì. It is just like a cat keeping a mouse which cannot escape. The Qì of mother and son mutually love each other in the womb and finally combine and generate a baby. Therefore, it is said: 'The sole Grand Ultimate contains the real Qì. The way of containing the real sole Qì is like a human carrying an embryo, giving birth when ten months have completed.'"[2]

To generate spiritual life, you need heaven Qì (Yángqì, 陽氣) and earth Qì (Yīnqì, 陰氣). When these two combine and interact, life is formed. To produce the golden elixir, you absorb Qì from food and air (Yángqì) and also from Original Essence (Yīnqì). Then Qì can be stored to a high level and the foundation of longevity established.

From the scientific point of view, what you are doing is storing electric charge in the Huángtíng, the second human brain.[3,4] This second brain connects to the upper brain via the spinal cord, which is central to the human nervous system and is highly conductive tissue. The two brains, though viewed as being separate, thus function as one. The upper brain generates thought (EMF), while the lower brain acts as a battery, supplying charge to the entire body. Whenever EMF is generated, the charge is led to the required area to activate the physical body, manifesting the mind and Qì into physical action.

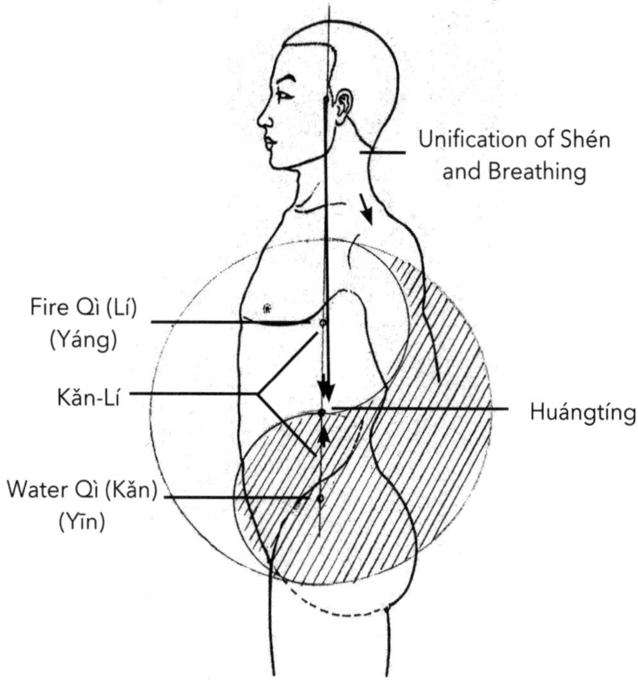

Figure 3-1. Conceiving the Spiritual Embryo

For strong and abundant Qì, you need a powerful, concentrated mind (high EMF) and a good battery able to store Qì in abundance. When both brains are healthy and functioning harmoniously, your immune system is rebuilt, extending life significantly.

The abundant Qì stored in the Huángtíng is led to the brain to nourish and activate its cells to a high enough functional level to raise up the spirit. This describes what happens when the Holy Embryo is formed and matured in the Huángtíng, and then led to the brain to grow up in the second stage of training.

What is the Huángtíng, and how can it store Qì and give birth to the Spiritual Embryo? This cavity was first called Yùhuánxuè (Jade Ring Cavity, 玉環穴) in the book *Illustration of Brass Acupuncture and Moxibustion* (*Tóngrén Yúxuè Zhēnjiǔ Tú,* 銅人俞穴針灸圖) by Dr. Wáng, Wéi-Yī (王唯一). Afterwards, the Daoist book *Wánglù Shíyú* (王錄識餘) said, "In the *Illustration of Brass Acupuncture and Moxibustion* it was recorded that within the body's cavities of viscera and bowels, there is a Jade Ring (Yùhuán). But I do not know what the Jade Ring is."[5] Later, the Daoist Zhāng, Zǐ-Yáng (張紫陽) explained the place which the immortals use to form the elixir, "The heart is on top, the kidneys are underneath, spleen is to the left, and the liver is to the right. The life door is in front, the closed door to the rear, they are connected like a ring, it is white like cotton, an inch in diameter. It encompasses the Essence and refinement of the whole body. This is the Jade Ring."[6] The life door in front means the Qì door opens to the front and is closed in the rear. To lead Yīn and Yáng Qì there, you should access this cavity from the front.

The Huángtíng connects with the Conception and Thrusting Vessels through Yīnjiāo (Co-7, 陰交). Through the Thrusting Vessel, it connects with the upper brain and with the Governing Vessel at the Huìyīn (Co-1, 會陰). The gut is the second brain, with a similar structure to the brain in the head, and is able to store a great amount of Qì.[3,4] The Huángtíng (Yellow Yard, 黃庭) is located between the sternum (Middle Dāntián), where Yáng Fire Qì is stored, and the Lower Dāntián, where Yīn Water Qì is stored. The fasciae in the Huángtíng area stores an abundance of Qì, increasing the amount available to the Holy Embryo.

Given that the gut is widely accepted as being a second brain with a similar structure to the upper brain, how can it create a spiritual embryo? Though scientists believe the second brain has the capability of memory, they are not sure whether it can think. If not, then no EMF can be generated, and the spirit cannot be grown here. Therefore, this place could only be used for the purpose of Yáng and Yīn Qì interaction and raising them to a high level.

In Yìjīnjīng training you generate Qì by converting Original Essence in the Internal Kidneys. However, this does not provide enough Qì for the Xǐsuǐjīng training. To remedy this shortfall, more Essence must be drawn from the External Kidneys (testicles) by stimulating them and converting the essence they produce into Qì. From the standpoint of modern medicine, part of the health benefit of Xǐsuǐjīng Qìgōng comes from its use of stimulation to increase the production of hormones. These are secreted by the endocrine glands, including the testicles. They are complex chemical compounds transported by the blood or lymph, with powerful and specific effects on the functions of the body.

Hormones can stimulate activity, thinking, and growth. They are directly related to the strength of your life force, determining the length of your life and your state of health. They can stimulate your emotions and lift your mood, or depress you physically and emotionally. Traced back far enough, they are the very original source of one's thinking and ideas, even generating the enthusiasm for energetic activity. If you generate these hormones and use them properly, you can energize yourself to a degree quite impossible for the ordinary person.

Many important hormones can now be produced synthetically, but taking synthetic hormones is an unnatural and discontinuous process, unlike generating them within your body. If the hormones come from outside, your body is subject to abrupt changes which produce unwanted side effects. However, when you produce the hormones yourself, your body adjusts to the gradual increase in production. Many hormones are obtained from certain foods, but without providing enough Qì to fill up the vessels. The Daoists say, "Food is better than medicine for increasing health. Using Qì to improve health is better than eating food."[7] Xǐsuǐjīng stimulates the production and secretion of hormones. These are used to increase the Qì, which in turn nourishes the brain and raises the spirit of vitality.

You can only develop a healthy spiritual baby when you have sufficient Qì. To form the embryo, you need at least one hundred days of proper diet, accurate Kǎn and Lí adjustment, correct stimulation of the sexual organ to increase the Essence (semen), and abstinence from sex, to build up a strong Qì body combining Yīn and Yáng. In Xǐsuǐ Qìgōng, the process of refining Essence and converting it into Qì during the first one hundred days lays the foundation (Bǎirì Zhújī, 百日築基). The spiritual Embryo will only be healthy if it has this firm foundation.

The testicle Essence is one of the main sources of a man's energy. When it is abundant, his vital energy is high and his life force strong. When he loses the balance between production and expenditure of semen, his emotions also lose their balance. This leads to depression and speedy degeneration of the body. Part of this Essence is needed by the brain, to stimulate thought and to energize the body for activity. When semen production is insufficient, the brain does not obtain enough Qì, and the spirit's control of Qì circulation weakens. This results in sickness.

So the first step in Xǐsuǐjīng training is to increase semen production and convert it into Qì faster and more effectively than the body normally does. With the average mature man, the supply of semen fills up naturally without stimulation. It usually takes two to three weeks to replenish the supply of semen once it is lost. When a man's semen is full, hormones stimulate the brain and generate sexual desire, energizing him and making him impatient and inclined to lose his temper.

The time needed for the semen to replenish itself varies from one man to another. If one has sex frequently, semen is replenished faster. However, if one abstains for a period of time, the testicles start to function more slowly. If one has sex too often, the semen level will be low most of the time, affecting the conversion of hormones into Qì. The four Qì vessels in the legs receive most of their Qì from the conversion of semen. If you have too much sex you will find your legs weaken through Qì deficiency in these vessels.

The body produces semen during sleep from midnight until morning, because Qì circulation starts in the head (Bǎihuì, Gv-20, 百會) and circulates down the front of the body, following the Conception Vessel and then Governing Vessel, reaching Bǎihuì again. The Huìyīn and Bǎihuì, which are connected by the Thrusting Vessel, are both major points of Qì flow at midnight. When Qì circulation reaches the Huìyīn, it stimulates the genitals and interacts with Original Qì from the Dāntián to generate semen Qì (Jīngqì, 精氣).

Healthy males usually have erections when they wake in the morning. This starts quite soon after birth. Of course, at this age boys cannot generate sperm, and they do not have sexual urges. Chinese medical society believes that once a boy is formed, his testicles continuously generate semen. This interacts with the Original Qì (Yuánqì, 元氣)

at the Dāntián and generates Semen Qì (Jīngqì, 精氣), which is transported to the brain, including the pituitary gland, to stimulate growth. When a boy's Yuánqì is healthy and strong, the interaction of semen and Yuánqì is also effective, and the boy grows normally. Once he reaches his teens, his testicles will also start to generate sperm. Normally, more is produced than is needed for growth, so Qì is full and abundant, making him healthy and strong.

Starting at midnight when you are sleeping and your body is relaxed, the Semen Qì from the testicles nourishes the brain and rebalances its energy. It is this rebalancing which generates dreams.

In Xǐsuǐjīng training, there are two general methods for stimulating semen production. One is Wàidān, using physical stimulation, and the other is Nèidān, using mental stimulation. The more the groin is stimulated, the more semen will be produced and the longer this organ will function normally. You must convert this semen into Qì more efficiently than is normally done by your body. If you do not effectively convert the excess semen into Qì, lead it to the brain, and spread it out among the twelve channels, the abundant semen will cause your sexual desire to increase and your emotions to lose their balance.

Theoretically, the method of Essence-Qì conversion is very simple. You lead the Qì from the four vessels in the legs upward to the Huángtíng cavity and also to the brain. This causes the Qì in these four vessels to become deficient, and more Essence must be converted to replenish the supply. In this case, you are consuming the extra Essence being generated. The process of leading the Qì upward is called Líànqì Shēnghuá (煉氣昇華), which means "train the Qì to sublimate." When the Qì is led up to nourish the brain, it is called Huánjīng Bǔnǎo (還精補腦), which means "return the Essence to nourish the brain."

The more you practice, the more efficiently you convert semen into Qì. There are two major styles of semen conversion, Buddhist and Daoist. Buddhists emphasize Nèidān conversion, which is generally much slower than the Daoists, who, in addition to Nèidān, also train Wàidān conversion. In Nèidān conversion, Yì and breathing are the keys to leading the Qì up. Coordinating posture and movements at the Huìyīn, the Qì is led up to the Huángtíng and brain.

Wàidān conversion also leads the Qì in the legs up to the Huángtíng and brain. Daoist methods of testicle stimulation are faster, because they increase semen production and Wàidān Essence-Qì conversion. They are called Gāowán Yùndòng (睪丸運動, Testicle Exercises) or Chílǎo Huánjī Yùndòng (遲老還機運動, Slowing Aging and Returning the Functioning Exercises). The more semen you have, the more Qì you can convert it into, and the more efficiently you can do so.

3-3. Purifying Qì and Converting It into Spirit (Líànqì Huàshén, 煉氣化神)

Ten Months of Pregnancy (Shíyuè Huáitāi, 十月懷胎)

During the first stage, the Spiritual Embryo is formed in the Huángtíng. This is the seed from which the baby grows. The second stage is Ten Months of Pregnancy (28 days for each Chinese lunar month), during which you provide it with purified Qì, just as a mother supplies nutrition and oxygen to the embryo. You train converting semen efficiently into Qì as the Spiritual Embryo grows and develops. If this process is insufficient, the baby's development will be deficient, and it may die. You are developing it into an entity with its own life.

You lead Yīn and Yáng Qì to the Huángtíng, where they interact harmoniously, forming the Spirit Embryo. In the second stage, you accumulate more Qì in your Huángtíng. It takes ten months of intensive practice to accumulate enough for the third stage of training, in which you activate extra brain cells and improve their function. This raises your spirit to a high level.

As the embryo grows, its spirit also develops to become a healthy, complete being. You nourish it with Qì and also with spirit, like a mother who focuses her spirit and concentration on her embryo to obtain a spiritually healthy baby. The mother's thoughts and habits are passed on to the baby. In the same way, the Spirit Embryo develops its spirit, and this stage of training is called Purifying the Qì and converting it into Shén. The Daoist Lǐ, Qīng-Ān (李清菴) said, "Shén and Qì combine to create the super spiritual quality. Xīn (心) and breath depend on one another to generate the Holy Embryo."[8] To endow the Embryo with spirit, you combine your Shén and Qì in the Huángtíng, giving the holy Embryo a supernatural, spiritual quality. Xīn is your Emotional Mind, and the breathing is the training strategy. Coordinate your emotions and breathing, and focus on this holy Embryo, so its spirit can grow and mature.

Some practitioners believe that once the Embryo is formed, it should be moved to the Upper Dāntián to grow, but this is a matter of choice. First you need plenty of Qì, then you use it to nourish the Embryo, and finally, you establish its spirit. With abundant Qì to activate and energize your brain cells and raise up your spirit, where the Embryo grows is not important. "When the elixir is accomplished in ten months, the holy Embryo is completed, and the real person appears."[9] After meditating for ten months, the Qì is abundantly stored in the Huángtíng. Then you lead it up to nourish your brain. You can now discard the mask you have been wearing, as this is the stage of Self-Recognition.

3-4. Refine Spirit and Return It to Nothingness (Líànshén Fǎnxū, 煉神返虛)

Three Years of Nursing (Sānnián Bǔrǔ, 三年哺乳)

Having carried the Spiritual Embryo for ten months, it is ready to be born. Qì has been stored in abundance at the Huángtíng, and the Embryo's Shén has been established.

You now lead the Embryo up to the Upper Dāntián to be born. The Upper Dāntián, with the Yìntáng cavity (M-HN-3, 印堂, third eye), is where you sense and communicate with Nature's energy, and with the spirit world. This place is called Shéngǔ (神谷, Spiritual Valley), as its physical structure looks like the entrance to a deep valley formed by the two lobes of the brain. When you communicate with the natural energy, it seems to be happening in a deep valley which reaches the center of your thinking and also far beyond what you can see.

The brain holds many mysteries which today's science still cannot explain. I believe the valley formed by the two brain lobes is the key to the length of brainwaves. Energy resonates in this valley and is transmitted outward like waves from the antenna of a radio station. The Upper Dāntián is the gate which allows us to communicate with Nature and for our thoughts to be passed to others.

If one can activate more brain cells through Qìgōng, one may increase the brain's sensitivity to a wider range of wavelengths. One may perceive things more clearly, and have a heightened sensitivity to natural energy. One might even intuitively sense the thoughts of others without oral communication. With abundant Qì and strong concentration, it is also possible to cure others using your mind and Qì. This is the stage of self-awareness and awakening.

Having led the Qì to activate the brain, the next obstacle is opening the gate of the third eye. This is obstructed by the skin, the skullbone, and the frontal sinus. They block much of the energy emitted or received by the brain, which is why this gate is considered closed. However, bones are semi-conductors. Through concentrated meditation, we can generate significant potential difference, or EMF, between the brain and the outside of the head. Once this potential difference reaches the threshold level, the bone becomes a conductor. Then you can communicate with the outside world without obstruction. The gate is called Xuánguān (玄關, Tricky Gate). When concentrated Qì opens, the process is called Kāiqiào (開竅, opening the tricky gate). Once this gate is opened, it stays open.

Another gate is located on top of the head, called Bǎihuì (Gv-20, 百會) in acupuncture or Níwángōng (泥丸宮) in Qìgōng, where your brain can communicate with natural energy. It is not the spiritual center, but simply a gate able to exchange Qì with nature. This gate is commonly used to absorb heaven Qì from the sun and stars, and earth Qì from the earth's magnetic field.

In this third stage of enlightenment meditation, you lead the abundant Qì to the brain to activate unused brain cells and thereby increase brain capacity. Then you concentrate the abundant Qì to open the gate. This means the spirit baby is born in the Upper Dāntián, and now you must nurse it. This is called Yǎngshén (養神, nurse the Shén), meaning to protect, care for, and nourish it as it develops. By increasing the brain's Qì level, you can sense and communicate with nature more effectively. As your spirit communes with nature, it becomes accustomed to staying with the natural energy and gradually forgets the physical body. Since the natural spirit cannot be seen, it is called "nothingness," which also refers to the absence of emotions and desires. Therefore, this stage of training is called Refining Shén and Returning it to Nothingness. Since your spirit body originated from physical and emotional nothingness, in this training, you are returning to nothingness. The Buddhists call this Sìdà Jiēkōng (四大皆空), or Four Large Are Empty. This means the four elements (earth, fire, water, and air) are absent from the mind, so that you are completely indifferent to worldly temptations.

You nurse your spirit baby for at least three years. Just like a real baby, it needs to be protected and nurtured until it can be self-sufficient. If it travels, it cannot go too far, like a small child gradually familiarizing itself with its new environment. This is the first stage of enlightenment or Buddhahood.

I would like to translate a Daoist song about this stage of cultivation.

The Song of Great Dào
大道歌
《遵身八箋・清修妙論箋》

The Great Dào is not far but in the body. Ten thousand material objects are empty, but human nature is not empty. If human nature is not empty, and can stay together in harmony with Qì, the Qì will return to the original ocean (Real Lower Dāntián), and longevity is unlimited. To keep the spirit staying in the body, do not leave even one object in Língtái (spiritual platform). If any object remains in the heart, the spirit will not be clear. This wastes the real essence and damages the tendons and bones (physical body). The spirit directs the Qì, and through Qì, the shape endures. Then you will live long without needing herbs. The techniques are easy, but the secrets are hard to meet. The correct way has always been changed and separated from the path. So even though a thousand or ten thousand people learn, not even one accomplishes the training. When the spirit leaves the body, immediately bring it back. When the spirit returns, the Qì will also return automatically. Practice thus every morning and evening, and the spiritual Embryo will be born naturally and automatically.

大道不遠在身中，萬物皆空性不空。性若不空和氣住，氣歸元海壽無窮。欲得身中神不出，莫向靈台留一物。物在心中神不清，耗散真精損筋骨。神御氣兮氣留形，不須藥物自長生。術則易知訣難遇，總然易了不專行。所以千人萬人學，畢竟終無一個存。神若出兮便收來，神返身中氣自回。如此朝朝並暮暮，自然赤子產靈胎。

The great Dào of longevity and enlightenment is within us, to be reached through cultivation. The mind should not be engaged in material objects which, after all, are empty and impermanent. Train to overcome the influence of objects generated from earth, fire, water, and air. Cultivate your true nature, and raise up your spirit. Once you harmonize with the Qì, it can be kept at the Real Lower Dāntián. Since you do not waste your Qì, you can live a long time.

Keep your mind pure, free from material objects around you and from emotional bondage. Keep your spirit in its spiritual center. If it wanders away, it leads Qì away and wastes it. When the spirit is kept firmly inside the body, the Qì will stay. When the Qì is abundant and stays, the body will be strong and healthy. This is the key to longevity. The key to producing the spiritual Embryo is to keep the spirit inside the body.

To develop the Spiritual Embryo, cultivate and raise your spirit, with the abundant Qì stored in the Real Lower Dāntián. But if your mind is swayed by material attractions, you cannot store enough Qì to generate the Spiritual Embryo. This is the stage of cultivating your true nature to be free from physical and emotional bondage.

3-5. Crushing the Nothingness (Fěnsuì Xūkōng, 粉碎虛空)

Nine Years of Facing the Wall (Jiǔnián Miànbì, 九年面壁)

At this stage, you see the spiritual world as more real than the physical. "Crushing nothingness" means destroying the illusion which connects the physical world with the spiritual plane. According to Buddhism, your spirit cannot separate from your physical body completely, because it is still connected to the human world by emotions and desires. Only if you free yourself from these bonds can your spirit separate and be independent. Nine years of meditation gives your spirit the time to experience the natural energy world and to learn to live independently. Then it can separate from your physical body and continue living without it. It lives in the natural energy and continues even when the physical body is dead.

The highest goal of a Buddhist monk is to reach enlightenment or Buddhahood. He develops his Shén to be independent and exist even after the body dies. His Qì energizes his brain so strongly that it interacts with the electrical charge in the air and generates a glow around his head. This may even occur in earlier stages. It is frequently shown in pictures of Buddha, especially when he is shown meditating in the dark. It is identical to the halo in pictures of Western saints.

This stage is called Líànshén (煉神), or train the spirit. Your spirit receives its education from the natural energy. This generally takes more than twelve years—in fact, usually many lifetimes. You strengthen your Baby Shén in every lifetime, and one day you reach enlightenment. However, many Buddhists and Daoists believe the entire training depends on one's understanding, and that if one could really understand it, one could reach enlightenment in virtually no time at all. I am inclined to agree with them. In virtually every field of endeavor, if one ponders and understands the principles, he finds ways to reach the goal far sooner than expected.

I would like to point out that there are many documents about the first two stages, but very little written about the later two stages of enlightenment training. However, if your desire is sincere and your mind focuses on the goal, you will understand what you need to do to reach the next level. No one can understand you better than yourself.

References

1. 胎指金丹，產金丹喻為懷胎。

2. 薛道光《悟真篇》註："嬰兒者，即丹也。丹是一，一是真一之氣，天地之母氣也。以母咽氣歸五內，以伏子氣，猶貓伏鼠而不走也。子母之氣相戀于胞胎之中，結成嬰兒之一。故曰：太一含真氣。言含真一之氣。如人懷胎，十月滿足，然後降生。"

3. "Complex and Hidden Brain in the Gut Makes Stomachaches and Butterflies," by Sandra Blakeslee, *The New York Times*, Science, January 23, 1996.

4. *The Second Brain: The Scientific Basis of Gut Instinct and a Groundbreaking New Understanding of Nervous Disorders of the Stomach and Intestine*, Michael D. Gershon, New York: Harper Collins Publications, 1998.

5. 王錄識餘云："銅人針灸圖，載臟腑一身俞穴有玉環，余不知玉環是何物。"

6. 張紫陽玉清金華祕文，論神仙結丹處曰："心上腎下，脾左肝右，生門在前，密戶居後，其連如環，其白如綿，方圓徑寸，密裹一身之精粹，此即玉環。"

7. 藥補不如食補，食補不如氣補。

8. 李清菴詩云："神氣和合生靈質，心息相依結聖胎。"

9.《金丹真傳・溫養》："丹成十月聖胎完，自有真人出現。"

Chapter 4

Five Regulatings

4-1. Introduction (Jièshào, 介紹)

Whether you practice Internal Elixir (Nèidān, 內丹) or External Elixir (Wàidān, 外丹) Qìgōng, there are five regulating processes to reach the final goal of practice. These are: regulating the body (Tiáoshēn, 調身), regulating the breathing (Tiáoxí, 調息), regulating the Emotional Mind (Tiáoxīn, 調心), regulating Qì (Tiáoqì, 調氣), and regulating the spirit (Tiáoshén, 調神). These five are commonly called Wǔtiáo (五調, Five Regulatings).

The Chinese word Tiáo (調), which I translate as "regulating", consists of two words, namely Yán (言), which means speaking or negotiating, and Zhōu (周), which means to be complete, perfect, or round. Tiáo means to adjust or to fine-tune a thing until it is complete and harmonious with others. It is like tuning the notes of a piano to be in harmony with one another. Tiao means to coordinate, cooperate, and harmonize by ongoing adjustment. All five aspects—body, breathing, mind, Qì, and spirit—need to be regulated until harmony is achieved.

The key to regulating is through feeling, which is the language of the mind and body. The deeper and more sensitively you feel, the more profoundly you can regulate, and vice versa. It requires significant effort to reach the finest stage of feeling and regulating. This training of inner feeling is called Gōngfū of self-internal-observation (Nèishì Gōngfū, 內視功夫, internal feeling or awareness). The more refined your Gōngfū, the deeper you harmonize with others.

At the beginning, your mind is focused on regulating and on making it happen, so it is not natural or smooth. Later it becomes regulating without regulating. "The real regulating is without regulating."[1] It is like learning to drive, with your mind on the road and the controls of the car. This is the stage of regulating. Once you are experienced, your mind does not have to regulate. You drive without driving, and everything happens naturally and smoothly. With the five Qìgōng regulatings, you practice until regulating is unnecessary. Then your feeling is profound, and regulating is achieved naturally and automatically.

Next we will discuss these five regulatings, and the importance of mutually coordinating them, as they pertain to meditation.

4-2. Regulating the Body (Tiáoshēn, 調身)

A tense posture in meditation affects Qì circulation, and disturbs the mind. "When shape (posture) is incorrect, Qì will not be smooth. When Qì is not smooth, the Yì (Wisdom Mind) is not at peace. When Yì is not at peace, then Qì is disordered."[2]

The purposes of regulating the body are to:

1. Find the most natural and comfortable posture for meditation. This allows the Qì and breathing to flow smoothly, so the mind relaxes and focuses on the raising the Spirit.
2. Provide the best conditions for self-internal-feeling. When your body is well regulated, your feeling can reach a profound level. When mind and body communicate, your judgment will be accurate, and your mind circulates Qì effectively.
3. Coordinate body and mind, using Yì (意, Wisdom Mind) and correct feeling.

Three Stages of Relaxation. Relaxation is a major key to success in Qìgōng practice. It opens your Qì channels, and allows Qì to circulate smoothly and easily.

Each stage has two aspects, mental and physical. Mental relaxation precedes physical relaxation. There are two minds, the Emotional Mind (Xīn, 心) and the Wisdom Mind (Yì, 意). The Xīn affects your feelings and the condition of your body. The Yì leads you to a calm and peaceful state, which allows you to exercise sound judgment. Your Wisdom Mind must first relax, so it can control the Emotional Mind and let it relax too. When the peaceful Wisdom Mind and Emotional Mind coordinate with your breathing, the physical body also relaxes.

There are three stages of relaxation. The first is superficial physical relaxation, which most people can achieve. Adopt a comfortable posture and avoid unnecessary strain. You may look relaxed, but you are still tense inside. Your mind does not have to reach a very deep level to achieve this stage.

The second stage involves relaxing the muscles, tendons, and ligaments. Your meditative mind feels deep inside the muscles, tendons, and ligaments. From this feeling you can gauge the level of your relaxation. This level opens your Qì channels to allow Qì to accumulate in the Real Lower Dāntián.

The final stage is relaxation which reaches the internal organs, the bone marrow, and every pore of your skin. Your mind must achieve profound calmness and peace to sense the organs and marrow, and to lead the Qì to any point in your body. You will feel light and transparent, as though your body has disappeared. You can also lead the Qì to strengthen your Guardian Qì (Wèiqì, 衛氣) to protect you from outside influences. You can adjust Qì in your organs to regulate Qì disorders, protecting them and slowing their degeneration.

An important aspect of Qìgōng training is leading the five Qì toward their origins (Wǔqì Cháoyuán, 五氣朝元). This involves adjusting Qì in the five Yīn organs, namely lungs, heart, kidneys, liver, and spleen. One can generally feel the lungs more easily, because they move when you inhale and exhale. Once you have relaxed them, you can feel your heartbeat. After that, the kidneys can be sensed more easily than the liver and spleen because liquid flows constantly through them. The liver will be next, and then the spleen. Because the liver is much larger than the spleen, it is easier to feel the blood move inside it.

Yīn and Yáng in Regulating the Body. To regulate the body into a desired state, you apply the concept of Yīn and Yáng in your practice, adjusting them using Kǎn (坎, Water) and Lí (Fire, 離). When your mind is calm, and breathing long and smooth, your body relaxes deeper and Qì can circulate smoothly. The deep calm mind and long breath are Kǎn (Water), making your physical body more Yīn, and your Qì body more Yáng. The physical body is cooler, while the Qì body is more assertive.

By contrast, when you are excited, with short and heavy breathing, your physical body will also be tense, hot, and energized. Qì stagnates so it can manifest into physical form. The excited mind and heavy breathing is Lí (Fire), making your physical body Yáng, and the Qì body more Yīn. The physical body is excited and the Qì circulation is slow and stagnant. Depending on your purpose, you regulate your body accordingly. To make your body more Yáng and build up external strength, use Lí. To internalize and make your Qì body more Yáng, use Kǎn.

When you practice Small Circulation meditation, since you are focusing on the Qì body instead of the physical, bring your physical body to the most relaxed Yīn state so Qì can be directed to circulate smoothly and abundantly.

Regulating the Body and the Spirit. When you meditate, relax your body as much as possible, so your mind can be calm, the Qì can circulate smoothly, and your feeling can be centered and balanced. Harmonize your mind and body, and build a firm root. Then the spirit can be raised. Relaxing the body is the first step in raising the spirit.

4-3. Regulating the Breathing (Tiáoxí, 調息)

Once regulating your body reaches the stage of regulating without regulating, you focus on the breathing. The body can be regarded as a battlefield, with Qì as soldiers, the mind as the general, and the spirit as fighting morale. Breathing is regarded as the strategy. When breathing methods are correct, Qì is led effectively. Since ancient times, Qìgōng breathing methods have been studied and practiced, and kept top secret by only being passed down orally in each style. Embryonic Breathing (Tāixí, 胎息) is the crucial key to storing Qì at the Real Lower Dāntián (Zhēn Xiàdāntián, 真下丹田) and to cultivating spiritual enlightenment. Embryonic Breathing is so important in Internal Elixir Qìgōng (Nèidān Qìgōng, 內丹氣功) that it is discussed in great detail in the previous book of this series, *Qìgōng Meditation—Embryonic Breathing*. It is briefly reviewed in Chapter 6 of this book. In this section, we will only summarize the general concepts of regulating breathing, its purpose, theory, and some techniques.

Purposes of Regulating the Breathing

1. **To convert nutrition, or food essence, into Qì efficiently.** The source of post-birth Qì is mainly from food. According to the biochemical formula, the more oxygen we inhale, the more efficient the biochemical reaction, and the more energy generated. The body converts this energy into heat, light, and bioelectricity (Qì).

$$\text{glucose} + 6O_2 \longrightarrow 6CO_2 + 6H_2O$$

$$\Delta G^{o\prime} = -686 \text{ Kcal}$$

2. **To improve metabolism, which is the efficiency of cell replacement.** Approximately one trillion cells die every day in a healthy person.3 To slow the aging process, they must be replaced each day, for which oxygen is one of the elements required. Without it, the new cells will be deformed and unhealthy. Dead cells (carbon) must also be disposed of. The respiratory system supplies the oxygen and removes the dead cells. Inhaling and exhaling deeply allows cell replacement to proceed smoothly.
3. **To serve the strategic purpose of regulating Yīn and Yáng.** Breathing is a Kǎn and Lí method with which you may adjust the body's Yīn and Yáng. Inhalation makes the body more Yīn, while exhalation makes it more Yáng.
4. **To coordinate and harmonize the body, mind, Qì, and spirit.** Breathing, as one of the five important regulatings, plays the important role of coordinating and harmonizing the others. Concentrating in a deep, profound inhalation can calm you and condense your spirit. Focusing in exhalation can raise the body's energy, excite the mind, and raise up the spirit. Correct breathing assists in leading Qì more efficiently.

Breathing and Qìgōng. There are Eight Qì Vessels (Mài, 脈), which function like reservoirs, and Twelve Primary Qì Channels (Jīng, 經), which function like rivers in your body. In addition, there are millions of tiny channels called Luò (絡) branching out from the twelve channels to the surface of the skin, to generate a shield of Guardian Qì (Wèiqì, 衛氣). This Qì is responsible for hair growth and for defending against negative outside influences. These tiny channels also enter the bone marrow (Suǐqì, 髓氣) to keep it healthy and producing blood cells. They also establish pathways for Qì exchange and communication between internal organs.

Qì circulates naturally and automatically without Qìgōng training. Qìgōng practice coordinates the mind and breathing, generating electromotive force to control the Qì circulation more efficiently. As one exhales, one expands the Qì and leads it from the primary channels to the skin, and the body becomes more Yáng. When one inhales, one draws in Qì and leads it from the primary channels to the bone marrow, and the body becomes more Yīn (Figure 4-1). When inhalation and exhalation are balanced, Yīn and Yáng are balanced.

As you get older, your breath becomes shorter, and less Qì is led to the skin and bone marrow. Qì stagnates there, and the skin starts to wrinkle, while the hair turns gray or falls out. Fewer blood cells are produced, and they are not as healthy as before. Because they carry less nutrition and oxygen through the body, you get sick more often and age faster. The first key to maintaining youth is regulating your breathing to control Kǎn and Lí, and thus the Yīn and Yáng of your body.

Table 4-1. General Rules of Breathing's Kǎn-Lí and Yīn-Yáng

Kǎn-Lí	Method	Consequence
Kǎn	Inhalation	Yīn*
Lí	Exhalation	Yáng*
Kǎn	Inhale, then hold the breath	Yīn
Lí	Exhale, then hold the breath	Yáng
Kǎn	Soft, slow, calm, and long breath	Yīn
Lí	Heavy, fast, and short breath	Yáng
Kǎn	Normal Abdominal Breathing (Buddhist Breathing)	Yīn
Lí	Reverse Abdominal Breathing (Daoist Breathing)	Yáng

*Yīn and Yáng are relative, not absolute. After defining a reference standard or level, compare them with each other.
Yīn: Cold, calm, body relaxed, and Qì body energized
Yáng: Hot, excited, physical body tense, and energized

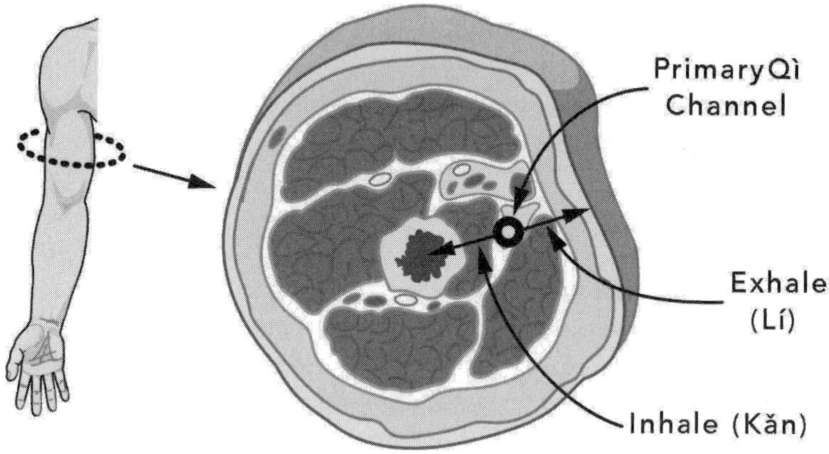

Figure 4-1. The Expansion and Condensing of Qì during Breathing

Breathing Methods

1. Normal Breathing (Píngcháng Hūxī, 平常呼吸)

Normal Breathing is also called Chest Breathing (Xiōngbù Hūxī, 胸部呼吸), in which the breath is controlled by emotion. Regulate it by relaxing the lungs. Concentrate until the practice is neutral, calm, and peaceful. The breathing can be long and deep while the body relaxes, and the heartbeat slows down. You may practice in any comfortable position, ten minutes each morning and evening, until one day you notice that your mind does not have to pay attention to the chest. Then concentrate on feeling the result of the training. When you exhale, you feel the pores of the skin open, and when you inhale, the pores close. It seems that all the pores are breathing with you. This is a low level of skin or body breathing. The feeling is very comfortable. When you can do this comfortably and automatically, you have regulated your Chest Breathing.

You should practice until you reach a level of regulating without regulating (Wútiáo Értiáo, 無調而調), which is known as "the real regulating". Then you will be practicing all the time, since you have built up a natural habit for your breathing. The most powerful Qìgōng practice is one which you have integrated into your lifestyle, including your breathing behavior.

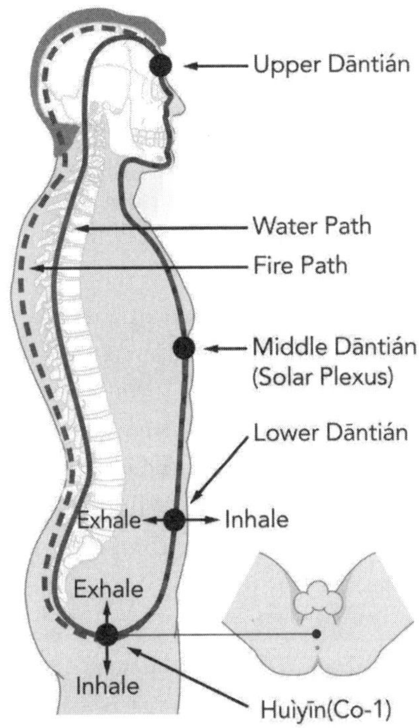

Figure 4-2. Normal Abdominal Breathing

2. Normal Abdominal Breathing (Zhèng Fùhūxī, 正腹呼吸)

Normal Abdominal Breathing is also called Buddhist Breathing (Fójiā Hūxī, 佛家呼吸). Control your abdominal muscles and coordinate them with the breathing. When you inhale, the abdomen expands, and when you exhale, it withdraws. Practice until the process becomes smooth, with the body relaxed. Concentrate on your abdomen initially to control the abdominal muscles. Afterwards the process becomes natural and smooth, and you are ready to build up Qì at the False Lower Dāntián (Jiǎ Xiàdāntián, 假下丹田, Qìhǎi, Co-6, 氣海).

Then coordinate your breathing with the movements of your Huìyīn (Co-1, perineum, 會陰). When you inhale, gently push the Huìyīn down, and when you exhale hold it up (Figure 4-2). You gently hold up the Huìyīn without tensing, and it remains relaxed. Tensing impedes Qì circulation and causes tension in the abdomen, which can generate other problems. Initially, use your mind to control the muscles of the abdomen and perineum. Later, your mind does not need to be there to make it happen, and you regulate without regulating. You feel a wonderful comfortable feeling at the Huìyīn, and the Qì is led more strongly to the skin than when you did "Chest Breathing." It will feel as though your whole body is breathing with you.

Table 4-2. Normal Abdominal Breathing

Body Neutral (inhalation and exhalation are equal length)
  Yīn: Inhalation (abdomen expands, Huìyīn pushed out gently)
  Yáng: Exhalation (abdomen withdraws, Huìyīn held up gently)
Body Yīn
  Inhalation longer (abdomen expands, Huìyīn pushed out gently)
  Exhalation (abdomen withdraws, Huìyīn relaxed)
Body Yáng
  Inhalation (abdomen expands, Huìyīn pushed out gently)
  Exhalation longer (abdomen withdraws, huìyīn held up strongly)

3. Reverse Abdominal Breathing (Fǎn Fùhūxī, Nì Fùhūxī, 反腹呼吸・逆腹呼吸)

Reverse Abdominal Breathing is called Daoist Breathing (Dàojiā Hūxī, 道家呼吸), which you start training once you have mastered Buddhist Breathing. It is called Reverse Abdominal Breathing because the movement of the abdomen is the reverse of Buddhist Breathing. The abdomen withdraws when you inhale and expands when you exhale (Figure 4-3). Buddhist breathing is more relaxed than Daoist breathing, which is more aggressive. Daoist breathing makes the body more Yáng, while Buddhist breathing makes it more Yīn.

Many people wrongly believe that reverse breathing is against the Dào, or nature's path. This is not true. It is simply used for different purposes. If you observe your breathing patterns, you notice we use reverse breathing in two types of situations.

First, when emotionally disturbed, we often use reverse breathing. When you laugh, you make the sound "Hā" (哈), using reverse breathing. Your abdomen expands, exhalation is longer than inhalation, Guardian Qì (Wèiqì, 衛氣) expands, and you get hot. This is the natural way of releasing excess energy from excitement or happiness. When you cry, you make the sound "Hēng" (哼) while inhaling, your abdomen withdraws, and inhalation is longer than exhalation. Guardian Qì shrinks and you feel cold. This is the natural way of preventing energy loss from inside your body. When you are sad, your spirit and your body's energy are low.

The second occasion in which we use reverse breathing is to energize the body, such as when pushing or lifting something heavy. You inhale deeply to take in more oxygen and then exhale while pushing the object, which is reverse breathing. When we are disturbed emotionally or have aggressive or strong intentions, we use reverse breathing naturally.

With practice, you can lead the Qì to the skin more efficiently than with Buddhist breathing. You can also lead it to the bone marrow to enhance the Marrow Qì (Suǐqì, 髓氣). Compare Normal Abdominal Breathing with Reverse Abdominal Breathing to see how Qì is led in these two different breathing strategies.

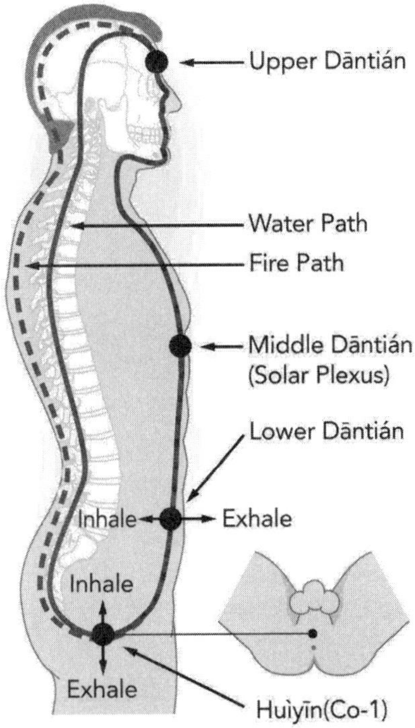

Figure 4-3. Reverse Abdominal Breathing

In Normal Abdominal Breathing, Qì circulates mainly in the primary Qì channels (Jīng, 經) connecting the internal organs to the extremities. Some also spread out through the secondary Qì channels (Luò, 絡) to reach the skin and bone marrow (Figure 4-4). Since most Qì remains in the primary Qì channels, the body is not energized and stays relaxed, enabling a state of deep relaxation. Normal Abdominal Breathing (Kǎn, 坎) makes the body Yīn, while Reverse Abdominal Breathing (Lí, 離) makes it Yáng.

In Reverse Abdominal Breathing, most Qì is led sideways through the Luò to the skin and bone marrow, while much less circulates in the primary Qì channels (Figure 4-5). Skin Breathing (Tǐxí, Fūxí, 體息・膚息) and Marrow Breathing (Suǐxí, 髓息) can be achieved more aggressively through Reverse Abdominal Breathing.

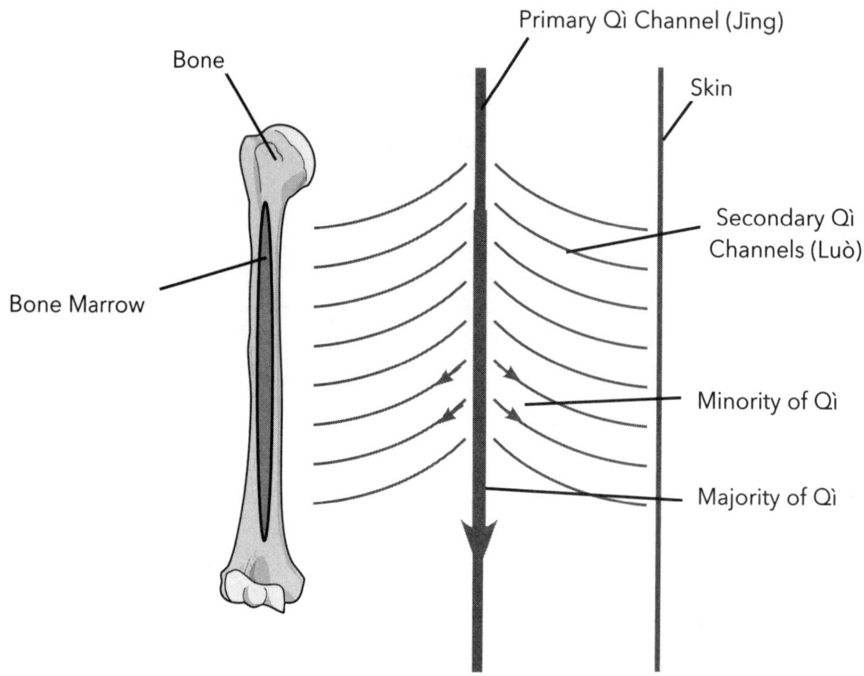

Figure 4-4. In Normal Abdominal Breathing, a Majority of the Qì Circulates in the Primary Qì Channels

Table 4-3. Reverse Abdominal Breathing
(Emotionally unsettled, the mind has Intention of Yīn or Yáng)

Body Neutral*
Yīn: Inhalation (abdomen withdraws, **Huìyīn held up gently**)
Yáng: Exhalation (abdomen expands, **Huìyīn pushed out gently**)
* Inhalation and exhalation are of equal length.

Body Yīn
Inhalation Longer (abdomen withdraws, **Huìyīn held up firmly**)
Exhalation (abdomen expands, **Huìyīn relaxed**)
* "Hēng" sound can enhance the body's Yīn.

Body Yáng
Inhalation (abdomen withdraws, **Huìyīn held up gently**)
Exhalation (abdomen expands, **Huìyīn pushed out firmly**)
* Hā sound can enhance the body's Yáng.

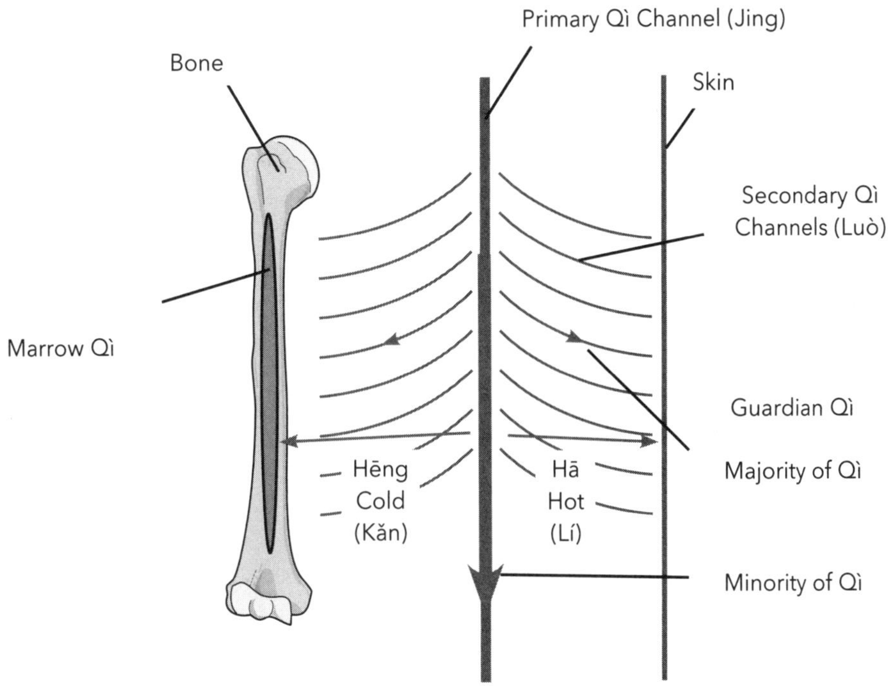

Figure 4-5. In Reverse Abdominal Breathing, a Majority of the Qì is Led to the Skin Surface and Bone Marrow

In Reverse Abdominal Breathing, when you inhale, you withdraw your abdomen and hold up your Huìyīn, while moving the diaphragm downward. Tension generated at the stomach area may cause pain, like when you laugh loudly or cry. So before practicing it, first practice Normal Abdominal Breathing for a while to relax and control the abdominal muscles. Use small movements at the beginning, before increasing the scale of abdominal movement.

4. Embryonic Breathing (Tāixí, 胎息)

Embryonic Breathing has always been a huge subject in Internal Elixir Qìgōng practice. It is the breathing method which allows you to store Qì in the Real Lower Dāntián (Zhēn Xiàdāntián, 真下丹田) and charge your biobattery to a high level. Your vital energy is raised, the immune system strengthened, and the body reconditioned. More importantly, once abundant Qì is stored, you can lead it upward through the spinal cord (Chōngmài, 衝脈) to nourish the brain and raise the spirit. This is the crucial key of spiritual enlightenment. Embryonic Breathing is also crucial in Skin Breathing and Marrow Breathing, which are closely connected to our immune system and longevity.

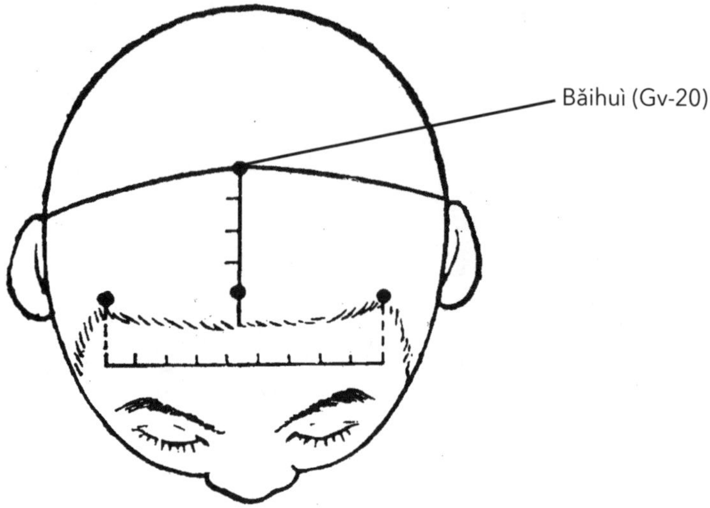

Figure 4-6. The Băihuì (Gv-20) Cavity

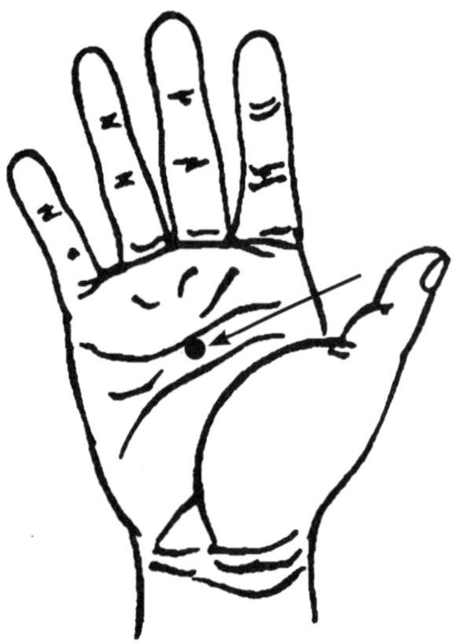

Figure 4-7. The Láogōng (P-8) Cavity

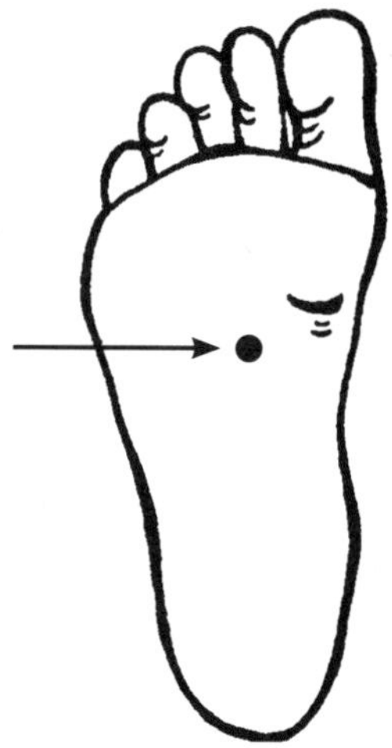

Figure 4-8. The Yǒngquán (K-1) Cavity

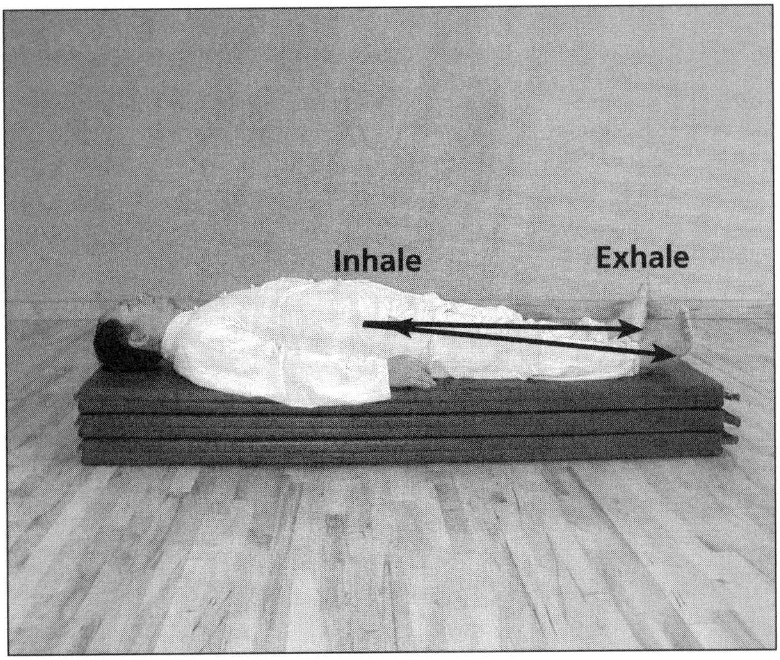

Figure 4-9. Yǒngquán Breathing with Normal Abdominal Breathing

Since Embryonic Breathing is also vital for Small Circulation, we discuss it separately in Chapter 6, together with Skin Breathing and Marrow Breathing. Again, for more detail, please refer to the previous book, *Qìgōng Meditation—Embryonic Breathing*.

5. Skin—Marrow Breathing (Fūsuǐxí, 膚髓息)

Skin Breathing (Fūxí, 膚息) is sometimes called Body Breathing (Tǐxí, 體息) Actually, Body Breathing involves breathing with the whole body, not just the skin. When you exhale, you lead Qì to the muscles and skin, and when you inhale, you lead Qì to the marrow and internal organs. You feel your whole body is transparent to Qì, as though it has disappeared. Skin-Marrow Breathing is closely related to Embryonic Breathing. When Qì is led to the Real Lower Dāntián, you are also leading it to the bone marrow, and when it is led to the Girdle Vessel (Dàimài, 帶脈), you are also leading it to the skin.

6. Five Gates Breathing (Wǔxīn Hūxī, 五心呼吸)

The five gates are: the head (Upper Dāntián and Bǎihuì, Gv-20, 百會), the two Láogōng (P-8, 勞宮) cavities on the palms, and the two Yǒngquán (K-1, 湧泉) cavities on the soles of the feet (Figures 4-6 to 4-8). Beginners use the Bǎihuì gate in the top of the head because there, it is easier to communicate with natural Qì. Later, the third eye (Tiānyǎn, 天眼) is used instead.

Having built up Qì at the Real Lower Dāntián, you harmonize your breathing and lead the Qì to the Yǒngquán cavities. For Yǒngquán breathing (Yǒngquán Hūxī, 湧泉呼

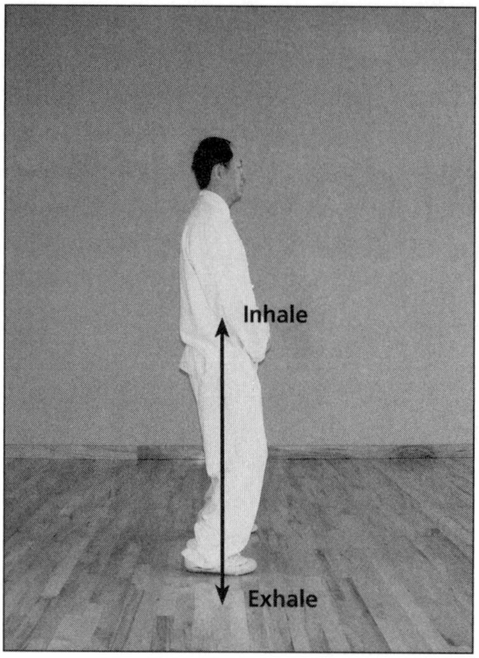

Figure 4-10. Yǒngquán Breathing with Reverse Abdominal Breathing

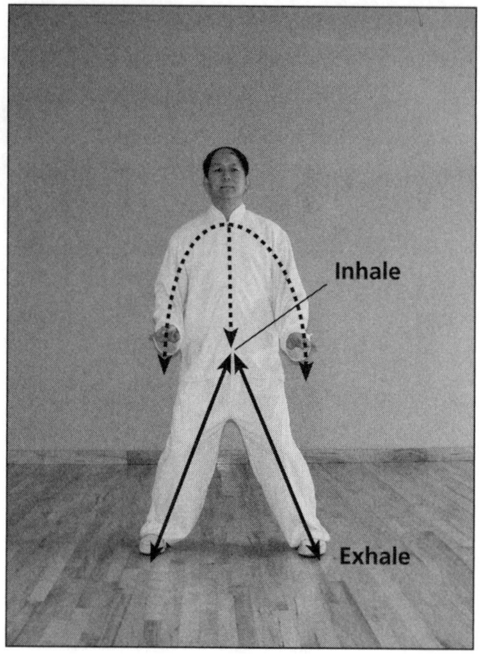

Figure 4-11. Four Gates Qì Breathing

吸) you may adopt any posture, even lying down and using Normal Abdominal Breathing. Inhale, leading Qì from Yǒngquán to the Real Lower Dāntián, and exhale, leading it back to Yǒngquán (Figure 4-9). When you inhale, the abdomen and Huìyīn (Co-1, 會陰) expand, and when you exhale, they withdraw. Even though the mind is involved, it does not aggressively lead the Qì, and relaxation is paramount.

To lead Qì to the Yǒngquán aggressively, Reverse Abdominal Breathing is more effective, and the best posture is standing. Inhale, leading Qì from the Yǒngquán cavities to the Real Lower Dāntián, and when you exhale, your mind leads the Qì back to the Yǒngquán, while you slightly squat down and imagine pushing your feet down into the ground (Figure 4-10). When you inhale, the abdomen withdraws while the Huìyīn is held up, and when you exhale, they expand.

Yǒngquán Cavity Breathing is also called Sole Breathing (Zhǒngxí, 踵息), as described by the well-known Daoist scholar Zhuāngzi (莊子) during the Chinese Warring States Period (403–222 BCE, 戰國): "The breathing of the ancient truthful persons (Zhēnrén, 真人, Daoists) was deep and profound. They used the soles to breathe, while seculars use the throat."[4] So Yǒngquán Breathing has been trained for more than two thousand years. For medical Qìgōng, Yǒngquán Breathing is one of the most effective methods to regulate abnormal Qì in three of the Yīn organs, namely the liver, kidneys, and spleen.

With Yǒngquán Breathing well established, and having reached the real regulating of no regulating, add the Láogōng Breathing at the center of your palms. These two gates regulate the heart and lungs. Use either Normal Abdominal Breathing or Reverse Abdominal Breathing. Inhale, leading Qì from the four gates to the Real Lower Dāntián, and exhale, leading it back again (Figure 4-11).

Four Gates Breathing is a common method of Grand Qì Circulation (Dàzhōutiān, 大周天). Once you reach a profound level, add the fifth gate, which elevates the practice into Spiritual Breathing (Shénxí, 神息).

7. Spiritual Breathing (Shénxí, 神息)

Spiritual Breathing is also called Fifth Gate Breathing (Dì Wǔxīn Hūxī, 第五心呼吸), Bǎihuì Breathing (Bǎihuì Hūxī, 百會呼吸), or Upper Dāntián Breathing (Shàng Dāntián Hūxī, 上丹田呼吸). It means to breathe through the third eye, and is crucial in opening the third eye for enlightenment.

Reaching the level of Spiritual Breathing presupposes regulating your body, breathing, mind, and Qì, and now the spirit. Your Qìgōng practice and the search for spiritual enlightenment has reached the final stage and is approaching maturity. According to *The Complete Book of Principal Contents of Life and Human Nature* (*Xìngmìng Guīzhǐ Quánshū*, 性命圭旨全書): "What is spiritual breathing? It means the maturity of cultivation."[5] That means cultivating the interaction of Kǎn and Lí has reached the stage of regulating without regulating, and all the cultivations have become natural. We will discuss this subject further in the forthcoming books on the subjects of Qìgōng Meditation and Spiritual Enlightenment.

There are some other breathing methods trained in Daoist Qìgōng, such as Turtle Breathing (Guīxí, 龜息) and Hibernation Breathing (Dōngmiánxí, 冬眠息). Since they are not related to Small Circulation, and I do not have profound understanding of their practice, they are not discussed here.

Final goals of regulating the breathing. *The Complete Book of Principal Contents of Life and Human Nature* (*Xìngmìng Guīzhǐ Quánshū*, 性命圭旨全書) says, "Regulate the breathing, you must regulate until the real regulating ceases. Train the spirit, you must train until the spirit of being without spirit."[6] Practice Embryonic Breathing until you achieve regulating without regulating. It is the same in cultivating your spirit. First aim for spiritual neutrality and enlightenment. Afterwards, no further enlightenment is necessary.

The Correct Theory of Becoming a Heavenly Fairy, A Frank Discussion of Taming the Breathing (*Tiānxiān Zhènglǐ·Fúqì Zhílùn*, 天仙正理・伏氣直論) states, "When ancient people talked about the way of regulating the breathing, it is to follow the rules of nature's to and fro (circulation) without stubbornly keeping the shape of to and fro. This means to match the breathing as if there were no breathing."[7] The goal of regulating the breath is to follow nature without stagnation and practicing until regulating becomes unnecessary.

Some Ancient Documents about Regulating the Breath

1. Questions from a Buddhist Guest about Lístening to the Heart (Tīngxīn Zhāikè Wèn, 聽心齋客問)

Expanding the bellows means to regulate the real breathing. When exhaling, the air exits, and when inhaling, the air enters. When exiting, then it is like the earth Qì's ascending, and when entering, it is like the heaven Qì's descending. This breathing is the same as the heaven and the earth. Isn't the space between the heaven and the earth just like the wind bellows?

鼓槖籥，曰調真息。呼則氣出，吸則氣入，出則如地氣上升，入則如天氣下降，與天地同。故天地間，其猶槖籥乎？

Tuóyuè (槖籥) means the bellows, used to assist air circulation. We know that breathing is a strategy in Qìgōng practice, able to make Qì circulate smoothly in the body. The lungs are the air bellows, while the Lower Dāntián is the Qì bellows. When the lungs take in air, the Qì sinks to the Lower Dāntián like the Qì descending in nature. When air is expelled by the lungs, the Qì in the Lower Dāntián rises up through the body like Qì ascending in nature. The human body is a small microcosm of heaven and earth. The tricky key to taking in the air and expelling it is the nose, while the piston of the Qì bellows in the Lower Dāntián is at the Huìyīn (Co-1, 會陰, perineum). Once you regulate your breathing to be natural (regulating without regulating), it is called Real Breathing (Zhēnxí, 真息).

2. An Essay about Regulating the Breath

(The Complete Book of Zhūzi, Sòng Dynasty)
(Tiáoxízhēn, 調息箴)
(朱子全書・宋・朱熹撰)

The tip of the nose has white, I observe it all the time and at all places. Allow it to be soft, gentle, and supple. When extreme calmness has been reached, it hisses like a spring fish in the pond. When action has reached its extremity, it is harmonized like the torpor of a hundred insects. Open and close harmoniously, and its marvelousness is unlimited. What else can preside? It is achieved by not presiding. The clouds in the sky and the heaven cycling as it is. Who dares to question it? Keeping in one place harmoniously. Then, can live one thousand two hundred years.

鼻端有白，我其觀之，隨時隨處，容與猗猗。靜極而噓，如春沼魚，動極而翕，如百蟲蟄。氤氳開闔，其妙無窮，誰其尸之？不宰之功。雲臥天行，非予敢議，守一處和，千二百歲。

The white at the tip of the nose means the air. Regulate the breath until it is soft, gentle, and supple. When I am extremely calm, inhaling deeply, then I exhale like a fish in the spring time. When I am extremely active, exhaling efficiently, then I retain it calmly and harmoniously like the torpor of insects. Breathing harmoniously this way, what else can compare? Success depends on regulating without regulating. Then it is like the clouds in the sky, and nature repeating its cycles; who else dares to contest with you? Keep the mind at the Real Lower Dāntián (Zhēn Xiàdāntián, 真下丹田) harmoniously, and you may live to be one thousand two hundred years old.

To obtain longevity, first regulate your breathing until no regulating is necessary. Second, keep Qì at its residence at the Real Lower Dāntián. This is Embryonic Breathing (Tāixí, 胎息).

3. Regulating the Breath[8]

(Original Truth of Using No Herbs; Qīng Dynasty; Wāng, Áng)
(Tiáoxí, 調息)

(勿藥元詮・清・汪昂輯)

Regulating the breath has been thoroughly studied by three groups: Buddhism, Daoism, and Confucianism. Upon reaching the great achievement, one may enter the Dào, and reaching the small achievement preserves health. Sanskrit documents from India teach looking at the tip of the nose, counting the breaths in and out internally. This is the beginning practice of Stopping Vision (Zhǐguān, attraction of visual objects). Zhuāngzi in his book Nánhuájīng said, "A sage breathes through the soles." Great Yì (Yìjīng, Book of Changes) explains in its trigram, "When it gets dark, gentlemen enter Yànxí (meditation or profound breathing)." Wáng, Lóng-Xī (王龍溪) said, "The ancient sages had deep breathing without sleeping. Therefore, it is said, when getting dark, enter the Yànxí." The method of Yànxí is, when it is getting dark, the ears do not hear, the eyes do not see, the four limbs are not moving, and the heart has no thoughts or cares. It is like a seed fire. Pre-Heaven Original Shén and Original Qì gather to nourish each other mutually. The real Yì is soft as cotton, opening and closing naturally. The self-being exists in the same body (space or dimension) as insubstantial emptiness, so it can live as long as insubstantial emptiness. Those worldly people (seculars) are bothered with daily management, the spirit is bound and tired. They depend on the single night's sleep to be used during the day. A point of spiritual light (self-subconscious spiritual being) all covered by the Post-Heaven's dirty Qì. This is, the Yáng falls into the Yīn.

調息一法，貫徹三教，大之可以入道，小用可以養生。故迦文垂教，以視鼻端，自數出入息，為止觀初門。莊子《南華經》曰：〝聖人之息以踵。〞大易隨卦曰：〝君子以向晦入晏息。〞王龍溪曰：〝古之聖人，有息無睡，故日向晦入晏息。〞晏息之法，當向晦時，耳無聞，目無見，四體無動，心無思慮，如種火相似，先天元神元氣，停育相抱，真意綿綿，開闔自然，與虛空同體，故能與虛空同壽也。世人終日營擾，精神困憊，夜間靠此一睡，始夠一日之用。一點靈光，盡為后天濁氣所淹，是謂陽陷于陰也。

The Qìgōng techniques of regulating breathing have been studied and practiced in three major philosophic schools, namely Buddhism, Daoism, and Confucianism. If you practice breathing correctly, you gain good health and longevity. In Buddhist and Daoist societies, through correct breathing practice, the Qì is stored and led up to the brain to nourish the Shén (神) for enlightenment. Entering the Dào (Rùdào, 入道) means to enter the path of searching for the truth. The Daoists who comprehend the truth of nature are called Truthful Persons (Zhēnrén, 真人).

Regulating the breathing in Buddhist society is considered crucial to regulating the mind. To stop the mind from continuous distraction and wandering in meditation, concentrate your breathing (look at the tip of the nose, Yǎnguānbí, 眼觀鼻) and count the breaths. Make the breathing deeper and calmer. Slowly, the thoughts connecting with the surroundings and with the past, present, and future, are stopped. In Buddhist meditation, this is called Stopping Vision (Zhǐguān, 止觀). "Use the eyes to look at the tip of the nose" does not mean to physically look at the nose. It simply means to gather your attention and to concentrate on your breathing.

As Zhuāngzi (莊子) said, "A sage breathes through the soles," namely Two Gates Breathing through the Yǒngquán (K-1, 湧泉) cavities. Later it developed into Four Gates Breathing, and finally reached the practice of Five Gates Breathing (Wǔxīn Hūxī, 五心呼吸). *Yìjīng* (易經) said, "When it gets dark, gentlemen enter the Yànxí (晏息, deep breathing meditation)." The best time for regulating the breath is after sunset. Then, nature and the body turn from Yáng to Yīn. If you practice regulating the breathing at this time, you can easily calm your body and mind to reach a profound level of meditation. This is also mentioned by Daoist Wáng, Lóng-Xī (王龍溪). He implies that ancient sages, through regulating the breathing, did not need more than a little sleep, since they obtained a deep level of rest from meditation.

The way of Yànxí (晏息) is to, after sunset, close the ears to the noises around you. Partially close your eyes to stop the vision and enhance your feeling. Keep the body extremely calm and relaxed. The mind should be without worries or cares. It is just like a tiny fire, little Yáng within Yīn, in the darkness. The subconscious Yīn mind awakens while the conscious Yáng mind is calm. Original Spirit (Yuánshén, 元神) is raised and harmonized with Original Qì (Yuánqì, 元氣). In this profound meditative state, your

Shén unifies with natural Shén. Ordinary people must rely on their night's sleep to overcome tiredness. Even during sleep, their minds are confused by dreams generated from emotions and desires, so mind and body degenerate quickly. In this way, the Yáng falls into the Yīn.

4. The Method of Regulating the Breathing[8]

(Original Truth of Using No Herbs; Qīng Dynasty; Wāng, Áng)
(Tiáoxífǎ, 調息法)

(勿藥元詮・清・汪昂輯)

The method of regulating the breathing is, do not be restricted by the timing, sit anywhere and anytime you wish. The body is balanced and upright, allow it to be comfortable and natural. Do not lean and bend forward. Loosen the clothes and ease the belt to regulate the body properly. Circle the tongue in the mouth several times. Gently and slowly breathe out dirty air, then gently and slowly breathe in through the nose. Repeat this, and when saliva is generated, swallow it. After biting the teeth a few times, the tongue touches the palate of the mouth. The lips and teeth are closed, and the eyes are closed like the new moon. Then gradually begin regulating the breathing. Do not pant and do not be coarse. Either count the exhalation or the inhalation, from one to ten, from ten to a hundred. Restrain your mind in counting and do not be disordered. If the mind and the breathing are in harmony, and random thoughts are no longer generated, stop counting and allow it to be natural. The longer you can sit, the more marvelous it will be. When you raise up the body, slowly and comfortably extend your arms and legs, not suddenly. If you practice this intelligently, various peculiar visions appear in the calmness. This can direct you to enlighten your mind and comprehend the Dào. It is not just for preserving health and extending life.

調息之法，不拘時候，隨便而坐，平直其身，縱任其體，不倚不曲，解衣緩帶，務令調適。口中舌攪數遍，微微呵出濁氣，鼻中微微納之，或三、五遍，或一、二遍，有津咽下；叩齒數通，舌抵上齶，唇齒相著，兩目垂簾，令朧朧然；漸次調息，不喘不粗，或數息出，或數息入，從一至十，從十至百，攝心在數，勿令散亂，如心息相依，雜念不生，則止勿數，任其自然，坐久愈妙。若欲起身，須徐徐舒放手足，勿得遽起。能勤行之，靜中光景，種種奇特，直可明心悟道，不但養身全生而已也。

From the same source as the previous one, this paragraph describes regulating the breathing. There are many methods, though the principles and theory remain the same. It is important to keep the body relaxed (regulating the body), keep the mind calm (regulating the mind), and breathe softly, deeply, and naturally (regulating the breathing). To regulate your breathing to a profound level, you must also regulate your body and mind. They must harmonize and coordinate with each other. The key to regulating the breathing is not to hold it, but to regulate it until it can be natural, smooth, and slender.

5. Four Demeanors of Regulating the Breathing[8]

(Original Interpretation of Using No Herbs; Qīng Dynasty; Wāng, Áng)
(Tiáoxí Sìxiàng, 調息四相)

(勿藥元詮・清・汪昂輯)

There are four demeanors in regulating the breathing. Those when they breathe, there is a sound, it is classified as wind breathing. If the wind persists, then Qì and mind are dispersed. Those when they breathe, there is no sound but the nose is obstructed, it is classified as panting breathing. If the panting persists, then Qì and mind are stagnant. Those when they breathe, there is no sound and no stagnation but to and fro has shape, it is classified as Qì breathing. If the mind focuses on Qì, then it is fatigued. Those when they breathe, have neither sound nor stagnation, the air exits and enters softly, as though it existed and as though it does not exist. Shén and breathing mutually rely on each other. This is the demeanor of real regulating of the breathing. When the breathing is truly regulated, then the mind is steady, and real Qì can circulate naturally. This allows you to capture the variations of nature. Every breath returns to its origin. This is the root of life.

調息有四相：呼吸有聲者風也，守風則散；雖無聲而鼻中澀滯者喘也，守喘則結；不聲不滯而往來有形者氣也，守氣則勞；不聲不滯，出入綿綿，若存若亡，神氣相依，是息相也。息調則心定，真氣往來，自能奪天地之造化，息息歸根，命之蒂也。

This paragraph explains how, from the demeanors of a meditator, we can tell how correct is his breathing. Those who breathe heavily make noise, indicating that Qì is dispersed. Those who breathe without smoothness and uniformity, their Qì circulation is stagnant. Those who pay too much attention to their breathing are fatigued. Only in those whose breathing is soft, slender, uniform, deep, natural, and smooth, is their Shén peacefully harmonized with Qì circulation. Original Spirit awakens, allowing you to return to the origin of your life.

6. Lǐzhēnrén's Sixteen Marvelous Secret Words of Longevity

(Eight Notes on Longevity; Ming Dynasty; Gāo, Lián)
(Lǐzhēnrén Chángshēng Yīshíliùzì Miàojué, 李真人長生一十六字妙訣)

(遵生八箋 ・明・高濂撰)

Once inhaling, immediately lift up (the perineum) to return Qì to the navel (Lower Dāntián). Once lifting, immediately swallow the saliva, to allow the water and fire to blend.

一吸便提，氣氣歸臍；一提便咽，水火相見。

Kǎn (坎) means Water Qì produced from Original Essence (Yuánjīng, 元精), while Lí (離) means Fire Qì generated from Post-Birth Essence, namely food and air. When these two blend, Shén can be raised to a higher level.

These words reveal the secret of how to cause Fire Qì and Water Qì to blend and interact. This secret is at the Huìyīn (Co-1, 會陰), or perineum. When you inhale, gently lift up your perineum, and lead Qì to the Lower Dāntián. Immediately after inhaling, swallow the saliva to lead Qì down to the Lower Dāntián. Reverse Abdominal Breathing should be used for this practice.

The above documents offer you some references. In Chapter 6, we discuss breathing techniques, especially Embryonic Breathing (Tāixí, 胎息), in more detail.

4-4. Regulating the Mind (Tiáoxīn, 調心)

Regulate the Emotional Mind (Xīn, 心) until it is under control. This is the most difficult subject to train in Nèidān Qìgōng. It sets your mind to deal with itself, and since everyone has his own way of thinking, it is also the most difficult subject to explain.

The methods of regulating the mind have been widely studied, discussed, and practiced in all Chinese Qìgōng societies, which include scholar, medical, religious, and martial arts groups. First we define the mind and then the purposes of regulating it. We discuss the Buddhist and Daoist points of view, and finally we analyze methods of practice.

Two Minds, Xīn and Yì 心・意. Chinese society describes two minds. Xīn, the Emotional Mind (heart, 心), is Yáng, making you confused, scattered, depressed, or excited. Yì, the Wisdom Mind (intention, 意), relates to rational and logical thought. It is Yīn, making you calm, concentrated, and able to feel and ponder deeply. The word Yì (意) consists of three words. Lì (立) on top means to establish, Yuē (曰) in the middle means to speak, and Xīn (心) at the bottom means the heart. So Yì means to establish communication while the Emotional Mind is under control.

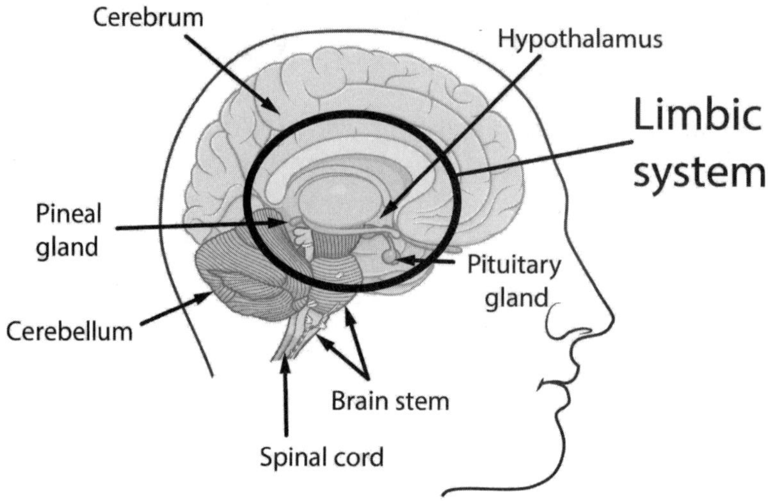

Figure 4-12. Brain and Emotions

Xīn and Yì are directed by different parts of the brain.[9,10] Magnetic resonance imaging (MRI) has determined that while the limbic system near the center of the brain governs emotional thinking, the prefrontal cortex just behind the forehead controls logic, judgment, and executive functions (Figure 4-12). For this reason it can be considered the seat of civilization, or perhaps a "mental traffic cop." It regulates many other parts of the brain, including the limbic system, and modulates emotional responses. However, while a person's limbic system is fully functional by the age of twenty, the prefrontal cortex takes longer to form and develop.

The Yì generated by the prefrontal cortex determines wise, clear thought and judgment, and calm, logical behavior, while the Xīn from the limbic system leads to confusion and emotional behavior. The key to making the prefrontal cortex mature earlier and faster than normal is to use it as early as possible. Learning mathematics, physics, philosophy, or listening to classical music, leads Qì to the front of the brain for faster development. Those who meditate to open the third eye focus their minds at the front of the brain and become wiser.

We use Yì to control, coordinate, and harmonize the Xīn. In scientific terms, we develop the prefrontal cortex to a powerful level, to control and direct the thinking generated by the limbic system of the brain.

Purposes of Regulating the Mind (Tiáoxīn Zhī Mùdì, 調心之目的). The purposes of regulating the mind vary from one school to another. Qìgōng practitioners in scholar and medical societies aim for a calm, peaceful, and harmonious mind so emotions do not disturb Qì circulation. Thoughts affect Qì circulation in the organs. Happiness and excitement affect the heart, while anger affects the liver. The kidneys are affected by fear and the lungs by sadness. (Table 4-4) Regulating your Emotional Mind to a state of harmony and peace benefits your health.

According to the ancient medical book *Thousand Golden Prescriptions for Emergencies* (*Bèijí Qiānjīn Yàofāng*, 備急千金要方), "Contemplate too much, then the spirit is tired. Obsess too much, then aspirations are dispersed. Too much desire, then the will is confused. Involved too much in affairs, then the body is fatigued. Talk too much, then Qì is deficient. Laugh too much, the internal organs can be injured. Worry too much, then the heart is fearful. Too much joy, then expectations stop. Too much happiness, then (one) makes mistakes and is disordered. Angry too often, then circulation in hundreds of vessels is unsteady. Too many favors, then bewitched and ignore regular affairs. Too much wickedness, then gaunt without happiness. Without getting rid of these twelve 'too much,' then the control of flourish and protection (spirit and health) are lost, and blood and Qì circulation disordered. This is the root of losing the life."[11] Wrong sentiments are the root of sickness. In medical and scholar Qìgōng, regulating the mind to be calm, neutral, and not disturbed by emotions is the main task of practice.

Daoist and Buddhist religious groups, having regulated the Emotional Mind to a peaceful state, also aim for Buddhahood and enlightenment. Having controlled the

	WOOD 木	**FIRE 火**	**EARTH 土**	**METAL 金**	**WATER 水**
Direction	East	South	Center	West	North
Season	Spring	Summer	Long Summer	Autumn	Winter
Climactic Condition	Wind	Summer Heat	Dampness	Dryness	Cold
Process	Birth	Growth	Transformation	Harvest	Storage
Color	Green	Red	Yellow	White	Black
Taste	Sour	Bitter	Sweet	Pungent	Salty
Smell	Goatish	Burning	Fragrant	Rank	Rotten
Yīn Organ	Líver	Heart	Spleen	Lungs	Kidneys
Yáng Organ	Gall Bladder	Small Intestine	Stomach	Large Intestine	Bladder
Opening	Eyes	Tongue	Mouth	Nose	Ears
Tissue	Sinews	Blood Vessels	Flesh	Skin/Hair	Bones
Emotion	Anger	Happiness	Pensiveness	Sadness	Fear
Human Sound	Shout	Laughter	Song	Weeping	Groan

Table 4-4. Emotion and Internal Organs

Emotional Mind and developed their Wisdom Mind to a profound stage, they search for the meaning of life and of nature.

Finally, martial arts Qìgōng practitioners raise up the spirit of vitality and build a highly concentrated mind to lead Qì efficiently and to develop the sense of enemy, which is critical in battle. While your mind is calm and clear, your spirit is raised to a state of high alert.

Whatever the goals of each school, the principles of training are the same.

1. To Harmonize Body and Mind (Shēnxīn Pínghéng, 身心平衡).

To achieve a calm meditative mind, first attend to the condition of your body. When it is tensed and energized, breathing is rapid and your mind is excited. Body and mind must coordinate and harmonize with each other. This is called the Balance of the Body and the Xīn (Shēnxīn Pínghéng, 身心平衡). *The Complete Book of Principal Contents of Life and Human Nature* (*Xìngmìng Guīzhǐ Quánshū*, 性命圭旨全書) said, "When the body is not moving, the Xīn is peaceful. When Xīn is not moving, the spirit abides by itself."[12] The first step in regulating the mind is to calm the body, so the mind can be calm. When the emotions are calm, the Wisdom Mind can function efficiently, and the spirit of vitality can be raised.

2. To Harmonize the Breathing and the Mind (Xīnxí Xiāngyī, 心息相依).

Regulating the Emotional Mind (Xīn) is done by the Wisdom Mind (Yì). Xīn is compared to a monkey or ape while Yì is compared to a horse (Xīnyuán Yìmǎ, 心猿意馬). A monkey is weak, but can be unsteady and disturbing, generating confusion and excitement. A horse, though powerful, can be calm, steady, and controlled.

Thousands of years of experience in meditation have discovered that, in order to "tame the monkey mind" and lead it into a cage, one needs a banana. This banana is the breathing. As you focus on your breathing, your Emotional Mind becomes restrained and calm. When your breathing becomes long, slender, soft, and calm, your mind becomes calm, and vice versa. Mind and breathing mutually affect each other, working harmoniously to reach a high level of meditation. This is called Xīn and Breathing Mutual Reliance (Xīnxí Xiāngyī, 心息相依).

The Complete Book of Principal Contents of Life and Human Nature (Xìngmìng Guīzhǐ Quánshū, 性命圭旨全書) says, "To conform with the Daoist's deep profound breathing, Xīn and breathing rely on each other mutually. When breathing is regulated, Xīn can be calm."[13] To have a calm Emotional Mind, first regulate your breathing through Daoist breathing methods.

Questions from a Buddhist Guest about Listening to the Heart (Tīngxīn Zhāikè Wèn, 聽心齋客問) explains, "The Xīn has been relying on affairs and objects for a long time; separated from its residence, it cannot be independent. Therefore, use Gōngfū of regulating the breath to restrain Xīn. Xīn and breathing can then mutually rely on each other. Regulating does not mean to use Yì, but only a thought of one inhalation and one exhalation. Once Xīn separates from its residence, it is without others and without self, and breathing cannot be regulated. Keep the breathing soft and continuous as though existing, yet not existing (regulating without regulating). After a long time, it will be become proficient naturally."[14] This paragraph explains that our Emotional Mind concerns itself with human affairs and objects around us and is influenced by them. Then it is confused and cannot be independent. The way to restrain it is to regulate the breathing, until the Emotional Mind and the breathing are mutually dependent on each other. You should not have an intention (Yì), but simply pay attention to the breathing. After you have practiced for a period of time, you will be able to breathe softly, naturally, smoothly, and continuously. The Xīn will stay at its residence without disturbance.

3. Use the Mind to Build Up, Store, and Lead Qì Circulation (Yǐyì Zēng, Cún, Yǐn Qì, 以意增、存、引氣).

In religious and martial Qìgōng, one of the main goals is using the mind to build up Qì, store it, and lead its circulation.

"Keep the Yì at the Dāntián" (Yìshǒu Dāntián, 意守丹田). To build up and store Qì in the Real Lower Dāntián (Zhēn Xiàdāntián, 真下丹田), practice Embryonic Breathing (Tāixí, 胎息), and keep your mind in this Qì residence. If your mind is away from this center, Qì is led away from it and consumed, without being stored and built up to a higher level.

"Use the Yì to lead the Qì" (Yǐyì Yǐnqì, 以意引氣). After building up abundant Qì, use your mind to lead it. In Nèidān practice, first lead Qì to circulate in the Conception (Rènmài, 任脈) and Governing Vessels (Dūmài, 督脈) to complete Small Circulation (Xiǎozhoutian, 小周天). Then lead the Qì to the extremities, skin, bone marrow, and brain for Grand Circulation (Dàzhōutiān, 大周天).

4. Raise the Spirit of Vitality for Enlightenment (Shéntōng, 神通).

Again, the final goal of Buddhist and Daoist Qìgōng is enlightenment or Buddhahood. To this end, build up and store Qì at the Real Lower Dāntián, then lead it up through the Thrusting Vessel (Chōngmài, 衝脈, Spinal Cord) to the brain, to nourish the brain and raise the spirit. The goal is to open the third eye. Having lied and cheated to conceal our secrets behind a mask through thousands of years, humans have closed our third eye. By doing so, we lost the power of telepathy and communion with the spirit of nature. To reopen this third eye, we must be truthful, not hiding anything, and then accumulate Qì in the front of the brain.

To raise the spirit to enlightenment, regulate your Xīn to an extremely calm, clear, and steady state. *Dào Scriptures* (道藏) said, "Xīn is the master of the whole body, the commander of a hundred spirits. When calm, wisdom is generated; when acting, confusion originates. Its steadiness and confusion are within the movement and the calmness."[15]

Let us summarize the Qìgōng methods practiced in Buddhist and Daoist society, first discussing the origin of thoughts. By recognizing the root of emotional disturbance and confusion, we can find ways to stop it.

The Origin of Thoughts (Qǐniàn Zhīyuán, 起念之源). Buddhists cultivate a neutral and empty state of mind, separate from the Four Greatnesses (Sìdà, 四大), the earth (Dì, 地), water (Shuǐ, 水), fire (Huǒ, 火), and wind (Fēng, 風) (Sìdà Jiēkōng, 四大皆空). They believe this renders their spirits independent, so they can escape from the recurring cycle of reincarnation.

Most thought is generated from emotions, by the seven passions and six desires. After thoughts pass through the Wisdom Mind, then action is taken. When a person's Wisdom Mind is strong, the action will be rational and reasonable. But if one's Emotional Mind is so strong that the Wisdom Mind cannot interpret the emotional thought before initiating action, the action will be emotional and irrational. For example, when you encounter a traffic jam, initially you feel no problem. If the jam lasts for an hour, your Emotional Mind becomes uneasy and impatient, turning into anger and frustration. Your Emotional Mind has been agitated and excited. But if your Wisdom Mind steps in and asks whether traffic will improve if you lose your temper, the answer is no. In this case your Wisdom Mind takes over to control your Emotional Mind.

Observing Thoughts (Guānniàn, 觀念). To prevent emotional thought from initiating, keep your mind in a neutral state, which is not the usual way of human nature. Old thoughts commonly linger in one's mind, and one keeps thinking about them, being constantly disturbed and agitated. This kind of thought is called Niàn (念), which means "the old thought always borne in mind." To stop this disturbing thought, first recognize it. Many people fear to face it and simply hide behind a mask, but sooner or later, it reappears to disturb them.

To keep the old thought from lingering in your mind, first be awakened. This step is called observing the thoughts (Guānniàn, 觀念). From this observation, you awaken. Zhìyóuzǐ (至游子) said, "Do not fear initiation of a thought, but be afraid of awakening too late."[16] Often, if emotional action has already taken place before your awakening, the mistake will have been committed. When you regret at this time, it is already too late to undo your action.

To reach a profound level of observing thoughts and understanding them is no easy task. There are three extents (Sānjiè, 三界) of this mental cultivation. Dào Scriptures (Dàozàng, 道藏) said, "The extent of desire, extent of color, and extent of colorlessness. When Xīn forgets worry and thoughts, it transcends desire. When it forgets the surrounding environment, it transcends color. When it sees nothing, it transcends colorlessness."[17] This is equivalent to the Buddhist saying that the mind should be separated from the Four Greatnesses: earth (Dì, 地), water (Shuǐ, 水), fire (Huǒ, 火), and wind (Fēng, 風) (Sìdà Jiēkōng, 四大皆空). This means the free thought, unbounded by surrounding objects.

Buddhists have three ways of observing thoughts, called "three observations" (Sānguān, 三觀). These are: observation of emptiness (Kōngguān, 空觀), observation of falsehood (illusion, Jiǎguān, 假觀), and observation of the neutral (neither empty nor illusory, Zhōngguān, 中觀).[18]

In Kōngguān (observation of emptiness, 空觀), you observe and then comprehend the meaning of events. After long pondering, you see everything bothering us emotionally is only temporary and small compared with our lifetime or with the age of the universe. All emotional disturbances are empty and meaningless. Our lives come from emptiness and end with it. What really matters is how truthful we are, so our spirit can grow. Every physical lifetime serves the education and growth of our spirit. Any disturbance is only empty thought. Once you grasp this, you can analyze the event from the truthful subconscious point of view.

A story may inspire your thinking about this. In ancient China, two monks walked down a muddy road which they found to be completely block at a certain point by a large puddle. A beautiful lady in a lovely gown stood at the edge of the puddle, unable to go farther without spoiling her clothes.

Without hesitation, one of the monks picked her up and carried her across the puddle, set her down on the other side, and continued on his way. Hours later, when the two monks were preparing to camp for the night, the second monk turned to the first and said: "I can no longer hold this back. I'm quite angry at you! We are not supposed to look at women, particularly pretty ones, never mind touching them. Why did you do that?" The first monk replied, "I left her at the mud puddle; why are you still carrying her?" Emptiness in your mind depends on how you think.

In Jiǎguān (observation of falseness, 假觀), you pay attention to tracing back the root of each event. You realize we fight for glory, dignity, love, wealth, and power, created from the illusion of the mind. We humans created all these emotions as a matrix and entered it. Afterwards, most of us do not enjoy it and constantly bear the pain of illusion. Each lifetime is like a show on stage, with everyone wearing a mask, playing their allotted role, and hiding their true spiritual identity. We lie, cheat, smile, and cry, without involvement of our real spiritual identity, which is truthful and pure. Events and problems are false, not real, being only an illusion of life. Once you comprehend this, all thoughts generated by the Emotional Mind become meaningless.

Ponder a story from Japanese Zen society, about a bold and handsome young Samurai warrior standing before an aged Zen master, asking, "Master, I have reached a high level of Zen theory and practice, but would like to ask a serious question."

The master humbly replied, "What question would you like to ask?"

"Please teach me about heaven and hell," the Samurai replied.

The master froze motionless for just a moment and then suddenly snapped his head in disgust and seethed, "Teach you about heaven and hell? I doubt you could even keep your own sword from rusting, you ignorant fool! How dare you suppose you could understand anything I might have to say?"

The old man went on, becoming more insulting, while the young swordsman's surprise turned first to confusion, then to dismay and hot anger. Master or no master, who insults a Samurai and lives? At last, teeth clenched and blood boiling in blind fury, the warrior drew his sword to end the old man's tirade and life.

The master looked straight into his eyes and said gently, "That is hell."

At the peak of his rage, the Samurai realized this was indeed his teaching, that the master had driven him into a living hell of uncontrollable anger and ego. The young man, profoundly humbled, sheathed his sword and bowed to this great spiritual teacher. Looking into the wise man's aged, beaming face, he felt more love and compassion than he had ever felt in his life. The master, sensing the changed demeanor, raised his index finger and said, "And that is heaven."

Emotional disturbances are created from false illusion in the mind. Do we create heaven and hell in our minds, and keep ourselves trapped in this matrix, or do heaven and hell really exist? Do we create God in our imagination or does God create man in His? What proof is there, and how truthful would it be?

In Zhōngguān (observation of neutral, 中觀), you neither deny the emptiness of the matter, nor its illusory existence. You may, through observation, lead your thoughts into the neutral point that all things are empty and also false. It is the observation of double reflections (Shuāngzhào, 雙照), or relative comparison.

In a small village in southern China lived the hardest worker in his community. Day and night he toiled, and year by year his riches grew. As time passed, his hoard of money increased, as did his concern for failure or loss. He worried about how to make more money and how to keep both friends and enemies away from the massive wealth he had accumulated.

He raised the fence around his house and strengthened the walls, with strong locks on the doors and bars on the windows, until the house resembled a jail. He felt safe and believed himself the happiest man alive as he counted his money all day.

A curious passerby peered in and saw him sitting there smiling as he counted. He called out, "Why are you so happy? It seems you're in jail!"

The man answered, "No! It's not that I'm in jail, it's that you are outside of it."

Many of us dream of money, making it our obsession. Invisible walls are built and personal jails created in which we enjoy ourselves, yet friendships are held at bay. What does it really mean to be happy, to be rich both materially and spiritually? The truly rich are those who know how to make money yet also know how to share with others. This sets you free from the bondage of material obsession.

A wealthy businessman from the north spotted a fisherman relaxing against his canoe and smoking a pipe. The businessman was dismayed, "Why aren't you sailing for fish?"

"I caught enough today already."

"The sun is still high in the sky, you could catch plenty more, couldn't you?" insisted the businessman.

"Why should I?" retorted the fisherman.

"Money! You would have more money!" the businessman exclaimed. "With a better engine on your boat, you could go to deeper water and catch more fish. Soon you could buy a better net and catch even more fish and make even more money. Finally, you may become rich enough to buy a fleet of new boats, even becoming as rich as me."

"And then what would I do?"

"Sit and enjoy your life."

"That is what I am doing now," said the fisherman.

When you desire something, know when to stop. Keep your mind neutral and see two ends instead of only one direction. To free yourself from emotional bondage, practice these three observations until you comprehend the meaning of life from the depths of your heart. You will see the reason for everything that happens, in the spiritual learning process, without dwelling on events. After watching a stage show that touches you emotionally, if you dwell on it emotionally, you are in emotional bondage. Instead, learn from it about the meaning of life, so your mind looks far instead of near.

Since we are all on the stage of life, each one carries a mask which allows us to fit in the show. However, deep inside we all know that it is only a show and not our true identity. Without a mask in this masked society, we could not survive.

My grandmother told me a story about a king, who always wore a stern and solemn mask whenever he met his officers. Because of this, his officials respected, loved, feared, and obeyed him, so he could rule the country effectively. One day his wife told him that what the officials respected and loved was not him, but his mask. To prove his wife wrong, he removed it. From then on, his officials could see his real face and discern his thinking from his facial expression. They started to fight each other in front of him, and even to dispute his policies and decisions. In a short time, the country fell into disorder. The king realized the power of the mask. He gave the order to chop off the heads of all those officials who had seen his face. He replaced the mask on his face and could once again rule the country effectively.

You can see why it is hard for many spiritual people (truthful persons) to survive in this masked society and why they shun lay society to go to the mountains.

Stopping Thoughts (Zhǐniàn, 止念). "Stopping thoughts" means to stop old thoughts which hang around in your mind. These can be emotionally troubling, disturbing your state of calm. Stopping thoughts also means to stop a new thought from being initiated. The emotionally disturbed mind is the origin of the body's Yáng fire. *The Complete Book of Principal Contents of Human Life and Temperament, Hēng Anthology (Xìngmìng Guīzhǐ Quánshū·Hēngjí,* 性命圭旨全書・亨集) says that "if a thought is initiated, then everywhere is fire. In the quiet place where thoughts cease, Spring can blossom."[19] Spring blossoming means the harmonization of the mind, body, breathing, and spirit.

To stop thoughts, first stop your inner observation from observing, which is the stage of Zhǐguān (止觀). Awaken and comprehend the root of thoughts through observation to find the way to stop them. Then, observation becomes necessary, because it is regulated.

Wéimó Classic (*Wéimójīng*, 維摩經) said, "To restrain the Xīn from emotional affinity is called stopping. To see deeply and reach far clearly, is called observation." It also said, "Every thought returns to its origin, is called stopping. Everything can be discriminated clearly, is called observation."[20]

The first phrase explains that to reach Zhǐguān, you first stop emotional affinity with the outside world. This is the meaning of "stopping" (Zhǐ, 止). When your mind is so clear and profound that you analyze the situation through observation, and can thus stop both the old thought and also the initiation of a new one, it is called observation (Guān, 觀).

The second phrase explains "stopping" (Zhǐ, 止) to be the bringing of all disturbing thoughts back to focus on the Dāntián where they originate. Pay attention to the Dāntián, either Upper Dāntián for Shén or Real Lower Dāntián for Qì, and coordinate with your deep breathing. Then all disturbing thoughts can be stopped and replaced with one thought. To see deeply to the root of reality is called observation (Guān, 觀).

Methods of Stopping Thoughts (Zhǐniànfǎ, 止念法). Buddhist and Daoist societies developed many methods of regulating thought. The first step is to restrain the wandering Emotional Mind from the attraction of the outside world. Close your eyes and focus on regular, deep, and soft breathing, which calms the Emotional Mind. As mentioned earlier, it is said, "The eyes observe (Guān, 觀) the breathing, and the breathing observes the Xīn. "[21]

Once you have reached Zhǐguān, you prevent new thoughts from initiating. Pay attention to your breathing, and keep your mind at the Dāntián. In Zhuāngzi, Secular

World (Zhuāngzi·Rénjiānshì, 莊子・人間世), it is said, "With a unified will, do not listen with the ears but with Xīn. Do not listen with Xīn, but with Qì. Listening ceases at the ears, and Xīn stops when harmony (Fú) is reached. What is Qì? It is insubstantial and exists in all objects. Only by following the Dào can you gather this insubstantial Qì, which is obtained from the purification of Xīn (Xīnzhāi)."[22]

To regulate your Emotional Mind (Xīn, 心), stop listening to the outside world, and pay attention to your Emotional Mind. Once you bring your thoughts from outside to inside your body, pay attention to Qì through breathing. Fú (符) means to match, harmonize, coordinate, or cooperate. Stopping the activity of Xīn is achieved through the coordination of breathing.

To gather Qì at the Real Lower Dāntián, first calm the Xīn. Xīnzhāi (心齋) means purified Xīn, and implies a calm and sincere mind. In this way Qì can be preserved at its residence. This is the way of Dào (道).

In the Anthology of Daoist Village (Dàoxiāngjí, 道鄉集), it is said, "Today, I would like to teach you the method of ceasing thought. For example, when my Xīn looks at the water, my thought will be on the water. When my Xīn looks at the moon, my thought will be on the moon. If my eyes focus on looking at the Qì cavity (Qìxuè, Dāntián), my Xīn will be on the Qì cavity."[23] This defines the key to stopping thought as paying attention to the Qìxuè (氣穴). Qìxuè means Upper Dāntián or Real Lower Dāntián. Once you pay attention to the breathing and keep your mind at the Dāntián, the thought disappears.

Cease Activity of Xīn (Xíxīn, 息心). The final goal in regulating the mind is stabilizing it from emotional disturbance, and keeping it from wandering about, also called Dìngxīn (定心). But first you must cease the activity of Xīn (Xíxīn, 息心). The Collection of Neutral Harmony (Zhōnghéjí, 中和集) states, "Carefully study the writings of those holy men in Three Teachings (Sānjiào, Three Schools), the word of ceasing, Xí, is the simplest and most straightforward. If you put Gōngfū in ceasing, you will not need much effort to reach Buddhahood and immortality. Cease the feeling of affinity (Xíyuán, 息緣) to reach the pivotal function of original Chán. Cease the Xīn (Xíxīn) to comprehend and understand the theory of Confucianism profoundly. Cease the breathing (Xíqì) to reach the marvelous Dào of condensing the Shén. These three ceasings are mutually required by each other without any conquest."[24]

Sānjiào (三教) means Three Teachings or Three Schools, namely Buddhism, Daoism, and Confucianism. All of them describe methods of ceasing (Xí, 息). Xí here means to stop or cease any action or prevent it from being initiated. Here it means regulating without regulating (Bùtiáo Értiáo, 不調而調). When regulating is no longer necessary, all regulating processes cease.

The key practice of Buddhists is to cease the affinity (Xíyuán, 息緣) which connects with secular affairs. Then the Emotional Mind will be calm and peaceful, the Shén of the subconscious mind will awaken, and Buddhahood can be achieved. This cultivation is called Chán (禪). *The Transliteration of Wisdom Garden* (*Huìyuàn Yīnyì*, 慧苑音義) said, "Chán, it means to calm down the Xīn to ponder."[25] It is the meditation of stabilizing the activity of Xīn.

The cultivation of "ceasing" in the Confucian school is to cease the Xin's activity, so the scholar philosophies can be comprehended. These include the relationships between humans, and between humans and nature. When these philosophies are understood, the mind can be peaceful and calm.

But to Daoists, "ceasing" means to cease regulating the breathing, by practicing Embryonic Breathing with the condensed mind. This is the necessary path to reach enlightenment.

Stabilizing Xīn (Dìngxīn, 定心). Regulating the mind to keep it calm and stable is called Dìng (定), the stabilization of Xīn. You bring mind and body into harmony, so you can ponder profoundly and finally comprehend the Dào. In *Four Books, Great Study* (*Sìshū. Dàxué*, 四書・大學), Confucius said, "Only knowing how to cease, can you then have steadiness (Dìng). When there is steadiness, your mind can be calm. Then you can be peaceful, and able to ponder. When you ponder, you will gain."[26] To Confucian scholar society, the final goal of meditation is to gain, or understand, the meaning of life and the laws of nature (Dào). To comprehend this deep philosophy, you go through necessary procedures. The first is to cease (Zhǐ, 止) the initiation of thought, so your mind becomes steady, controlled, calm, and peaceful, and clear for you to ponder. Through deep pondering, you comprehend the reasons for events.

How do we define Dìng (stabilization, 定)? In *Theory of Evaluating Wisdom* (*Zhìdùlùn*, 智度論), it is said, "Regulate the Xīn to where it should be. Cease worry and condense (stabilize) the Xīn. When Xīn is steady at one place without moving, it is called steadiness (Dìng). Regulate the Xīn to accept the solution through observation. This is called acceptance (Shòu, 受). To regulate the violence of the Xīn, to straighten its curve (intricacy) and stabilize its dispersion, this is called regulating, straightening, and stabilizing. To regulate the actions of Xīn and allow it to be as it should, is called regulate the Xīn to where it should be. To cease the mind's affinity and worry, so as to condense and focus the thought of Xīn, is called cease worry and condense the Xīn. "[27]

In Buddhist meditation, Dìng (steadiness of the Xīn and the body, 定) is always emphasized. Entering this steadiness is called Rùdìng (入定). First cut off all emotional disturbance and keep your mind at the Upper and Real Lower Dāntián. The Upper Dāntián (brain) is the residence of the Shén, while the Real Lower Dāntián (second brain) is the residence of Qì. When Qì is kept at its residence, the body can be calmed without stimulation or excitement. When Shén is condensed at its residence, the mind becomes calm and clear.

Learn to face your Emotional Mind, analyze and understand it, and remove the mask from your face. Only when these affinities of Xīn can be removed, can your mind be kept steady at one place. This is the way to reach steadiness (Dìng, 定).

The final goal is profound stabilization of Xīn, called Great Steadiness (Dàdìng, 大定). Dàdìng means, "When Xīn for Buddhism is clear and bright, it is called Dàdìng."[28] The mind is peaceful and calm, the body extremely relaxed, as Shén and body harmonize and coordinate with each other. This defines the steadiness and the calmness of both mental and physical bodies. Once you reach this stage, you have established a firm foundation for cultivation of spiritual enlightenment.

I would like to share a Samurai story with you.

A boy of ten was playing in his house when a Samurai swordsman entered and started killing people. The boy hid behind a large clothes cabinet, and through a gap he saw clearly what was happening. The swordsman was his father's political enemy, and the boy was the family's only survivor. The swordsman finished his killing, then left without searching the cabinet.

The boy traveled the country searching for the best Zen master. He swore he would become the most famous and skillful Samurai swordsman, so he could avenge the murder of his family. He found a master and practiced day and night, with vengeance in his heart.

By his early twenties, he became one of the best-known Samurai swordsmen in Japan. He traveled to every corner of Japan, searching for his enemy. But after twenty-five years of searching, all efforts were in vain, and his enemy seemed to have disappeared from society.

His disappointment great, one day he entered a deep valley where only a few tribesmen lived. He came to a small river, where an old man was rebuilding a bridge, slowly and strenuously moving wood piece by piece. The original bridge had been swept away by a torrent, and the villagers had to travel far downstream to cross the river.

Talking to the old man, he could not believe his eyes. The old man was the one who had killed his family more than thirty years before. Without hesitation, he drew his sword to cut off his head. Before doing so, he explained why. The old man freely admitted to killing his family, but had one final request.

"This bridge is the only hope for the village. Allow me to finish building it before killing me," the old man asked.

Since the old man's request was good, he agreed to permit him to finish the bridge. But he would watch him day and night, so he could not run away. The avenger built a tent next to the old man and watched him build the bridge. Progress was slow and time-consuming, and after six months, he joined in to help the old man finish the bridge, to hasten the day of his revenge.

Eating together, talking and helping each other, in time they became good friends. The bridge was completed in the third year. On completing the job, the old man came to the Samurai's tent. He had washed his body clean. He knelt before the avenger, and said, "It is time for you to take my life to avenge your family."

The Samurai found he could not draw his sword for revenge. He knelt in front of the old man and said: "My first life was hatefulness, like hell. My second life is kindness and peace, like heaven. I cannot kill you, otherwise I would also kill my second life." So they traveled together and treated each other like father and son.

4-5. Regulating the Qì (Tiáoqì, 調氣)

The purposes of regulating Qì are 1. Producing Qì (Shēngqì, 生氣); 2. Nourishing and protecting Qì (Yǎngqì, 養氣); 3. Storing Qì (Xùqì, 蓄氣); and 4. Transporting Qì (Xíngqì, 行氣). Next, we discuss the theory and key practices of these four.

1. Producing Qì (Shēngqì, 生氣)

There are three ways to produce Qì, namely herbs, breathing, and massage.

Herbs. Qì originates primarily from the biochemical reaction of the food we eat and the oxygen we inhale, which releases energy. Different foods produce different quantity and quality of energy, so herbs have been thoroughly researched in Chinese medical science. Different herbs are used to regulate the body's energy status.

Qì from food and air is called Post-Heaven Qì (Hòutiānqì, 後天氣) or Fire Qì (Huǒqì, 火氣), because food and air are not pure and clean. The Qì generated from them can cause emotional disturbance and physical problems. This is the main cause of fire in our mental and physical bodies.

Abdominal Breathing. Through deep abdominal breathing, oxygen and carbon dioxide are exchanged efficiently, promoting the body's metabolism. The energy from the biochemical reaction is stronger. Deep abdominal breathing also helps convert abdominal fat into Qì, increasing the quantity of Qì in the body.

This kind of breathing is called Pre-Heaven Breathing (Xiāntiān Hūxī, 先天呼吸) and the Qì produced is called Pre-Heaven Qì (Xiāntiānqì, 先天氣), which is clean and pure, able to calm down your mind and make your physical body healthy.

Massaging the Abdomen. The *Muscle/Tendon Changing and Marrow/Brain Washing Classic* describes the correct way to massage the abdomen. Wrong techniques make the body, especially the intestines, too Yáng, triggering constipation. If Qì is increased too rapidly, it can also go up and damage the heart. If you do not know the techniques, you should not attempt to increase Qì in this way. Abdominal breathing is much safer than massage. To know more about Muscle/Tendon Changing and Marrow/Brain Washing Qìgōng, please refer to the book, *Qìgōng—The Secret of Youth*, by YMAA.

Other than these three methods, you may also strive to maintain your hormone level (Original Essence, Yuánjīng, 元精). Hormones act as catalysts in regulating the body's metabolism and expediting biochemical reactions, so Qì can be produced smoothly and abundantly.

2. Protecting and Nourishing Qì (Yǎngqì, 養氣)

Protecting means to preserve and keep, and nourishing means to cultivate and raise up. After generating Qì, maintain it and cultivate it to a stronger level. It is like raising a child: after you have generated life, you protect it and raise it so it can grow stronger.

Protect Original Essence. Protect Qì by protecting your Original Essence (Yuánjīng, 元精). A man should regulate his sexual activities, abuse of which weakens the kidneys. According to Chinese medicine, this is the primary cause of losing Qì for men.

Also regulate your lifestyle. If you are fatigued mentally or physically, the consumption of Qì increases, so regulate your mental and physical activities. Get enough sleep and rest, and keep a regular daily schedule.

Regulate the Breathing. To keep the Qì in the body, breathe deeply and softly without holding your breath. Breathing too fast increases the heartbeat, tensing the body and mind, and consuming Qì.

But maintaining physical strength requires exercise, during which the breath and the heartbeat speed up. The key is knowing when to stop and how much exercise is needed to maintain health. Yáng exercise is necessary to maintain physical life, and Yīn rest is also required to preserve and restore life, through conservation of Qì. Both are equally important, and you need both.

When you exercise, breathe properly without holding your breath. You need a large quantity of oxygen to convert glucose into the energy required. Holding the breath too much consumes Qì.

Regulate the Xīn. Mental fatigue, especially emotional disturbance, uses up Qì. To protect your Qì, the most important key is regulating your Emotional Mind. In a neutral state, Qì can stay at its residence without manifesting, so it is preserved and protected. There is a document which emphasizes regulating the mind to preserve Qì, which I will translate next and offer some commentary.

Stone Tablet with One Hundred Words (Lǚ, Yán)[8]
《百字碑》(Bǎizìbēi)
(古今圖書集成・博物匯編神異論；呂岩作)

When cultivating Qì, do not just talk about preserving it. When calming down the mind, it should be doing without doing. If you know the origins of movement (Yáng) and stillness (Yīn), there is nothing for you to ask anyone else. Face the real reality, you must deal with daily affairs, but you should not be infatuated by them. Then your temperament can be steady and self-controlled, and Qì will naturally be preserved. Then the elixir can be conceived, and Kǎn and Lí can interact under control within the kettle. Interaction of Yīn and Yáng initiates the repeated cycle, and this will bring a natural derivation of new life, enlightened like thunder. White clouds move upwards, and sweet dew sprinkles Xūmí (fullness of human virtue). I drink the wine of longevity by myself, how can others know how free and unfettered I am? I sit down to listen to songs by the instrument without strings. I comprehend clearly the pivotal function of natural creation. These sentences offer the ladder to ascend to Heaven (enlightenment).

養氣忘言守，降心為不為。動靜知宗祖，無事更尋誰？
真常須應物，應物要不迷。不迷性自住，性住氣自回。
氣回丹自結，壺中配坎離。陰陽生反復，普化一聲雷。
白雲朝頂上，甘露洒須彌。自飲長生酒，逍遙誰得知？
坐聽無弦曲，明通造化機。都來十二句，端的上天梯。

Cultivating Qì is not just about maintaining it. Most important is to regulate your Xīn (Emotional Mind). This must be regulated until no more regulating is necessary and it becomes natural. Your mind becomes clear and your judgment neutral and accurate. Whether active or still, you know where the origins are. If you know clearly what is happening, why do you need to ask anyone else? To live in this human world, you deal with necessary affairs, but without being lured by money, glory, power, pride, jealousy, or other human desires and emotions. If your mind is separated from these temptations, it can be calm and steady. Qì returns to its origin (Real Lower Dāntián), forming the elixir (Spiritual Embryo). You control life easily through adjusting Kǎn and Lí. Through Kǎn and Lí, the Yīn and Yáng of your spirit and body is regulated as you wish. Through cultivating Yīn and Yáng, when the time is ripe, you open your third eye for enlightenment like a clap of thunder. When this happens, you have no doubt about your life, which will be like pure white clouds floating in the sky and sweet dew upon Xūmí (須彌). Xūmí is the Daoist term for the spiritual being in the fullness of human virtue. You live long and enjoy life to the fullest. You communicate with nature like listening to a song without sound, understanding its pivotal functions.

Gather and Exchange Qì with Nature and Partners. Energy from the sun, moon, earth, trees, and any other source of natural energy can nourish the body. By meditating at dawn facing the sun, one absorbs solar energy to enhance the body's Qì. Practicing Qìgōng facing the moon a couple days before it is full is also a good way of absorbing Qì. Orienting a house by coordinating the sun's and earth's magnetic fields is known as Fēngshuǐ (wind-water, 風水), which determines good energy for living. Using natural energy to nourish one's Qì is very important in Qìgōng practice.

To harmonize and balance Qì, and to nourish one another, many Daoists use partners to exchange Qì through meditation or special Qìgōng practices. This is known as Dual Cultivation (Shuāngxiū, 雙修), which is also described in *Qìgōng—The Secret of Youth*, and *Qìgōng Grand Circulation for Spiritual Enlightenment*.

3. Storing Qì (Xùqì, 蓄氣)

After conserving, protecting, and cultivating Qì, you must store it in the biobattery at the Real Lower Dāntián. You lead the Qì there and keep it there.

To keep the Qì there, you keep your mind there. When your mind strays, you are leading Qì away and consuming it. Keeping the mind at this center is called Yìshǒu Dāntián (意守丹田), achieved through Embryonic Breathing (Tāixí, 胎息). There is a document which explains the importance of Embryonic Breathing, which I translate here with commentary. For more on the subject, refer to my previous book, *Qìgōng Meditation—Embryonic Breathing*.

Classic of Embryonic Breathing[8,29,30]

《胎息經》(Tāixíjīng)

The embryo is conceived from the concealed Qì. Qì is developed through (regulating) the breath of the embryo. When Qì is present, the body may live. When Shén abandons the body and the shape disperses, death follows. Knowing the spirit and Qì makes long life possible. Firmly protect the insubstantial emptiness (Spiritual Embryo) to cultivate spirit and Qì. When spirit moves, the Qì moves. When spirit stops, the Qì stops. For a long life, spirit and Qì must coordinate harmoniously with each other. When Xīn is not infatuated by thoughts coming or going, then Spirit and Qì will not exit and enter, and will thus remain naturally. To practice intelligently is the true way.

胎從伏氣中結，氣從有胎中息。氣入身來為之生，神去離形為之死。知神氣可以長生，固守虛無以養神氣。神行則氣行，神住則氣住。若欲長生，神氣相住。心不動念，無來無去，不出不入，自然常住。勤而行之，是真道路。

Nobody knows when or by whom this classic was written, but it has been passed down for generations and is considered one of the most important documents about Embryonic Breathing.

The Holy Embryo (Shèngtāi, 聖胎) or Spiritual Embryo (Shéntāi, 神胎) is conceived from Qì stored at the Real Lower Dāntián. To obtain this concealed Qì, practice Embryonic Breathing. Once you have stored it abundantly, your life force becomes strong, bringing you good health and longevity. But to manifest this Qì as physical life force, you need a strong spirit, to focus the circulation and manifestation of Qì. Without this living spirit, you lose your health and die. One who cultivates his spirit and Qì lives a long and healthy life. The first part of the classic explains how to regulate the relationship between physical life, Qì, and Shén.

Keep your mind firmly at the Real Lower Dāntián, called Xūwú (虛無), which means "nothingness." Your mind remaining at the Real Lower Dāntián, is the state of Wújí (No Extremity, 無極), the state of no discrimination, or nothingness. Only here can you really be in a neutral state of mind. Clear out emotions and desires. This is described in *Dào Dé Jīng* as, "Approach the nothingness to its extremity, and maintain calmness with sincerity."[31] The mind leads the Qì. When actively thinking, you are leading Qì away from its residence and consuming it. To store abundant Qì, you must conserve, protect and build it. These three important things are emphasized in Internal Elixir Qìgōng (Nèidān Qìgōng, 內丹氣功).

To build up abundant Qì, you not only keep your mind at the Real Lower Dāntián, but also practice Embryonic Breathing. To manifest Qì efficiently for daily life, you need a strong and highly-controlled Shén. Qì consumption is limited and efficiency high. The key to longevity is to coordinate and harmonize Shén and Qì. To keep Shén pure and strong, calm the Xīn. Xīn is like a monkey, while Yì is like a horse (Xīnyuán Yìmǎ, 心猿意馬). To keep the monkey steady, restrain it in its "cage," the Wújí state. This is crucial to success.

4. Transporting Qì (Xíngqì, 行氣)

Having preserved, protected, cultivated, and stored Qì, you need to circulate it efficiently. "Use your mind to lead the Qì" (Yǐyì Yǐnqì, 以意引氣). The key to this is "leading" (Yǐn, 引). The mind should not be in the Qì, but ahead of it. If your mind pays attention to the Qì, it stagnates. If you want to move from where you are standing, your mind must be on the spot you wish to move to. If your mind stays at the place where you are standing, no movement can take place. "The Yì should not be on the Qì, if on the Qì, then stagnant"[32]

The methods of leading and what you wish to accomplish depend on how extensively and profoundly you grasp the theory, the principles of Yīn and Yáng, and the goal of your training. There are five common goals for a Qìgōng practitioner, which vary according to the depth of the training.

Connection of the Yì and Qì. Before you can connect your Yì with the Qì, you must recognize the existence of the Qì, originating from the feeling of its existence. Qì is energy that cannot be seen, only felt. You train to establish a sensitive feeling for it. When this feeling focuses on the inner body, it is called Gōngfū of Inner Vision (Nèishì Gōngfū, 內視功夫).

After this, you establish the connection between the Yì and the Qì. This feeling is like a piece of rope you hold connected to a cow's nose. Without this rope, you will not be able to lead the Qì.

Once you have established this connection, then you must also know how much effort and force you need to lead the cow. Too strong or too weak, the cow will either resist or stay still. This coordination is called Harmonization of the Yì and Qì (Yìqì Xiànghé, 意氣相合).

Leading Qì To or Away From a Specific Spot in the Body. Once you can lead the Qì, you lead it from one place to another in the body for different purposes. For healing, you may lead it to a deficient place for Qì nourishment (Bǔ, 補). You can also lead stagnant Qì away from a specific place for releasing (Xiè, 洩). If your kidneys are deficient in wintertime, you can lead Qì to them for nourishment. If you have a joint injury, you can lead Qì away to ease the pain and relax the joint, to expedite the healing process.

Qìgōng practitioners also lead Qì above the diaphragm to energize and excite the mind and body (Yáng), and lead it below the diaphragm to cool down (Yīn). One leads Qì to the Láogōng (P-8, 勞宮) cavities and to the fingertips for healing, by exchanging Qì with a patient. Qìgōng martial artists lead Qì to the Yǒngquán (K-1, 湧泉) cavities to establish a firm root for combat.

There are many applications once you can efficiently lead the Qì with your Yi. The more you practice, the better the results will be. Success depends on your Yì, how strong it is and how much you focus in meditation.

Small Cyclic Heaven Circulation. For a healthy and resilient body, one builds up Qì, then circulates it in the Conception and Governing Vessels (Rènmài, Dūmài, 任脈・督脈). This is called Small Cyclic Heaven Circulation (Xiǎozhōutiān, 小周天) or simply Small Circulation. When Qì circulation is abundant in these two vessels, the Qì in the Twelve Primary Qì Channels can be regulated smoothly. This maintains abundant Qì supply to the whole body, making it strong and healthy.

Grand Cyclic Heaven Circulation. Once you have accomplished Small Cyclic Heaven, you have a firm foundation for Grand Cyclic Heaven (Dàzhōutiān, 大周天) practice. This includes: A. Twelve Primary Qì Channels Grand Circulation, B. Martial Arts Grand Circulation, C. Mutual Qì Exchange Grand Circulation and D. Spiritual Enlightenment Grand Circulation.

Since these are such large subjects, we introduce their theory and practice in separate books. Martial Arts Grand Circulation is discussed in the book *The Essence of Shaolin White Crane*.

Spiritual Enlightenment. Even though Spiritual Enlightenment practice is part of Grand Cyclic Heaven Circulation, due to its profound theory and difficulty in practice, it is discussed separately. It is of more interest to Buddhists and Daoists aiming for Buddhahood or spiritual enlightenment.

In Spiritual Enlightenment Grand Cyclic Heaven Circulation, you practice Embryonic Breathing to store Qì at the Real Lower Dāntián, and condition the biobattery there. Then lead Qì up through the spinal cord (Chōngmài, 衝脈) to energize brain cells and activate their function. When the energy level of the brain reaches a certain level, the Qì moves along the Spiritual Valley (Shéngǔ, 神谷) to reopen the third eye for enlightenment. We will discuss this in more detail in *Qìgōng Grand Circulation for Spiritual Enlightenment*.

Jade Pendant Inscription of Transporting Qì[29,30]

(Xíngqì Yùpèi Míng, 行氣玉佩銘)

When transporting Qì, if deep, then accumulate. If Qì is accumulated, it can be extended. When extended, it can be sunk downward. If sunk downward, then steady. If steady, then firm. If firm, then able to germinate. Having germinated, it can grow. When growing, it retreats. When retreating, it returns to heaven. The foundation of heaven is the top (Upper Dāntián) and the foundation of earth is the bottom (Real Lower Dāntián). Following these rules, one may live, otherwise one dies.

行氣，深則蓄，蓄則伸，伸則下，下則定，定則固，固則萌，萌則長，長則退，退則天。天几舂在上，地几舂在下，順則生，逆則死。

When circulating Qì in the body, deep breathing relaxes the body and calms the mind. Qì circulation can be deep and Qì storage abundant. Only then can Qì be strong enough to be distributed everywhere in the body. “Transport Qì as though through a pearl with a nine-curved hole, even the tiniest place will be reached.”[33] The body’s metabolism becomes smooth, natural, and healthy. Abundant Qì is led down and stored in the Real Lower Dāntián to stabilize and strengthen one’s life.

Leading and storing Qì in the Real Lower Dāntián is the process of Embryonic Breathing (Tāixí, 胎息). It returns mental and physical life to its origin, the Wújí state (無極). Then new life can germinate and grow. After fulfilling the purpose of Qì manifestation, retreat and return to the origin, the Real Lower Dāntián. This process is the way of the heavenly cycle (Dào, 道). Conserving and storing Qì at the Real Lower Dāntián, you manifest it efficiently in your life. Having completed the manifestation, you return the Qì and conserve it again at the Real Lower Dāntián. Manifesting Qì to the maximum depends on how thoroughly you purify your spirit and raise it up to govern the Qì circulation. The head is the heaven (Tiān, 天) while the abdomen is the earth (Dì, 地) in Qìgōng practice. The Upper Dāntián is the residence of the spirit, while the Lower Dāntián is the residence of Qì. Store Qì at the Real Lower Dāntián and keep your spirit high and focused at the Upper Dāntián to achieve longevity.

4-6. Regulating the Spirit (Tiáoshén, 調神)

Before you read this section, you are advised to re-read the definition of Shén in Chapter 3, to understand the profound meaning of ancient documents and the methods of cultivating Shén.

Here we discuss two important Qìgōng terminologies, Spiritual Valley (Shéngǔ, 神谷) and Valley Spirit (Gǔshén, 谷神), which appear in many ancient documents. We then introduce the five keys of training to regulate the Shén, followed by two main training keys. Finally we summarize the goals of Shén training.

Valley Spirit and Spirit Valley (Gǔshén Yǔ Shéngǔ, 谷神與神谷)

In Chapter 6 of *Dào Dé Jīng* (道德經・六章), it is said, "The Valley Spirit (Gǔshén) does not die, so it is called Xuánpìn. The key to reaching this Xuánpìn is the root of heaven and earth. It is very soft and continuous as if it were existing. When it is used, it will not be exhausted."[34]

The spirit (Shén, 神) resides at the space between the two hemispheres of the brain. It resembles a valley between mountains, trapping energy and generating resonant vibrations which correspond with the energy outside the valley. The Shén in this valley is called Valley Spirit (Gǔshén, 谷神) and the valley is called Spiritual Valley (Shéngǔ, 神谷). The Shén residing in this valley governs the energy vibration of the whole body and thus the Qì status and its manifestation. When this Shén is strong, Qì manifesting in your life will be strong, and your life will be long and healthy.

Xuán (玄) means original (Yuán, 元). Pìn (牝) refers to female animals and means mothers. Therefore, Xuánpìn means the Origin or Root of Líves. When the Valley Spirit is centered (condensed) and functions actively, the life force is strong. Xuánpìn (玄牝) is called Tàijí (太極, Grand Ultimate) in *Yìjīng* (Book of Changes). This Tàijí is the Dào (道) of lives in the great nature. Xuánpìn can be summarized as "The root of creation, variation, bearing, and raising of millions of lives. It is the mother of millions of objects in heaven and earth. It is another name for Dào."[35]

The door to reaching this Xuánpìn is through natural Shén (heaven and earth). This is very soft and continuous as though existing, and yet not existing. It cannot be seen, but is felt through cultivation. When used, it will not be exhausted.

To reach this natural Shén, you must open your third eye, called Tiānmù (heaven eye, 天目) or Yùmén (jade gate, 玉門) by religious societies, and Yìntáng (M-HN-3, seal hall, 印堂) by medical society. Wǔdāng's Illustration of Cultivating Truth (Wǔdāng Xiūzhēn Tú, 武當修真圖) said, "The place under the Míngtáng (明堂) (medical Ézhōng [M-HN-2], 額中, center of forehead), above the midpoint of the line connecting the two eyebrows, where the spiritual light emits, is named heaven eye (Tiānmù, 天目)."[36] It is also mentioned in the document *Seven Bamboo Slips of the Bamboo Bookcase* (*Yúnjí Qīqiān*, 云笈七籤), "The space between the two eyebrows is the Jade Gate (Yùmén, 玉門) of Níwán (泥丸)."[37] Níwán (泥丸) is a Daoist term meaning "Mud Pill," referring to the brain, or Upper Dāntián. The lower center of the Spiritual Valley (Shéngǔ, 神谷) between the two hemispheres of the brain is called Níwángōng (泥丸宫), or Mud Pill Palace (Figures 4-13 and 4-14).

To regulate Shén means to cultivate it until it reaches the supernatural divine state. In Daoist society, there is a song which says, "There is a Shén in every human body. There is a supernatural divine light (Língguāng, 靈光) which can be developed in this Shén. This supernatural divine light alone can shine into thousands of valleys. Its Dào of variations is unlimited, spreading millions of ways."[38] Once you cultivate Shén to an enlightened level, it can reach everywhere in the universe.

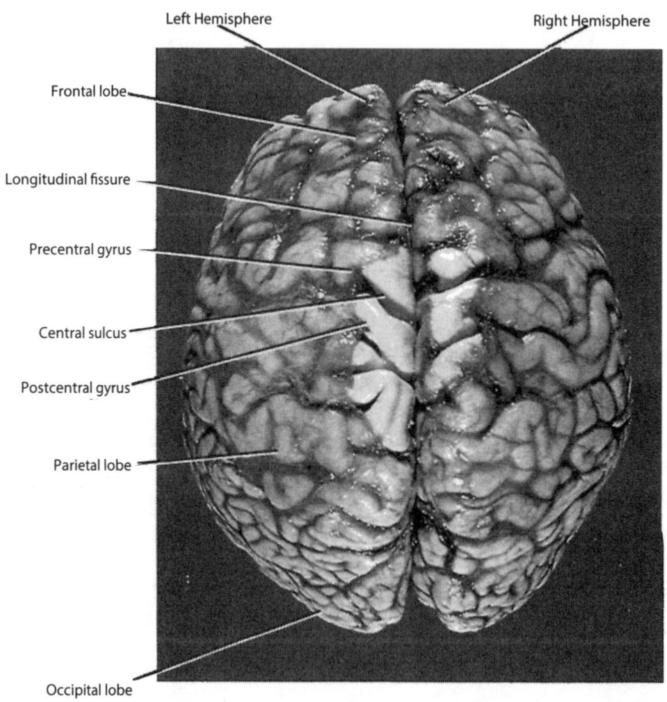

Figure 4-13. The Brain Encompasses Two Hemispheres

There is a song in Buddhist society which says, "Do not search far for Buddha since he is in the Spiritual Mountain. Where is the Spiritual Mountain? It is actually in your mind. Everyone should have a pagoda at Spiritual Mountain, under which to cultivate his being."[39] Pagoda (Tǎ, 塔) implies good deeds you have done, and the comprehension of nature you have accumulated in spiritual cultivation.

To conclude this subsection, I will translate a few ancient documents about Shén. Keep reading them repeatedly, and you will suddenly comprehend the meaning of spiritual cultivation.

Observing Vessels
(Màiwàng, 脈望)

The brain is the Upper Dāntián, the palace where the Original Shén (Yuánshén) resides. If one grasps this Original Shén and makes it stay at this Original Palace, then the golden Qì arises automatically, and the Real Breathing can be stabilized naturally. If one way is opened, then hundreds of ways will all be opened. When the big gate is opened, then hundreds of gates are all opened.

腦為上田，元神所居之宮，人能握元神，棲于本宮，則金氣自升，真息自定，所謂一竅開而百竅齊開，大關通則百關盡通也。

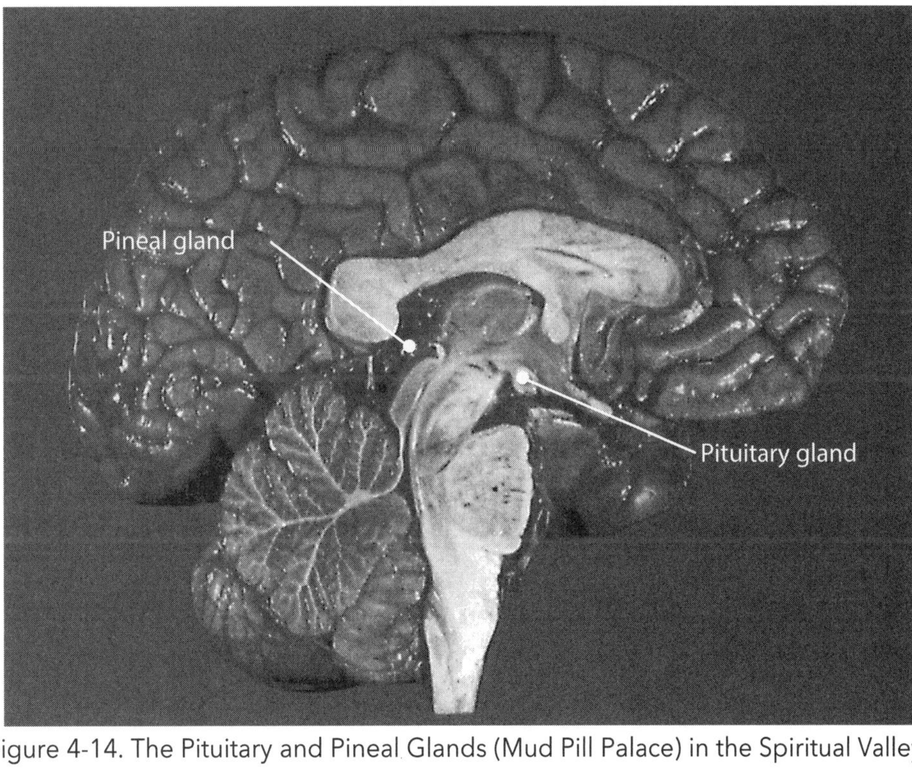

Figure 4-14. The Pituitary and Pineal Glands (Mud Pill Palace) in the Spiritual Valley

The brain is the Upper Dāntián (Shàng Dāntián, 上丹田), the residence of the Shén. The Shén resides at the Upper Dāntián since birth and is called Original Shén (Yuánshén, 元神). The document Detailed Outline of Galenical (Běncǎo Gāngmù, 本草綱目) said, "brain is the residence of Original Shén."[40] If you condense your Shén and contain it in its residence, the Qì in your body will be conserved. Keep your mind calm and peaceful, and avoid being distracted by human affairs and emotional disturbances. Then Qì storage at the Real Lower Dāntián (Zhēn Xiàdāntián, 真下丹田) will be abundant and can be led up to nourish the brain and Shén. The breathing becomes slender, soft, and steady. This clears away obstacles to Qì in the entire body, and brings health and longevity.

Concealed Secret of Féng's Family
(Féngshì Jǐnnáng, 馮氏錦囊)

There is a crux in the body named Xuánpìn, which enables life to live by receiving Qì. This is the residence of Shén, where the Three Origins (Sānyuán) are gathered. It is the cavity where Jīng (essence), Shén (spirit), Hun (soul), and Pò (vigor) meet. It is the root where the Golden Elixir (Jīndān, Qì) returns to, and where the immortals conceive their Holy Embryo.

身中一竅，名曰玄牝，受氣以生，實為府神，三元所聚，精神魂魄會于此穴，乃金丹還返之根，神仙凝結聖胎之地也。

This document describes the Spiritual Valley (Shéngǔ, 神谷), or Mud Pill Palace (Níwángōng, 泥丸宮), where the Shén resides. When Shén is present, and the body is nourished by Qì, there is physical life. When Shén departs from the body, there is death. To nourish this Shén, gather the Three Origins (Sānyuán, 三元), namely Jīng (Essence, 精), Qì (氣), and Shén (Spirit, 神) at this place. Then Shén can be raised to a high level.

Pò (魄) is the vital spirit supported by Qì while one is alive. When one dies, the Po becomes Hún (Soul, 魂), meaning the spirit after death. Jīndān (金丹) means Golden Elixir and implies precious Qì. When this precious Qì is led up to nourish the Shén, you can reach immortality. Remember the song which says, "There is a Shén in every human body. There is a supernatural divine light (Língguāng, 靈光) which can be developed in this Shén. This supernatural divine light alone can shine into thousands of valleys. Its Dào of variations is unlimited, spreading millions of ways."[38] Once you cultivate Shén to an enlightened level, it can reach everywhere in the universe.

Songs of Valley Spirit—1

(Gǔshénggē–Yī, 谷神歌 - 一)

I have an interior insubstantial empty valley. When talking about it, it seems to be there, again it seems not to be there. When talking about it, even if it were not there, we could not ignore it. When talking about it, even if it were there, it could not be resided in.
Valley, valley, so marvelous. Shén, Shén, it is the real Great Dào. Keep it, protect it, you can be on the list of those without death. Cultivate and refine it, you can be called an immortal divine (Xiānrén).

我有一腹空谷虛，言之道有又還無，言之無兮不可舍，言之有兮不可居。
谷兮谷兮太玄妙，神兮神兮真大道，保之守之不死名，修之煉之仙人號。

This song describes the importance of the Spiritual Valley (Shéngǔ, 神谷) and how crucial it is for the cultivation of Valley Spirit (Gǔshén, 谷神). This Spiritual Valley is between the two lobes of the brain (Níwángōng, 泥丸宮). It cannot be seen, only felt. In it, the Valley Spirit resides. To reach the Dào of enlightenment, you must feel the existence of the Spiritual Valley, keep the Shén there firmly, and cultivate it. This is the way to reach immortality. Xiānrén (仙人) are those who have attained spiritual immortality and enlightenment.

Songs of Valley Spirit—2

(Gǔshénggē–Èr, 谷神歌 - 二)

When the Valley Spirit obtains its Yī (one), the Líng (ingenuity) can be developed. When the Spiritual Valley obtains its Yī (center), fullness can be achieved. If one keeps this oneness, then from this alone one may achieve longevity.
It is not too difficult to obtain longevity. However, it cannot be achieved if one neglects the body. If trained and the accomplishment achieved, the ordinary bones are changed naturally.

神得一以靈，谷得一以盈，若人能守一，只此自長生。
長生本不遠，離身還不見，煉之功若成，自然凡骨變。

Yī (一) here means one, singularity, or simplicity. If the Shén can condense into oneness at its residence without dispersing, the powerful spiritual vibration enables you to develop Líng (靈), which means ingenuity, intelligence, dexterity, cleverness, and comprehension.

When the Spiritual Valley obtains this concentrated Shén, the coherent resonant energy becomes full and strong, and the Qì is governed effectively by the Shén. To attain longevity, also heed your physical health and not just mental and spiritual cultivation. The key is both the physical and the mental. Only if these two balance each other and have a strong foundation can you lead a long, healthy life. Daoists usually cultivate both body and mind. This dual cultivation is called Xìngmìng Shuāngxiū (性命雙修) and means Dual Cultivation of Temperament and Lífe.

Songs of Valley Spirit—3
(Gǔshéngē–Sān, 谷神歌 - 三)

If Valley Spirit does not die, you have gained the gate to Xuánpìn. Exit and enter as softly as the Dào exists within. When cultivating Shén to return it to the insubstantial nothingness at midnight, use the river to transport the Qì to Kūnlún.
The dragon is singing and the tiger is also shouting, the wind and the clouds meet and the old yellow lady is screaming. The fair lady in the fire is shy and charming. Look inward to see the baby in the water.

谷神不死玄牝門，出入綿綿道若存，修煉還虛夜半子，河車搬載上崑崙。
龍又吟、虎又嘯，風雲際會黃婆叫，火中姹女正含嬌，回觀水底嬰兒俏。

Xuán (玄) means Original (Yuán, 元), and Pìn (牝) means mothers. So Xuánpìn (玄牝) means the origin or root of lives, the key to longevity. To keep the Shén at its residence, follow the Dào, softly, gently, and persistently. Cut off external distractions and emotional disturbances, gradually and gently. If you try to force it, the Emotional Mind will be even more disturbed. To lead the Qì up through the Thrusting Vessel to nourish the brain, you must train at midnight, because Qì is strongest at that time.

Dragon (Lóng, 龍) and Tiger (Hǔ, 虎) means Yīn and Yáng Qì in the body. The Old Yellow Lady (Huángpó, 黃婆) is the matchmaker who brings Yīn and Yáng together. Through interaction of Yīn and Yáng, the spiritual baby embryo is conceived. Huángpó is the Shén and the breathing, which bring Yīn and Yáng together.

The baby (Yīngér) and the shy lady (Chànǚ) meet the old yellow lady (Huángpó), and son and mother meet each other with the same Yì (mind). In the Golden Palace (Jīndiàn) and Jade Hall (Yùtáng), there are twelve doors. Golden Male (Jīngōng) and Wooden Mother (Mùmǔ) are just coming.
After passing layers of key doors, immediately lock the gate. Inspect cows in the Big Dipper (Dòuniú), and immediately start the fire. Advance the fire to eliminate Yīn and initiate the sole Yáng. Thousand years of peach have started to bear fruit.

嬰兒奼女見黃婆，兒女相逢兩意合，金殿玉堂門十二，金公木母正來過。
重門過后牢關鎖，點撿斗牛先下火，進火消陰始一陽，千歲仙桃初結果。

The baby (Shén) and the shy lady (Qì) are now brought together by the old yellow lady (Huángpó, 黃婆, mind and breathing) in harmony with each other. They are led up from Huángtíng (黃庭) to the Upper Dāntián, passing through twelve doors (throat area). Original Essence and Shén become one. Yīngér (嬰兒) means baby (son) and implies the Spiritual Embryo. Chànǚ (the shy lady, mother, 奼女) implies Qì. This means the Xīn has been calmed and unified with the Shén at Huángtíng (黃庭). The baby embryo is conceived and led to the Upper Dāntián.

Jīndiàn (金殿) is also called Jīnshì (金室), or Golden Palace, and implies the lungs. Yùtáng (玉堂) means Jade Hall, the palate of the mouth. Twelve doors means the throat area. Jīngōng (金公) means Golden Male, or Original Essence (Yuánjīng, 元精), and Mùmǔ (木母) means Wooden Mother, or liver. Líver belongs to wood in the Five Elements (Wǔxíng, 五行). It is related to Shén and produces heart fire (Xīn, 心). When Shén and Xīn are harmonized, the mind is calm and the spirit condenses.

After passing the throat to the Upper Dāntián, immediately confine the Spiritual Embryo there. Dòuniú (斗牛) means Big Dipper, which implies the process of condensing Shén at the Upper Dāntián. After long practice, the Spiritual Embryo can be born.

The Golden Bird (Jīnniǎo) flies on the east coast of the curved river (Qūjiāng). The Jade Rabbit (Yùtù) shines with clear light on the west coast. The bird and the rabbit walk to the tip of the mountain. The fair lady in the furnace takes off her blue cloth. After taking off the blue cloth, the pure clean body is exposed. The baby is then led to the layers of curtains. After ten months of strong and heavy emotion, a boy is born. Say he can live long and will not die.
I advise you to practice and cultivate. If the Valley Spirit does not die, the goal of immortality can be achieved. Comprehend the theory and carefully adopt those marvelous details. One day, I will reach the Immortal Land (Yíngzhōu) with you.

曲江東岸金烏飛，西岸清光玉兔輝，烏兔走歸峰頂上，爐中姹女脫青衣。
脫卻青衣露素體，嬰兒引入重幃里，十月情濃產一男，說道長生永不死。
勸君煉，勸君修，谷神不死此中求，此中悟取玄微處，與君白日登瀛洲。

Qūjiāng (曲江) means Curved River (Intestines, Real Lower Dāntián). Jīnniǎo (金烏) means Golden Bird (Original Spirit, Yuánshén, 元神). Yùtù (玉兔) means Jade Rabbit (Original Essence, Yuánjīng, 元精). The first sentence means Original Spirit and Original Essence become one, being led up to the furnace, or Upper Dāntián. The lady takes off her blue clothes, to give birth to the baby. Blue clothes imply manifestation of Shén via the liver. The Líver's color is between blue and green in Chinese medicine. Shén is manifested through birth of the spiritual baby.

The baby is born after ten months of pregnancy and kept behind the curtain for nursing. It is the beginning of eternal spiritual life. Yíngzhōu (瀛洲) is the holy mountain in the east sea where dwell the immortals of Chinese legend.

Thesis of Valley Spirit's Immortality[29]

(Gǔshén Bùsǐ Lùn, 谷神不死論)

（紫清指玄集・宋・白玉蟾撰）

What is the valley? It means Heavenly Valley (Tiāngǔ). What is Shén? It means the Original Spirit of the body. The Heavenly Valley has the capability of creation and variation, though it holds the insubstantial nihility. A valley on earth contains millions of objects and has mountains and rivers. Humans have the same natural disposition as heaven and earth, therefore we also have a valley. There is a real oneness conceived in this valley where the Original Spirit (Yuánshén) resides. There are nine palaces in the head which correspond with the nine heavens above. Among them, there is a palace at the center called Níwán (Mud Pill), or Huángtíng (Yellow Yard), also called Kūnlún, or Tiāngǔ (Heavenly Valley). The names are numerous. It is where the Original Spirit resides. It is empty as a valley, and Shén lives in it. This Shén is called Gǔshén (Valley Spirit).

谷者，天谷也。神者，一身之元神也。天之谷，含造化，容虛空；地之谷，容萬物，載山川。人與天地同所稟也，亦有谷焉。其谷藏真一，宅元神，是以頭有九宮，上應九天，中間一宮，謂之泥丸，亦曰黃庭，又名崑崙，又名天谷，其名頗多，乃元神所住之宮，其空如谷，而神居之，故謂之谷神。

The space between the two hemispheres of the brain is called Heavenly Valley (Tiāngǔ, 天谷). The head is regarded as Heaven, while the perineum (Huìyīn, Co-1, 會陰) is considered the Sea Bottom (Hǎidǐ, 海底). This Heavenly Valley has many other names, such as Spiritual Valley (Shéngǔ, 神谷), Yellow Yard (Huángtíng, 黃庭), Mud Pill (Níwán, 泥丸), or Kūnlún (崑崙).

It is named Spiritual Valley because the Shén lives there. It is called Yellow Yard since it is an important place for cultivation. (The Huángtíng at the stomach area where the Spiritual Embryo is conceived is also called Yellow Yard.) It is named Mud Pill due to the appearance of the pineal and pituitary glands. It is called Kūnlún because that is one of the highest mountains in China.

Though the Spiritual Valley is empty and does not contain material objects like the valleys on the earth, which contain rivers, trees, and many other objects, it has the capability of creation and variation. Daoists believe there are nine layers of spiritual cultivation, with a palace in each. The brain also has nine palaces corresponding to the nine palaces of heaven. Among them, the center one is most important. This is where the Original Spirit (Yuánshén, 元神) resides. This central palace is called Níwángōng (Mud Pill Palace, 泥丸宮). When you concentrate your mind there, the pineal and pituitary glands are activated by the abundant Qì. This significantly enhances production of melatonin and human growth hormone (HGH), two hormones crucial to longevity and vitality.

When Shén exists, there is life. When Shén goes, there is death. Being attached to objects (human affairs) during daytime and to dreams at night, Shén cannot abide peacefully at home. Yellow corn unripened, the dream not yet awakened, the whole life's glory, splendor, wealth, and rank. A hundred years of sorrow, worry, happiness, and joy, isn't it happening just as in a dream? Once dead, life cannot reverse. Shén roams and cannot return. Life and death are parted, the path between life and death is cut off. Thus we see that if Shén does not live, one cannot live by oneself, and if the Shén is dead, one will also be dead naturally. If Shén abides in its valley without dying, how then can one die? The reason Valley Spirit (Gǔshén) does not die is because of Xuánpìn.

神存則生，神去則死。日則接于物，夜則接于夢，神不能安其居也。黃粱未熟，南柯未寤，一生之榮辱富貴，百歲之悲憂悅樂，備嘗于一夢之間，使其去而不還，游而不返，則生死路隔，幽明之途絕矣。由是觀之，人不能自生而神生之，人不能自死而神死之。若神居其谷而不死，人安得而死乎？然谷神所以不死者，由玄牝也。

If your mind is always distracted by human affairs and emotions, your Shén cannot stay at its residence. Human life is short and passes like a dream. If you waste time longing for glory, power, and wealth, neglecting to cultivate your Shén and keep it steady at its residence, you wake up one day to the realization that everything you have longed for is only a dream. To have immortal Shén, keep the Valley Spirit at the Spiritual Valley. Lǎozi said, "If the Valley Spirit (Gǔshén) does not die, it is called Xuánpìn (玄牝). The door to reach this Xuánpìn is the root of heaven and earth. It is very soft and continuous as though it existed. When used, it will not be exhausted."[34]

What is Xuán? It is Yáng and is the heaven. What is Pìn? It is Yīn and is the earth. However, Xuán and Pìn two Qì(s), all have profound implications. Without meeting those holy men to give instruction in the oral secrets, it cannot be understood easily. The Inner Classic of the Yellow Emperor said, "Original Shén resides in the Heavenly Valley. Protect it, then cultivation can be real." There is a Heavenly Valley called Níwán at the top of the body which is the residence of concealed Shén. A corresponding valley named Jiànggōng (heart) in the middle of the body is the residence of concealed Qì. Another divine valley called Guānyuán (Key Origin) at the bottom of the body is the residence of concealed Jīng.

玄者，陽也，天也；牝者，陰也，地也。然則玄牝二氣，各有深旨，非遇聖人，授以口訣，不可得而知也。《黃帝內經》云：'天谷元神，守之自真。' 言人身中上有天谷泥丸，藏神之府也；中有應谷絳宮，藏氣之府也；下有靈谷關元，藏精之府也。

Xuánpìn (玄牝) here means the interaction of Yīn and Yáng, to initiate life. Xuánpìn is the mother of life (creation and variations). It is difficult to understand and cultivate Yīn and Yáng Qì, and make them interact with each other. Usually, you need an experienced teacher to personally direct you on the right path.

This document mentions three valleys in the body to cultivate. The Spiritual Valley (神谷, Upper Dāntián) where the Valley Spirit resides is in the head. In the chest is the Jiànggōng (Middle Dāntián, 絳宮) which collects Post-Birth Qì converted from food and air. The third valley is Guānyuán (Lower Dāntián, 關元) where Pre-birth Original Qì is converted from Original Essence (Yuánjīng, 元精). These valleys conceal the essence of life.

The Heavenly Valley is a mysterious palace, the residence of Original Shén, the home of human natural spiritual disposition, and the vital way of spiritual cultivation. Holy men follow the rules of heaven and earth and know the origin of variations. They protect the Shén and keep it at this mysterious palace, and store Qì abundantly at the residence of Pìn. Shén and Qì mutually interact, enabling you to accomplish the cultivation of the real Dào naturally, unified with the Dào, and to enter the domain of being without death and without life. Therefore, it is said that when the Valley Spirit does not die, it is called Xuánpìn. Those holy men know how to apply their cultivation in Xuánpìn, know how to create and convert in a trance. When the Qì of Xuánpìn enters this root (Real Lower Dāntián), if you hold the breath too much, it becomes urgent. If you allow breathing to act freely, then it is out of control. So keep it very soft and continuous without any gap or interruption.

天谷，玄宮也，乃元神之室，靈性之所存，是神之要也。聖人則天地之要，知變化之源，神守于玄宮，氣騰于牝府，神氣交感，自然成真，與道為一，而入于不死不生，故曰谷神不死，是謂玄牝也。聖人運用于玄牝之內，造化于恍惚之中，當其玄牝之氣，入乎其根，閉極則失于急，任之則失于蕩，欲其綿綿續續，勿令間斷耳。

Spiritual Valley (Shéngǔ, 神谷) is also called Mud Pill Palace (Níwángōng, 泥丸宮). The Original Shén (Yuánshén, 元神) residing in this palace is powerful and marvelous, and is the origin of creation and variations. It directs your mind and thinking and is the Tàijí (Grand Ultimate, 太極) of the human universe.

Those who obtain the Dào follow both human and natural Tàijí and can thus know the Way of Nature. They unify and resonate their Shén with the natural Shén at its residence, and nourish it continuously with Qì. This is the way to achieve immortality of the Shén, called Xuánpìn (玄牝), the mother of creation and variations.

Keep Shén there through correct breathing, soft as a baby. Have a baby's heart (pure mind) without external attraction, which allows you to feel internally. Only then can you have soft breathing, as if it were there and as if it were not there, being regulated without being regulated. Lǎozi said, "When concentrating the Qì to reach its softness, can it be as soft as a baby?"

What is the meaning of "as if it were existing?" It means retaining it by following nature. After retaining Shén (at its residence) for a long time, it will be tranquil naturally. After practicing breathing for a long time, it will be stabilized naturally. When the temperament has become natural, then it can be used marvelously. Then no need to try hard or force it urgently, and "When used, it cannot be exhausted." Xuán and Pìn are the two origins at the top and bottom, and are the correct paths for the Qì mother to ascend and descend. Those worldly seculars do not know these roots or study their origin and say the nose and mouth are Xuán and Pìn. If the nose and mouth are Xuán and Pìn, how can they be called the doorways of Xuánpìn? This is all because these people cannot comprehend the marvelousness of training. How can they understand if they are not great holy men?

若存者，順其自然而存之，神久自寧，息久自定，性入自然，無為妙用，未嘗至于勤勞迫切，故曰用之不勤。即此而觀，則玄牝為上下二源，氣母升降之正道明矣。世人不窮其根，不究其源，便以鼻為玄，以口為牝。若以鼻口為玄牝，則玄牝之門又將何以名之？此皆不能造其妙，非大聖人安能究是理哉！

This last paragraph talks about Lǎozi's concept in spiritual cultivation. In *Dào Dé Jīng* (道德經), Chapter 6, it said "The Valley Spirit (Gǔshén, 谷神) does not die, then it is called Xuánpìn. The key to reaching this Xuánpìn (玄牝) is the root of heaven and earth (nature). It is very soft and continuous as if it were existing. When used, it will not be exhausted."[34]

The meaning of "as if it were existing" (Ruòcún, 若存) is to practice keeping the Shén at its residence and maintaining and conserving Qì at the Real Lower Dāntián until it becomes natural, namely regulating without regulating (Bùtiáo Értiáo, 不調而調).

Xuánpìn (玄牝) is the interaction between Shén at the Upper Dāntián and Qì at the Real Lower Dāntián, namely unification and harmony of Shén and Qì. This is the mother of creation and variations, and the way to achieve immortality. Many seculars falsely believe Xuánpìn to be the nose and the mouth (breathing).

Five Trainings of Shén (Lìànshén Wǔzé, 煉神五則)

There are five trainings to regulate Shén: 1. Raising the Shén (Yǎngshén, 養神), 2. Protecting the Shén (Shǒushén, 守神), 3. Firming the Shén (Gùshén, 固神), 4. Stabilizing the Shén (Dìngshén, 定神), and 5. Focusing the Shén (Níngshén, 凝神). These are called Líànshén (煉神). Lían (煉) means to refine, train, or discipline. There are also two training keys and two purposes of training Shén.

Raising the Shén (Yǎngshén, 養神). Yǎng (養) means to nourish, raise, or nurse. Yǎngshén is the main training task for Scholars and Buddhists. Shén needs to be nourished with Qì. Fire Qì from food and air can raise up Shén easily, but also increases emotional disturbance, leading Shén away from its residence. Using Yì nourished by Water Qì to raise up your Shén is harder, but this Shén is stronger and more concentrated than that from Fire Qì. Adjust Xīn (Yáng) and Yì (Yīn) to raise up your Shén properly so it is raised but not excited and stays at its residence.

Raising the Shén correctly is like raising a child. You need great patience and perseverance. One way is to restrain his attention from the seven emotions and six desires. The other is to let him keep this contact with his human nature, yet educate his wisdom to make clear judgments, which is a long process, demanding understanding and patience. Raising Shén is not about increasing emotional excitement. This scatters the Yì, and Shén becomes confused and loses its center. Yǎngshén builds a strong spiritual center and helps it control your life.

Protecting the Shén (Shǒushén, 守神). After raising your Shén, keep it at its residence and train it. A child needs to keep his mind with his family instead of straying outside and running wild. Then you can educate him.

Shǒu (守) means to keep and protect. The training involves keeping Shén at its residence, which is much harder than raising it up. Shǒushén training uses the regulated mind to direct, nurse, watch, and keep the Shén there. It is like keeping your child at home instead of letting him leave home and run wild. Be patient and control your temper, regulating your Xīn and Yì. If you lose your temper, you only make the child want to leave home again. Once you have regulated your Xīn and Yì will you be able to keep your Shén effectively.

Firming the Shén (Gùshén, 固神). Gù (固) means to coalesce and to firm. After keeping Shén at its residence, you firm and coalesce it (Gùshén). Gǔshén means training Shén to stay at its residence willingly. After you control your child in the house, make him want from his heart to stay. Only then will his mind be steady and calm. To reach this, you need more love and patience until he understands the importance of staying home and growing up normally. This third step of Shén training is to make the Shén willing to stay at its residence in peace, by regulating thoughts and emotions.

Stabilizing the Shén (Dìngshén, 定神). Dìng Shén (定神) means to stabilize and calm the Shén. When your child is at peace, he will not be attracted to external distractions. Regulate your Shén to calm it down, so it is energized but not excited, with the mind peaceful and steady.

Condensing the Shén (Níngshén, 凝神). Níng (凝) means to condense, concentrate, refine, focus, and strengthen. The first four processes which raise up, keep, firm and stabilize, are the foundations of Shén cultivation. After this, you condense and focus your Shén into a tiny spot. This is where you train the Shén to a higher spiritual state. When focused in a tiny point, it is like a sunbeam focused through a lens. The smaller the point, the stronger the beam. Here is translation and commentary of an ancient article on condensing the Shén.

Anthology of Daoist Village

(Dàoxiāngjí, 道鄉集)

What does it mean to condense? It means to gather. What is Shén? It is the righteous thought in the Xīn. What is Xí (profound breathing)? It is to induce Pre-Heaven Real Qì (Original Qì). It has no shape or appearance. Pre-Heaven Qì is generated at the point of extreme nihility and sincere calmness. Xuè cavity (Real Lower Dāntián) is the original root of producing Pre-Heaven Qì. Why condense Shén at this Qì cavity? It is to place and condense righteous thought there and not allow Shén to be distracted and move away. When Shén is condensed, fire (Qì) can be gathered. When fire is gathered and led downward, water rises automatically. This is mutual coordination of fire and water, to condense Shén at the Qì cavity. What is Xí? It is breathing. What is Xí-Xí (Continuous Breathing)? Breathing very soft and unbroken. What is Guī (Returning)? Reversing the path of life and returning to its origin. What is Gēn (Root)? Root and foundation of life. Every breath is soft and continuous and returns it to this root. Breathing is not separate from the basic foundation of producing Qì. It is as though existing yet forgotten and seems to be there yet not there. This is how Embryonic Breathing was practiced since ancient times, following the natural way. If Shén condenses at the Qì cavity, breathing is also stabilized at this original root.

夫凝者聚也，神者心中之正念也。息者，先天之真氣也。無形無象，生于虛極靜篤之時，穴即生先天氣之本根。所以凝神氣穴者，即將我心中之正念，凝聚于氣穴，不令神往外馳。神凝則火聚，火聚于下，水自上升，此水火調濟之要訣。亦凝神氣穴之妙諦也。息者，呼吸也。息息者，綿綿不斷之義也。歸者，返回也。根者，基本也。息息歸根，即呼吸不離生氣根本。若存若忘，似有似無，昔所謂胎息者是也。須知此息，本乎自然，神既凝于氣穴，息也定于本根。

This describes mutual unification, coordination, and harmonization of Shén with Pre-Heaven Qì (Xiāntiānqì, 先天氣, Original Qì), which is conceived at the Real Lower Dāntián. Shén is fire (Yáng, son) while Pre-Heaven Qì (mother) is water (Yīn). Lead Shén down to unite with Pre-Heaven Qì, so mind and body can be calm and peaceful. Then Qì stays at its residence and is stored there.

Reach this goal through soft, slender, and continuous breathing, focusing your Shén at the Real Lower Dāntián. This is crucial in Embryonic Breathing, the root of life, so the Spiritual Embryo can be conceived. Regulate Shén through training Embryonic Breathing, the crux of Internal Elixir Qìgōng (Nèidān, 內丹). Refer to the previous book, *Qìgōng Meditation—Embryonic Breathing* for more detail.

Two Training Keys (Líànxí Èrjué, 練習二訣)

Remember, there are two keys in regulating Shén: 1. Mutual dependence of Shén and breathing (Shénxí Xiāngyī, 神息相依), and 2. Mutual harmony of Shén and Qì (Shénqì Xiànghé, 神氣相合).

Mutual Dependence of Shén and Breathing (Shénxí Xiāngyī, 神息相依). After Shén has been trained to a high degree, put it to work. The first assignment is coordinating with your breathing. In Qìgōng training, breathing is considered as the strategy. When this is directed by your Shén, it obtains optimum results. This strategy is called Shénxí Xiāngyī (神息相依), which means Shén and breathing are mutually dependent. Shénxí (神息) means Shén breathing. Your Shén and breathing become one, and Qì is led efficiently. This daunting task requires you to have regulated your body, breathing, and mind.

Anthology of Daoist Village[8]
(Dàoxiāngjí, 道鄉集)

> *"Be calm, then focus on the Real Lower Dāntián. Where your eyes focus, Xīn should follow. When Xīn and eyes have reached the place and ceased, then Xīn and breathing should accord with each other and gradually enter the Great Steadiness (Dàdìng)." "Shén is stabilized in coordination with breathing. Breathing is peaceful in coordination with Shén. When they accord with each other, the Great Steadiness can be reached."*
>
> 〝能靜時觀照下田，目之所在，心亦隨之，心目得其所止，而后心與息依，漸入大定。〞又〝神依息而定，息依神而安，互相依附，始歸大定。〞

"Eyes focus" means the Yì (意). Ancient documents often say, "The eyes observe (Guān, 觀) the nose (breathing), and the nose observes the Xīn."[21] Restrain your eyes, and focus on breathing, through which Xīn can be observed and regulated.

Qìgōng society often says, Xīn-ape and Yì-horse (Xīnyuán Yìmǎ, 心猿意馬). Xīn means heart, related to emotional disturbance. Use the Yi-horse to govern the Xin-monkey, with breathing as the strategy. With Xīn under control, stabilize Shén at its residence. Shén and breathing mutually harmonize and accord with each other. This is called the Great Steadiness (Dàdìng, 大定).

In Buddhist society Dàdìng means, "When Xīn for Buddhism is clear and bright, it is called Dàdìng."[28] The mind is at peace and the body extremely relaxed. Shén and body harmonize and coordinate with each other.

Mutual Harmony of Shén and Qì (Shénqì Xiànghé, 神氣相合). The second Shén training key uses Shén to direct the circulation and distribution of Qì, called Shénqì Xiànghé (Shén and Qì combine, 神氣相合). In battle, the fighting spirit of the soldiers determines their ability to fight and to execute strategy. Shén is the Son (Zǐ, 子), while Qì is the Mother (Mǔ, 母). When mother and son unite in harmony with each other, it is called Mǔzǐ Xiànghé (mutual harmony of mother and son, 母子相合). Some ancient documents describe the practice:

All Application Secrets of Real Holy Embryonic Spirit
(Methods of Transporting Qì)
(Zhūzhēn Shèngtāi Shényòng Jué, 諸真聖胎神用訣)
(御氣之法)

Go to the top to Níwán (Mud Pill Palace) and to the bottom to Mìngmén (Real Lower Dāntián). Two sceneries follow each other mutually, to save the remaining days and increase longevity. If Shén does not control exhaling, then breathing is not complete. If Shén does not govern inhaling, the breathing is not complete either. Coordinate and harmonize Shén and Qì mutually, in every breath, then the embryo can be conceived from concealed Qì, and Qì can be produced through Embryonic Breathing. Embryonic Qì coalesces internally and never dies.

上至泥丸，下至命門，兩景相隨，可救殘老矣。若呼不得神宰，一息不全，吸不得神宰，亦一息不全。若能息息之中，使神氣相合，則胎從伏氣中結，氣從有胎中息，胎氣內結，永不死矣。

Níwán (泥丸) implies the Upper Dāntián. The Spiritual Valley (Shéngǔ, 神谷) between the two hemispheres of the brain is called Níwángōng (Mud Pill Palace, 泥丸宮), referring to the pineal and pituitary glands. When these two glands produce abundant hormones, they promote smooth metabolism. Vital force is strong and Shén high. Mìngmén (Life Door, 命門) here means the Real Lower Dāntián instead of the Mìngmén cavity of acupuncture. The Real Lower Dāntián stores Qì, the life force.

Circulate Qì, controlled by Shén, through the Upper Dāntián and the Real Lower Dāntián. Shén and Qì mutually coordinate and harmonize with each other, through Embryonic Breathing, so the Spiritual Embryo can be conceived. Two Poles become one. This is the Wújí state, the initiation of life.

Ten Books of Cultivating Truth: Shortcut of Miscellaneous Writing (Xiūzhēn Shíshū·Zázhe Jiéjìng, 修真十書・雜著捷徑)

Qì is nourished by Qì, and Qì then meets Shén. When Shén and Qì are not separated, then it is true cultivation. The son does not leave the mother, nor the mother the son. When son and mother stay together, then live long without dying.

氣養于氣，氣會于神，神氣不散，是為修真。子不離母，母不放子，子母共守，長生不死。

To accumulate abundant Qì, you must find the extra Qì and store it at the Real Lower Dāntián (Zhēn Xiàdāntián, 真下丹田) by keeping your Shén there. When Shén and Qì unite in harmony, the Spiritual Embryo (Shèngtāi, 聖胎) can be conceived. Shén and Qì, like son and mother, will not part from each other. This is the way to reach longevity.

Marvelous Applications of Maintaining the Shape and Cultivating Internal Truth by Great Teacher Dámó (Dámó Dàshī Zhùshì Líúxíng Nèizhēn Miàoyòng Jué, 達摩大師住世留形內真妙用訣)

Without keeping the son and mother (Shén and Qì) together, even though Qì is stored internally through breathing, nevertheless Shén is constantly labored externally, becoming dirty and confused. Once Shén is dirty, the original harmonious Qì gradually disperses and cannot stay. Daoists often make this mistake, not knowing that shape and Shén are the core of practice. If one does not keep Qì and Shén internally but keeps them externally, their residences will be dangerous and gradually rotten. Non-Daoists labor their Shén and fatigue their thinking. There is not even a respiration leading Qì and Shén to the Qìhǎi (Real Lower Dāntián). If they expect longevity, isn't it too far to be reached?

若不知子母相守，氣雖呼吸于內，神常勞役于外，遂使神常穢濁而神不清。神既不清，即元和之氣漸散而不能相守也。道人常用之，而不知根本以形神為主。若人不知守于內而守于外，自然令宅舍虛危，漸見衰壞矣。況非道之人，勞神役思，無一息神氣注于氣海之中，而欲望其長生，豈不遠乎！

Shén and the Qì must combine and not separate from each other. First stop the mind from all outside distractions and emotional disturbances, lest your Shén become dirty. Through correct Embryonic Breathing, keeping Shén and Qì at the Real Lower Dāntián, you attain longevity.

Chapter of Clear Understanding (Mao, Ri-Xin; Sòng Dynasty)

(Lĭăomíngpiān, 宋・毛日新；了明篇)

Qì follows Shén and Shén follows Qì. Shén and Qì mutually follow each other and penetrate into Níwán. Keep Jīnguān locked and sealed constantly. Once having caught Jīnpǐn, then internal joy. Practice this Gōngfū diligently and establish strong will, throughout the day (twelve timings). When Yīn ends and Yáng has completed, Shén can leave the body. When this Gōngfū has been accomplished, your name will be on the list of immortality.

氣隨神，神隨氣，神氣相隨，透入泥丸裡。長把金關牢鎖閉，捉得金品，暗地添歡喜。下辛勤，須發志，十二時中，莫把功夫棄。陰盡陽全神出體，功行成時，名列神仙位。

This poem describes the mutual dependency of Shén and Qì. Once Shén and Qì enter Níwángōng (Upper Dāntián, 泥丸宮), keep it there firmly. Jīnguān (Golden Gate, 金關) means Upper Dāntián. Jīnpǐn (Golden Material, 金品) implies the Spiritual Embryo. Shíèrshí (twelve timings, 十二時) are the traditional Chinese divisions of the day.

Secrets of Applying Qì with Concentrated Shén[29]

(Yòngqì Jíshén Jué, 用氣集神訣)

(延陵先生集新舊服氣經・唐・延陵先生集)

Shén is gathered from insubstantial and made peaceful with substantial. Shén is wisdom of the Xīn. When Xīn is peaceful without desire, Shén can be like a king with harmony and righteous Qì. Having reached this stage, let Shén be free without restraint, the longer the better. Practice ceaselessly, so Qì in the body reaches extreme peace. This is delightful for heaven, so you live long. When outside the body (material world) is substantially empty, then it is also (delightful) for heaven. When inside the body is empty and comprehensive (without emotional bondage or desire), then it is also (delightful) for heaven. Practice for a long, long time, then enlightenment can be attained. All these secrets are understood internally. After practicing for a long time, understanding is deep and refined, matching the enlightenment of heaven. Then Qì can develop from Jīng internally. Dào can be reached, and this Dào will correspond with Dé (the virtue of nature). The completeness of the Dé is that, when it is used, it manifests Rén (benevolence). When divided (expanded), it demonstrates Yì (righteousness).

神集于虛，而安于實。神，心中知者也。安而無欲，則神王而氣和正。如此之時，則一任所之，唯久彌善。行之不已，體氣至安，謂之樂天，樂天則壽。身外虛空亦天也，身內虛通亦天也，習之久久，乃明生焉。密自內知之，久習彌廣而精，上合于明，明則內發于精，如是乃至于道，道應于德。德之成矣，用而為仁，分而為義。

Shén is insubstantial and cannot be seen. However, it can be felt and condensed to a high spiritual level. Though insubstantial, it must be in accord with the material world of secular society. Shén is related to the Wisdom Mind (Yì, 意) and the Emotional Mind (Xīn, 心). The Emotional Mind brings confusion and excitement, while the Wisdom Mind directs you to focused thinking and decisions. Shén can be raised and condensed, so the Emotional Mind under control becomes peaceful and calm. This results in harmonization of Shén and Qì's circulation, the stage of unification of Shén and Qì (Shénqì Xiànghé, 神氣相合). Practice often to achieve regulating without regulating, bringing health and longevity. Your mind becomes neutral and bright, clear and wise, reaching far and wide. Internally wise, externally you apply the Dào (道) of nature in action, which is called "Dé" (德). When Dào and Dé are applied in human society, it is benevolence (Rén, 仁) and righteousness (Yì, 義).

Jīngqì leaves from the head in daytime and resides at the abdomen (Real Lower Dāntián) at night. Therefore, respect the head and the abdomen. Settle the colors (materials) externally, while respecting righteousness within. Whenever there is an opportunity (for taking advantage), there is no slightest thought (of taking it). All in the mind is goodness. Thus, Shén and Qì engage the quality and harmonize into a single body. This is called Great Smoothness (Dàshùn). Heaven will protect (you) and (make you) auspicious without any disadvantage. This is because all the marvelous (manifestations of nature) have their roots. The Shén's insubstantial nothingness, inside Xīn, connects with its system. The Qì firmly concealed in the intestines should be nourished warmly and patiently. In daily life, close your eyes and observe the internal origin of the Qì. Whenever an event causes disturbance of the Líng (spiritual mind), close your eyes gladly and observe the Xīn internally. Reject it as though saying, "My Shén and Qì are concealed and developed from my body, making me able to reach the Dào." Then heaven will bestow auspiciousness, because heaven is the Líng of the insubstantial Qì. Use it to reach the ultimate of the Dào.

> 精氣晝出于首，夜栖于腹，當自尊其首，重其腹。色庄于外，敬直于中，應機無想，唯善是與，此神氣事質，合吾一體，謂之大順，天保祐之，吉無不利。凡妙本有所，神在心中之虛，上通其系，氣藴腸中之實，恆宜溫養之。平居常宜閉目內視氣源，每行一事利于生靈，則欣然閉目，內視其心，謝之若曰：'吾身之神氣，明發于吾形，使吾達道也。'如是則天降之吉。故天者，虛氣之靈，吾能用之，道極于斯矣。

In daytime, brain function leads Qì upward, and at night, during sleep, Qì returns to the Real Lower Dāntián for recharging. When you cultivate immortality, you must cultivate both Shén at the top (quality) and Qì at the bottom (quantity).

Many distractions cause emotional disturbance and increase desire. Whatever your thoughts and actions, let them be in the goodness of the Dào (道) and Dé (德). You feel righteous and enlightened internally, your spirit in harmony and at peace. This follows the way of nature, and nature will protect you.

Two Purposes of Regulating the Shén (Tiáoshén Èrzhǐ, 調神二旨)

There are two main purposes of regulating the Shén in Qìgōng practice. For secular society, it is to improve health and extend life, but for Buddhists and Daoists, the goal is to reach Buddhahood or enlightenment.

Health and Longevity. Yì is related to Shén. When Yì is strong and concentrated, Shén can be raised high. The most popular and essential purpose of Qìgōng practice is to attain health, using Yì to lead the Qì (Yǐyì Yǐnqì, 以意引氣). If concentrated Yì raises Shén, Qì circulates smoothly, and the body is healthy. Small Circulation meditation increases the Qì circulating in the Conception and Governing Vessels, and in the Twelve Primary Qì Channels.

Qìgōng also enhances longevity. It raises the spirit up to a high level, then uses it to govern the Qì (Yǐshén Yùqì, 以神馭氣) and to enhance Qì circulation in the bone marrow and brain. Qì is compared to soldiers in battle, while Shén is their fighting spirit. When the general's spirit is high, the morale of his soldiers is also high, and his orders are carried out effectively. In the same way, Qì nourishes the bone marrow and brain. Healthy marrow enhances production of blood cells, promoting metabolism and leading to longevity.

The following ancient document describes this process.

Historical Record: Autobiography of Tàshǐgōng
(Shǐjì, 史記・太史公自序)

How can one be alive? It is because of the existence of the Shén. How can this Shén be relied on to exist? It is because of the shape. When the Shén is greatly used, then exhausted. When the shape is greatly labored, then worn out. When shape and Shén are separated, they die. The dead cannot be revived, and those who are separated cannot be reunited. Therefore, holy men take spiritual cultivation very seriously. Shén is the root of the life while the shape is its vehicle.

凡人所生者，神也；所托者，形也。神大用則竭，形大勞則敝，形神離則死，死者不可復生，離者不可復反，故聖人重之。由是觀之，神者，生之本也，形者，生之具也。

Buddhists regard the spirit as the root of human life, while the physical body is only the vehicle for its cultivation. To reach Buddhahood, they cultivate the spirit more than the body. But Daoists regard the cultivation of the spirit and the body as being equally important. It takes many years to cultivate the Shén to reach enlightenment. If the physical body is weak and unhealthy, your life will be too short for spiritual cultivation.

To Buddhists, the material world does not exist, so there is nothing to be cultivated or considered. The Buddhist document, *Altar Classic of the Sixth Ancestor* (*Líùzǔ Tánjīng*, 六祖壇經) said, "Bodhi does not have a tree originally, nor is there a shining mirror in front. There are no objects there originally, so how can they be contaminated by dust or mud (objects or emotions)?"[41] Bodhi means an enlightened mind. Buddha was enlightened under the Bodhi tree. Shining mirror means a pure and clean Shén. When you cultivate Shén, the material world disappears, so there is no tree or mirror stand. With no material concept in your mind, how can it be cleaned of secular emotions and desires?

A Daoist document, *The Thesis of Nourishing Life* (*Yǎngshēnglùn*, 養生論), contrasts this, "Utter and receive Qì (Tǔnà, 吐納) through breathing, absorb food to nourish the body, thus allow the shape (physical body) and Shén to be harmonized. This means the mutual coordination of external and internal."[42] Tǔnà (吐納) means uttering and receiving, an ancient term for cultivating Qì through breathing.

Enlightenment. To spiritual cultivators, the final goal of regulating Shén is reaching enlightenment. That means comprehending the meaning of nature and human life, then unifying the human spirit with nature to become as one. This is the final goal of the unification of Heaven and Man (Tiānrén Héyī, 天人合一).

To reach this, one must open the third eye for communication. First build up abundant Qì at the Real Lower Dāntián. This is led up through the Thrusting Vessel to activate the brain and enhance the resonance of the Spiritual Valley. When spiritual energy reaches a certain level, the third eye reopens.

To reach this high level of cultivation, first regulate your mind. If it is trapped in emotional bondage, how can you build up your spirit and keep it neutral? Buddhists and Daoists define four steps in spiritual cultivation.

Four Steps to Cultivate Spiritual Enlightenment (Péishén Sìjiē, 培神四階)

Self-recognition (Zìshì, 自識). First set your spirit free from emotional bondage, otherwise the spirit stays in the emotional mud of secular society. Once the spirit is free from this bondage, it can reach the neutral state and finally unify with the natural spirit. Self-recognition (Zìshì, 自識) means observing the heart (Guānxīn, 觀心), that is, observing the initiation of thoughts and emotions to discover your true identity.

Important Script of Similar Contents (*Tóngzhǐ Yàochāo*, 同指要抄) said, "All religious styles, throughout generations, all considered observing the Xīn (Guānxīn, 觀心) as the most important in cultivation."[43]

The Complete Book of Principal Contents of Human Life and Temperament (*Xìngmìng Guīzhǐ Quánshū*, 性命圭旨全書) said, "When learning the Dào, first comprehend your own Xīn. The deep hidden place of your own Xīn is the hardest place to find. Once you have found it and no other place can be found, you realize that a secular's Xīn can be just like a Buddha's."[44] This describes the difficulty of discovering your true self hiding behind the mask. Once you have discovered this hidden Xīn, you recognize it and cultivate it. This cultivated Xīn can reach the same level as Buddha.

Self-awareness (Zìjué, 自覺). Having recognized your true identity, ponder deeply, and clearly discriminate truth from illusion. From discriminating between truth and falsehood, awareness arises. Your mind establishes contact with events and phenomena in your life. The feeling of self-awareness can be profound.

To Buddhist society, this is the stage where observation is stopped. It is the beginning of regulating the temperament and spirit towards goodness. *Anthology of Daoist Village* (*Dàoxiāngjí*, 道鄉集) said, "The real meaning of Buddhahood which has been handed down is: observation is stopped. What is observation? It means to place my vision warmly on the ultimate goodness. What is stop? It means to focus my real intention on the ultimate goodness."[45] Buddhist society has three observations (Sānguān, 三觀): 1. Observing Emptiness is observing the emptiness of all natural laws and events, 2. Observing Falseness is observing the falseness of all natural laws, 3. Observing Between is observing the non-emptiness and non-falseness of natural laws, keeping the neutral viewpoint. It also means double observation.[18] Zhǐguān (Stop Observation, 止觀) is the way to reach Guānzhǐ (observation is stopped, 觀止). Observe and analyze events and occurrences. Once you see through the events in your mind, nothing troubles you. This is the stage of Guānzhǐ, reached by cultivating your mind to the stage of ultimate goodness. Pay attention to all goodness, then nothing bothers you. You are kind, righteous and gentle, with no inner conflict. You are free from the affinity of emotions and desires.

Extreme calmness and peace within are the key to this self-awareness, reached through practicing Embryonic Breathing (Tāixí, 胎息), as described in the book, *Qìgōng Meditation—Embryonic Breathing*.

Self-awakening (Zìxǐng, 自醒) (Zìwù, 自悟). Through Embryonic Breathing, you reach self-awakening. Your mind is clear and allows you to comprehend accurately the truth of your life and nature. This stage is called entering the observation (Rùguān, 入觀). Entering means to comprehend the observation and the temperament (Wùxìng, 悟性).[46] This is the stage of enlightenment and Buddhahood (Fó, 佛), called understanding the heart and seeing through the temperament (Míngxīn Jiànxìng, 明心見性). Comprehension is no longer necessary (Líǎowù, 了悟).

How is Buddhahood defined? It means to achieve awareness and wisdom, to awaken through understanding and observation, to awaken through knowing the reasons behind natural laws, and to discriminate them clearly. It is like being awakened from sleep and is called "awakening through realization." Comprehend vexations through observation so they are not harmful. It is like observing and sensing "thieves" (contaminated thoughts) in secular society, so it is called awakening through observation.[47] Thesis of Buddha Ground (Fódìlùn, 佛地論) said, "All laws and all manifestations of nature can bloom and be awakened by themselves. We can also bloom and be awakened from emotional bondage, like being awakened from sleep and like the blooming of the lotus flower. This is called Buddha."[48]

To Buddhists, we are born and grow in emotional mud (Chéntǔ, 塵土, human matrix). We create dignity, glory, pride, happiness, sadness, jealousy, and desire. We lie and cover our faces with masks, and we all experience significant spiritual pain living in this human matrix. The mud makes us blind and deaf, and nothing is clear in our minds. The conscious mind is active, while the sub-conscious Shén is asleep. We are dreaming in the human matrix and not awakening.

Nevertheless, each of us has a lotus seed, our Original Shén. Through meditation, it buds and grows from deep in the mud. The subconscious mind grows, and after long practice, the lotus flower emerges from the matrix, and you see everything clearly. To awaken your Shén, bring all thoughts to your Shén center and keep the Shén there. This Upper Dāntián or Spiritual Mountain (Língshān, 靈山), in which there is the Spiritual Valley (Shéngǔ, 神谷), is where the Valley Spirit (Gǔshén, 谷神) lives.

Remember the song which says, "Do not search far for Buddha since he is in the Spiritual Mountain. Where is the Spiritual Mountain? In your mind."[39]

In a state of extreme calmness and emptiness, your mind is clear to comprehend the truth of nature. *The Righteous Rules of Heavenly Immortality: Straight Discussion of Two Qì Pre-Heaven and Post-Heaven* (Tiānxiān Zhènglǐ. Xiāntiān Hòutiān Èrqì Zhílùn, 天仙正理・先天后天二氣直論) said, "Those who apply Qì, how do they know it is true pre-heaven practice? When calmness (Jìng, 靜) and emptiness (Xū, 虛) have reached their extremities, there is no single slight thought involved in consciousness. This is the true pre-heaven practice."[49] Pre-Heaven truth (Xiāntiān Zhīzhēn, 先天之真) means the truthful state before birth, where the mind is simple and pure, extremely calm and sincere. However, how do you know you have reached this state in practice? When there is not even the smallest thought existing or initiating in your mind. Your subconscious mind (Pre-Heaven truthful mind) awakens to activity.

Qìgōng society classifies the conscious mind as Yáng, generated by the brain since birth. The subconscious mind is Yīn and is born with you. The conscious mind and memory are generated from conditioning by the environment and are not truthful. A thick facade covers the falseness of this conscious mind. However, the subconscious mind is truthful, connected with spiritual memory, which is active only when your body is calm and activities of your conscious mind have ceased.

To return to the Pre-Birth stage, cease physical and mental activity. Then the subconscious mind acts, and directs you to the true path of spiritual cultivation.

Freedom from Self-Bondage (Zìtuō, 自脫). The last stage of spiritual cultivation is to free yourself from physical, mental, and spiritual bondage. Once you have awakened spiritually, you see clearly who you are and how you want to be. Free yourself from the bondage of the human matrix. In Buddhist terms, the third eye opens. The lotus grows, and the flower emerges from the mud. Your spirit is reunited with the spirit of nature.

Freedom from Material Bondage. Set yourself free from the bondage of your physical body and all material attractions around you. Your body is only recycled material, and beauty is only temporary. Material concerns trigger mental bondage. Take care of this recycled material, protect it and nourish it, but free yourself from attaching to it.

What you need from the material world is enough energy supply for your physical strength, without sinking into the mud of materialism and losing the feeling of your life. Most material things you own will last longer than you, and you own them only as long as you live. If you pursue material enjoyment, your mind stays focused on materialistic concerns. To set yourself free from material bondage, the first step is to gain enough for comfortable living. Any extra beyond that entangles you deeper in the mud. To reach profound spiritual cultivation, Buddhists believe you must cultivate a neutral state separate from the four emptinesses of earth, water, fire, and wind (Sìdà Jiēkōng, 四大皆空, material world). They believe this is crucial to reaching Buddhahood.

Freedom from Mental Bondage. Mental bondage means the thoughts generated from the emotional matrix, and desires for both the mental and material worlds. Again, human suffering is caused by the seven passions and six desires (Qīqíng Líùyù, 七情六慾). The seven passions are happiness (Xǐ, 喜), anger (Nù, 怒), sorrow (Āi, 哀), joy (Lè, 樂), love (Ài, 愛), hate (Hèn, 恨) and desire (Yù, 慾). The six desires are the sensory pleasures derived from the eyes, ears, nose, tongue, body, and mind.

We humans, in order to survive in the harsh reality of this world, lie and trick each other. Truth within is hidden behind the mask we wear, decorated with glory, dignity, and honor, which are tools to enslave the souls and bodies of others. Lust for wealth and power has become the common core education for the next generation. A human emotional matrix has been created and all of us suffer within it.

To escape from this matrix, first awaken deep in your heart. With a neutral and open mind, see through the matrix we have created. The truth should always be in your mind, else the search for the Dào will be in vain. Ponder the words of Michael Faraday (1791–1867): "The philosopher should be a man willing to listen to every suggestion, but determined to judge for himself. He should not be biased by appearances, have no favorite hypothesis, be of no school, and in doctrine have no master. He should not be a respecter of persons, but of things. Truth should be his primary object. If to these qualities be added industry, he may indeed hope to walk within the veil of the temple of Nature." Once you have this truth in your mind, you have achieved a peaceful mind, and your spirit can awaken and be cultivated.

Freedom from Spiritual Bondage. You need to be free from mental bondage before setting out to escape from spiritual bondage. The spirit is overshadowed and blinded by traditional religious doctrines, based on the emotions of the past.

The various religions bind us in their spiritual religious matrix, created by those considered holy men in the past. The concepts of God, heaven, and hell were created in the human mind, and worship was initiated. As time passed, we have been led deeper and deeper away from the truth, and trapped in human-created spiritual bondage. Lǎozi, Chapter 1, said, "Dào, if it can be spoken (described), then it is not the true everlasting Dào. Name, if it can be named, then it is not the true everlasting name."[50] We humans, before really knowing the Dào, have already talked about Dào. Even if we know the true path to search for it, we still cling stubbornly to the old path and dare not change it.

To achieve this true Dào, we must continue to search for it, talking and exchanging opinions. Always keep in mind that the Dào we are talking about may not yet be true. Having seen the truth, we should not be afraid to face it, challenging our old thoughts and beliefs, and daring to accept mistakes and to dream about the future. Science should search for the true Dào, helping us to escape from the traditional religious matrix.

Escape from the traditional matrix and free yourself from spiritual bondage and doctrines. Awaken your subconscious spiritual mind, by bringing your mind and spiritual feeling to the day you were conceived. From this Daoist principle were derived the theory and techniques of Embryonic Breathing.

To return to the embryonic state, first get rid of the human emotional matrix. Focus the mind on the pineal and pituitary glands at the Mud Pill Palace (Níwángōng, 泥丸宮). Where there are brain cells, that is where conscious thought and the human matrix can be created. However, the lower center of the Spiritual Valley has no brain cells, so no matrix can be generated. Through this center, where the subconscious mind resides, we can resonate or communicate with the natural spirit. By calming the activity of the brain through absence of thought, we bring our spiritual awareness to a high level.

For strong resonance between your spirit and the natural spirit, you need strong spiritual energy at this Mud Pill Palace. Store abundant Qì at your Real Lower Dāntián (Zhēn Xiàdāntián, 真下丹田), and lead it up to nourish the Mud Pill Palace, raising spiritual energy up to a high level. Spiritual cultivation is discussed in more detail in my previous book, *Qìgōng Meditation—Embryonic Breathing*.

Once you bring your spiritual energy to a very high level, you reopen your third eye, called Tiānyǎn (heaven eye, 天眼) by Daoist society and Yìntáng (M-NH-3, sealed hall, 印堂) by Chinese medicine. Having reopened the third eye, your spirit can unite with the natural spirit without obstacle. This is the final stage of spiritual cultivation, the Unification of Heaven and Man (Tiānrén Héyī, 天人合一).

References

1. 真調為無調而自調。
2. 形不正，則氣不順。氣不順，則意不寧。意不寧，則氣散亂。
3. 解剖生理學 (*A Study of Anatomic Physiology*) 李文森編著。華杏出版股份有限公司。 Lǐ, Wén-Sēn, Táipéi, 1986.
4. 《莊子・大宗師》：〝古之真人，・・・其息深深。真人之息以踵，眾人之息以喉。〞
5. 《性命圭旨全書・火候》：〝神息者，火候也。〞指文火安神定息，任其自如，謂之神息。即〝不得勤，不得怠者，是皆神息之自然火候之微旨也。〞
6. 《性命圭旨全書・蟄藏氣穴，眾妙歸根》：〝調息要調真息息，煉神須煉不神神。〞
7. 《天仙正理・伏氣直論》：〝古人托名調息者，隨順往來之理而不執滯往來之形，欲合乎似無之呼吸也。〞
8. *Chinese Qìgōng Dictionary* (中國氣功辭典), by Lǚ, Guāng-Róng (呂光榮), 人民衛生出版社, Běijīng, China, 1988.
9. "Teens' Troubles Tied to Brain," Michael Lasalandra, *Boston Herald*, June 12, 1998.
10. "Inside the Teen Brain," by Shannon Brownlee, pp. 44-54, *U.S. News*, August 9, 1999.
11. 《備急千金要方・卷二十七・養性》：〝多思則神殆，多念則志散，多欲則志昏，多事則形勞，多語則氣乏，多笑則臟傷，多愁則心懾，多樂則意溢，多喜則忘錯昏亂，多怒則百脈不定，多好則專迷不理，多惡則憔悴無歡。此十二多不除，則榮衛失度，血氣妄行，喪生之本也。〞
12. 《性命圭旨全書・亨集》：〝身不動而心自安，心不動而神自守。〞

13.《性命圭旨全書・蟄藏氣穴，眾妙歸根》：〝合真人深深之息，則心息相依，息調心靜。〞

14.《聽心齋客問》：〝心依著事物已久，一旦離境，不能自立。所以用調息功夫，拴系此心，便心息相依。調字亦不是用意，只是一呼一吸系念耳。至心離境，則無人無我，更無息可調，只綿綿若存，久之，自然純熟。〞

15.《道藏・坐忘論》：〝夫心者一身之主，百神之帥，靜則生慧，動則生昏，欣迷動靜之中。〞

16.《至游子・集要篇》：〝不畏念起，惟畏覺遲。〞

17.《道藏・重陽立教十五論》：〝欲界、色界、無色界，此乃三界也。心忘慮念，即超欲界；心忘諸境，即超色界；不著空見，即超無色界。〞

18.〔三觀〕：一・空觀：觀諸法之空諦。二・假觀：觀諸法之假。三・中觀：一觀諸法亦非空，亦非假，即中也。二觀諸法亦空亦假，即是中，謂為雙照之觀。

19.《性命圭旨全書・亨集》：〝一念動時皆是火，萬緣寂處即生春。〞

20.《維摩經》：〝系心于緣謂之止，分別深達謂之觀。〞〝念念歸一為止，了了分明為觀。〞

21. 眼觀鼻，鼻觀心。

22.《莊子・人間世》：〝若一志，無聽之以耳而聽之以心；無聽之以心而聽之以氣。聽止于耳，心止于符。氣也者，虛而待物者也。唯道集虛，虛者心齋也。〞

23.《道鄉集》：〝余今傳汝止念之法。譬如我心看水，此念即在水上；我心看月，此念即在月上；設想此眼光專看氣穴，我心即在氣穴矣。〞

24.《中和集》：〝諦觀三教聖人書，息之一字最簡直。若于息上做功夫，為佛為仙不勞力。息緣達本禪之機，息心明理儒之極，息氣凝神道之玄，三息相須無不克。〞

25.《慧苑音義・上》：〝禪那，此云靜心思慮也。〞

26. 孔子曰：〝知止而后有定，定而后能靜，靜而后能安，安而后能慮，慮而後能得。〞

27.《智度論》：〝正心行處，見慮凝心，心定于一處而不動，故曰定；正受所觀之法，故曰受；調心之暴，直心之曲，定心之散，故曰調直定；正心之行動，使合于法之依處，故曰正心行處；息止緣慮，凝結心念，故曰息慮凝心。〞

28.《管子・內業》：〝佛心澄明，謂之大定。〞指腦神安靜，形體放鬆，神形相對協調與穩定。

29. *The Great Completion of Chinese Qìgōng* (中國氣功大成), by Fāng, Chūn-Yáng (方春陽), 吉林科學技術出版社, Jílín, China, 1989.

30. *The Complete Book of Nourishing the Life in Chinese Daoist Qìgōng* (中國道教氣功養生大全), by Lǐ, Yuǎn-Guó (李遠國), 四川辭書出版社, Chéngdū, Sìchuān China, 1991.

31. 《道德經・十六章》："致虛極，守靜篤。"

32. 意不在氣，在氣則滯。

33. 行氣如九曲珠，無微不到。

34. 《道德經・六章》："谷神不死，是謂玄牝。玄牝之門，是謂天地根，綿綿若存，用之不勤。"

35. "指造化生育萬物之根本，亦即天地萬物之母，即道之別稱也。"

36. 《武當修真圖》："明堂下，兩眉連線中點上方。有神光出，而曰天目。"

37. 《云笈七簽》："兩眉間為泥丸之玉門。"

38. "人人身中有一神，一神中有一靈光，靈光獨耀超千谷，道化無窮徹萬方。"

39. "佛在靈山莫遠求，靈山只在汝心頭。人人有個靈山塔，好向靈山塔下修。"

40. 《本草綱目》："腦為元神之府。"

41. 《六祖壇經》："菩提本無樹，明鏡亦非台，本來無一物，何處惹塵埃。"

42. 《養生論》："呼吸吐納，服食養身，使形神相親，表裡既濟也。"

43. 《同指要抄》："一代教門，皆以觀心為要。"

44. 《性命圭旨全書・涵養本源，救護命寶》："學道先須學自心，自心深處最難尋。若還尋到無尋處，方悟凡心即佛心。"指覺悟之心。

45. 《道鄉集》："佛之真傳，在于觀止。""觀者何？將我目光，溫煦于至善地之義也。""止者何？將我真意止于至善地之義也。"

46. 入觀：觀為觀想之義。入為悟性，即悟真理。

47. 即覺或智之意。如覺悟、覺察、覺知諸法之事理，而了了分明。如睡夢之寤，謂之覺悟。覺察煩惱，使不為害，如世人之覺之為賊者，故云覺察。

48. 《佛地論》："于一切法，一切種相，能自開覺，亦開覺一切有情，如睡夢覺醒，如蓮花開，故名佛。"

49. 《天仙正理・先天后天二氣直論》："夫用此氣者，由何以知先天之真也。當靜虛至極時。亦未涉一念覺知，此正真先天之真境界也。"

50. 老子・第一章："道、可道，非、常道；名、可名，非、常名。"

Part III. Small Circulation Meditation

(Small Cyclic Heaven or Microcosmic Meditation)

Chapter 5

Theoretical Root of Small Circulation Meditation

5-1. Introduction (Jièshào, 介紹)

There are six general purposes of Small Circulation Meditation:

1. Search for a peaceful mind.
2. Improve physical and mental health.
3. Find the center of self-being.
4. Comprehend the meaning of life.
5. Search for spiritual freedom.
6. Comprehend the meaning of the universe.

Through Small Circulation Meditation we rebuild the body from weak to strong and train the mind to be calm and focused. The Qì in the Eight Vessels and Twelve Primary Qì Channels becomes abundant, strengthening the immune system. Small Circulation is the first step in Internal Elixir practice, the foundation of Muscle/Tendon Changing and Marrow/Brain Washing Qìgōng.

There are various styles of Small Circulation, each with a different name. In Buddhist society it is called Turning the Wheel of Natural Law (Zhuǎnfǎlún, 轉法輪). Every style has its own theory and method. Study and compare them, and take the best from each.

There is a Chinese story about six blind men who touch an elephant to know what it looks like. The first one touches the elephant's ear and says, "An elephant is like a large fan." The second one touches the side of its body and says, "No, it is like a wall." The third one describes the leg, "No, the elephant is like a pillar." The fourth one touches the nose and shouts, "The elephant is like a large moving branch of a tree." The fifth one touches the ivory, and says, "It is a large horn sticking out of a huge mouth." The sixth one who touches the tail says loudly, "An elephant is a large swinging broom sticking out of the wall." If they were to put all of the information together, they would have a reasonable description of the elephant. This story shows we should not stubbornly insist there is only one viewpoint, as we often see only part of the story.

When you practice, don't waste time in just theoretical research. Practice and theory should go together. From practice, you gain experience, and from theory, you have a clear guideline for practice. Some people hesitate due to the danger involved, accomplishing nothing and simply wasting time. Be cautious but determined, and learn from the experience of others, and you will find the right path.

A priest staying in a church is told the dam wall has broken, and the church will be flooded. He refuses to leave, and says God will save him. As water enters the church and rises quickly, he climbs up on the roof and prays for mercy and a miracle to save him. A boat comes to rescue him, but he refuses, waiting for God's miracle to save him. The boat leaves as the waters keep rising. Another boat comes to rescue him, but is again rejected. A third rescue boat receives the same answer. The waters engulf the church, and the priest drowns.

When he arrives in Heaven, he blames God for not working a miracle to save him, but God says, "I sent three boats to save you but you rejected them all." Will you wait for the perfect theory, or grasp the opportunity while you can?

When Buddha traveled the countryside, he came to a river. An old Qìgōng master lived there, who asked him, "You are the Buddha? If so, can you do the same thing I can? I cross the river by walking on top of the water." Buddha said, "That is very impressive. But how long have you practiced it?" The old man replied, "It took me nearly forty years to achieve it." The Buddha looked at him and said, "It took you forty years! It takes me only a few coins to cross it on the ferryboat."

Often we spend too much time on unimportant things. Treat your time preciously and use it efficiently. Get rid of your dignity. If you take your dignity too seriously, you will not find a sincere teacher willing to teach from the heart.

A young Samurai swordsman entered the house of a famous Zen master. He looked at the master, bowed and said, "Master! I have reached a deep level of Zen, both in theory and practice. I have heard you are great so I come here to bow to you and hope you can teach me something."

The Zen master looked at this proud young man. Without a word, he went into the back room and brought out a teapot and a teacup. He placed the cup in front of the young man and started to pour the tea into the cup. The tea filled the cup quickly and soon began to overflow. The young man looked at the old man with a confused expression. He said, "Stop, master! The teacup is overflowing."

The old Zen master put the teapot down and smiled at him. He said, "This is you. You are too full already. I cannot teach you. If you wish to learn, you must first empty your cup." Can you be as humble as an empty cup?

When you find a good qualified teacher or source of learning, treat it preciously, so you don't miss the opportunity of learning. This chance may not come again. Traditionally, it was very difficult to find a qualified teacher. Even if you found one, you would not necessarily be accepted.

Today, it is easier to collect information since there are so many books and videos available. But the guidance of an experienced teacher is generally crucial to reach the final goal. Subtle advice can save you a great deal of time and effort. When you are lost in a big city, even though you have read the map, guidance from a passerby could save a lot of effort.

A young man had already spent more than seven years searching for a good master. He came to where a great teacher lived deep in the remote mountains with a few students. He was received kindly and expressed his intention of learning from the master. The master looked at him for a while, then brought out a teapot and a teacup. He poured tea into the cup, stopping when the tea reached the brim. He put the tea pot down with a smile, hinting to the young man that the place was already full. He could not accept another student.

The young man looked at the cup and realized what it meant. He lowered his head in sadness. Noticing a rice straw on the floor, he picked it up and carefully stuck it into the tea. The tea did not overflow. He looked at the master's face with hope, showing him, "Look, there is still space for me. The tea did not overflow."

Through this silent communication, the old master realized that the young man was one of those rare intelligent ones who could comprehend the profound feeling of the art. He accepted him with delight. It is very difficult to find an intelligent student able to comprehend the art deeply and to develop it. When a teacher finds this kind of student, it will be like a precious pearl in his hands.

In the next section, I review the history of Small Circulation practice. Then I summarize those acupuncture cavities related to the practice in section 5-3. We discuss the theory of Small Circulation in section 5-4. In section 5-5, crucial obstacles to Small Circulation, The Three Gates, are explained. We discuss different Small Circulation paths in section 5-6. Finally, an illustration of Internal Elixir meditation passed down from the Chinese Táng Dynasty (618–907 CE, 唐代) is introduced and interpreted.

5-2. Small Circulation—Past and Present (Xiǎozhōutiān Zhī Guòqù Yǔ Xiànzài, 小周天之過去與現在)

After more than 1500 years of study and development, the practice of Small Circulation Qìgōng meditation has gradually evolved, from initial limited knowledge to a stage which allows practitioners to have a clear understanding of the practice.

Small Circulation Practice in the Past

The practice of Small Circulation (Small Cyclic Heaven, Xiǎozhōutiān, 小周天) probably started in China around 500 CE, when Dámó's *Muscle/Tendon Changing and Marrow/Brain Washing Classic* (*Yìjīnjīng, Xǐsuǐjīng*; 易筋經・洗髓經) became available. There are a few reasons for this conclusion:

1. There are almost no Chinese documents available about the subject from before 500 CE.
2. Small Circulation is a necessary prerequisite to reach advanced accomplishment in Muscle/Tendon Changing.
3. Dámó (483–536 CE, 達摩) was originally from India. When he arrived in China during the Liáng Dynasty (502–557 CE, 梁朝), Indian Yoga had already existed for 800 years. Small Circulation practice was an advanced level of practice in Indian Yoga, called Microcosmic Orbit Meditation.
4. Daoist practice of Small Circulation was originally from Buddhist society, called Turning the Wheel of Natural Law (Zhuǎnfǎlún, 轉法輪). Even though Buddhism was imported into China during the reign of the Míng Emperor of the East Hàn Dynasty (58–76 CE, 東漢明帝), documents on Qìgōng spiritual enlightenment practice were very scarce. It was not until Dámó arrived, that actual Qìgōng practices were passed down.

Later, theory and practice of Small Circulation and Grand Circulation meditation were studied, researched, and developed in China. They blended with traditional Chinese Daoist theory based on the *Dào Dé Jīng* (道德經), written by Lǎozi (老子) (604–531 BCE), and a new understanding and practice developed. The most important influence from *Dào Dé Jīng* was the theory of Embryonic Breathing (Tāixí, 胎息). Without it, reaching the final goal of spiritual enlightenment would be very difficult.

With the addition of Chinese medical knowledge of Qì meridians and vessels, the theory and practice of Small Circulation were revised continuously and reached a profound level during the Qīng Dynasty (1644–1912 CE, 清朝). Many documents were written about Small Circulation during this period. I present some of them here with commentary.

A Small Cyclic Heaven of Yīn-Yáng Circulation Antithetic Writing of Regulating the Path
(Wú, Shī-Jī; Qīng Dynasty)
陰陽循環一小周天
(理瀹駢文・清・吳師機著)

It (Small Circulation) is actually called "Small Cyclic Heaven of Yīn-Yáng Circulation." Close the eyes and sit quietly. The nose inhales clean air. Expand the abdomen to enable internal Qì to descend to the Lower Dāntián under the navel. Transport Qì past Huìyīn and up the Governing Vessel. Pass the Tailbone (Wěilǘ), Squeezing Spine (Jiájí, between the shoulder blades) and Jade Pillow (Yùzhěn), Three Gates. Reach Bǎihuì (Gv-20) cavity on top of the head, follow the face to the tongue and connect with the Conception Vessel, descend down along the front of the chest, finally reach the Dāntián and again circulate through the original path. Where there is a problem (Qì stagnation or pain), inhale and think of the place, and exhale to lead the Qì back to the Dāntián. This strengthens the body and repels sickness. It is also named Sānmèiyìn.

全稱為陰陽循環一小周天。閉目靜坐，鼻吸清氣，鼓腹使內氣下降臍下丹田，運氣過肛門，沿督脈尾閭、夾脊、玉枕三關，到頭頂百會穴，順面部至舌與任脈接，沿前胸而下，至丹田復順原徑路循行。患在何處，收氣即存想其處，放氣則歸於丹田。可強身卻病。又名三昧印。

This document, which was written by Wú, Shī-Jī (吳師機) in 1864, discusses a few key points. First, to meditate, close your eyes to cut off the connection between your eyes and your surroundings. Second, to circulate the Qì smoothly, sit quietly with your body calm and relaxed. This is the pre-condition for Qì circulation. Third, breathe correctly. Breathing is the strategy of Qìgōng practice. When breathing correctly, Qì can be guided efficiently. Fourth, generate and accumulate Qì at the Lower Dāntián. Without abundant Qì stored there, the path of Qì circulating in the Conception and Governing Vessels cannot be widened, so regulating the Qì in the Twelve Primary Qì Channels will not be effective. Fifth, the path of Qì circulation is from the Lower Dāntián, via the Huìyīn, past the tailbone (Wěilǘ, 尾閭; Chángqiáng, 長強), Jiájí (夾脊; Língtái, 靈臺) and Yùzhěn (玉枕; Nǎohù, 腦戶), the Three Gates (Sānguān, 三關), then over the head, and down the front center line back to the Lower Dāntián. Small Circulation practice is the foundation of Muscle/Tendon Changing, which can change your body from weak to strong. It is also called Sānmèiyìn (三昧印) in Buddhist society, or Sānmódì (Samadhi, 三摩地) a special Buddhist term which means steadiness of the mind and body (Dìng, 定).

Small Cyclic Heaven
(Original Truth of Using No Herbs)
(Wāng, Áng; Qīng Dynasty)
小周天
(勿藥元詮・清・汪昂輯)

First, stop the Niàn (the thoughts lingering in the mind), calm the body and the heart, face east, and sit with crossed legs (Jiāzuò). The breathing is peaceful and harmonious. Use Sānmèiyìn and maintain it under the navel. Knock the teeth sixty-six times and gather your spirit in the whole body. The tongue circles the mouth sixty-six times both internally and externally, while you also circle both eyes following the circles of the tongue. The tongue touches the palate, count the breathing calmly until it reaches three hundred and sixty times. Wait until the spiritual water (saliva) is full, rinse (the mouth) several times. Use Four Secret Words (Sìzìjué), lead Qì from the Conception Vessel, past the grain path (Huìyīn), and reach the tailbone (Chángqiáng). Use Yì to transport, slowly lead Qì up to the central gate, Jiájí (Língtái cavity). Gradually speed up. Close your eyes and look up, inhale but do not exhale through the nose, thrust through Yùzhěn (Nǎohù cavity). Use the eye to lead it forward and pass Kūnlún (Bǎihuì), down to Quèqiáo (magpie bridge, tongue), then divide the saliva and send it down the Chónglóu (throat), enter Lí palace (heart, Middle Dāntián), and finally reach the Qìhǎi (Lower Dāntián). Pause for a moment, use the same method and repeat it three times. Divide the saliva in the mouth into three gulps and send it down. This is what is called "reversed flow of heavenly river water."

先要止念，身心澄清，面東跏坐，呼吸平和，用三昧印，按于臍下；叩齒三十六通，以集身神；赤龍攪海，內外三十六遍；雙目隨轉運，舌抵上齶，靜心數息，三百六十周天畢，待神水滿，漱津數遍；用〝四字訣〞，從任脈撮過穀道到尾閭，以意運送，徐徐上夾脊中關，漸漸速些；閉目上視，鼻吸莫呼，衝過玉枕，將目往前一忍，直轉崑崙，倒下鵲橋，分津送下重樓，入離宮，而至氣海；略定一定，復用前法，連行三次，口中之津，分三次咽下，所謂天河水逆流也。

This document was written by Wāng, Áng (汪昂) in 1682 CE during the Qīng Dynasty (1644–1912 CE, 清朝). The Qì path is the same as in the previous document, but it also describes the preparation for Small Circulation.

Niàn (念) is the thought lingering your mind and hard to get rid of. Jiāzuò (跏坐) is a special Buddhist meditation term which means to sit with crossed legs. Sānmèiyìn comes from Indian "Samadhi" and means great steadiness of the mind and body. Sìzìjué (四字訣) means Four Secret Words, namely Cuō (撮), Dǐ (抵), Bì (閉), and Xī (吸). Cuō means to condense, to focus, to concentrate. It implies the concentration of the mind and Qì. Dǐ means to press up, namely the tongue is pressing up against the palate of the mouth. Bì means to close, as in close or hold up the Huìyīn (perinium). Xī means to suck in, as in "leading the Qì up the spine in coordination with inhalation."

Quèqiáo (鵲橋) means Magpie Bridge, or tongue, which bridges the Conception and Governing Vessels. Chónglóu (重樓) means layers of stories, namely the throat area. Lígōng (離宮) means Lí Palace, or heart. In the Eight Trigrams (Bāguà, 八卦), Lí represents fire, and the heart belongs to fire in the Five Elements (Wǔxíng, 五行). Qìhǎi (氣海) is the Lower Dāntián (Xià Dāntián, 下丹田), which belongs to water, and is called Kǎn palace (Kǎngōng, 坎宮) in the Eight Trigrams.

To lead the Qì from Huìyīn (Co-1, 會陰, perineum, sea bottom) up the back to the crown is called Reversed Flow of the Heavenly River Water (Tiānhéshuǐ Nìliú, 天河水逆流).

> *Sit quietly for a while. Let the left and right hand each rub the Lower Dāntián one hundred and eight times, including the navel. Then cover the navel with clothes to keep the wind off. Rub the back of the thumbs until they are warm, and wipe the eyes with them fourteen times to get rid of (excess Yáng) heart fire. Rub the nose thirty-six times to moisten the lungs. Rub the ears fourteen times to nourish the kidneys. Rub the face fourteen times to strengthen the spleen. Cover the ears with the hands and beat the heavenly drum (Míngtiāngǔ). Raise the hands up gradually as if worshipping heaven, and repeat three times. Slowly exhale dirty air and inhale clean air. Hold the shoulders, move and shift the tendons and bones a few times. Rub Yùzhěn gate twenty-four times, rub kidney eyes one hundred and eight times, and also the center of each foot one hundred and eight times.*
>
> 靜坐片時，將手左右擦丹田各一百八下，連臍抱住，放手時將衣被圍住臍輪，勿令風入；次將大指背擦熱，拭目十四遍，去心火；擦鼻三十六遍，潤肺；擦耳十四遍，補腎；擦面十四遍，健脾。雙手掩耳鳴天鼓，徐徐將手往上，即朝天揖，如此者三，徐徐呵出濁氣四、五口，收清氣；雙手抱肩，移筋換骨數遍；擦玉枕關二十四下；擦腰眼各一百八下，擦足心各一百八下。

This document describes the recovery Qìgōng exercises right after Small Circulation meditation. Míngtiāngǔ (鳴天鼓) means to "beat the heavenly drum." Cover the ears with the palms, using the fingers to tap the base of the skull and the two major neck muscles. Refer to the YMAA book, *Eight Simple Qìgōng Exercises* (the Eight Pieces of Brocade, Bāduànjǐn, 八段錦).

These documents briefly describe the practice of Small Circulation, but without giving detail of how to build up Qì and the attendant dangers. The basic theory remains the same, though with different approaches to the final goal.

Small Circulation meditation is commonly practiced in Chinese martial arts society, as the foundation of Muscle/Tendon Changing, which strengthens martial power significantly. The common procedures as learned from a master are:

1. **Build up abundant Qì.** A master would teach how to build the Qì to a very high level at the Lower Dāntián through abdominal breathing. The student would spend up to ten years building this Qì and conditioning the Lower Dāntián.
2. **Circulate Qì in the Small Circulation path.** Since Qì is already abundant, it can be dangerous without correct technique. The crucial keys were often kept secret by the master, namely to control the Huìyīn cavity in coordination with breathing, and to touch the tongue to the palate of the mouth. Only when the student had earned his trust were these secrets revealed. There are three places, called Three Gates (Sānguān, 三關), which are dangerous in practice. The student would obey the master's orders step by step to get through these three gates. The danger in being unable to control this abundant Qì is that it can enter the wrong path, called "entering the fire" (Zǒuhuǒ, 走火). We discuss these three gates and their dangers in detail in section 5-5.

An important point is that Embryonic Breathing (Tāixí, 胎息) is the Yīn side of Internal Elixir (Nèidān, 內丹) practice. It is the crucial key in practicing Marrow/Brain Washing and is unknown in secular society. Even in Buddhist and Daoist monasteries, only a few monks reach a level profound enough to understand it. Whenever stored Qì is built up to an abundant level at the False Lower Dāntián, the excess is immediately distributed through the Conception and Governing Vessels and the Twelve Primary Qì Channels. The body, including the twelve internal organs, grows stronger. This is the fundamental concept of Muscle/Tendon Changing.

With Small Circulation training accomplished, the body and the manifestation of martial power are significantly enhanced. But too much Muscle/Tendon Changing training can also cause a serious problem called Energy Dispersion (Sàngōng, 散功). When the physical body has been over-energized, it can lead to high blood pressure and stroke. To balance this, practice the Yīn side of training, Marrow/Brain Washing Qìgōng. The first step is Embryonic Breathing (Tāixí, 胎息), described in detail in the previous book in this series, *Qìgōng Meditation—Embryonic Breathing.*

Modified Practice in Present Day

Though Small Circulation has been known in Indian Yoga, Chinese Buddhist Chán (Japanese Zen 禪), and Chinese Daoist societies, still only a few Qìgōng practitioners dare to practice it, due to the following reasons:

1. **Lack of understanding of theory and practice.** There is very little information available to read and study.
2. **Dangers during practice.** The Three Gates (Sānguān, 三關) are dangerous.
3. **Lack of an experienced teacher.** Often experience is essential for guidance, especially when there is a problem.

The following practice methods have developed from my personal practice, teaching, and study over more than 25 years. I believe this new approach has reduced the danger to the minimum.

1. **Teach theory first.** Theory is like a map of a city. Without it, the student can easily get lost, especially in today's environment where he does not live and practice together with the master. Most practitioners in the past did not know the theory, but this has now been understood and revealed. For any beginner, understanding the theory has become crucial for successful practice.
2. **Teach Embryonic Breathing first.** To prevent too much Yáng developing and the problem of energy dispersion, a student should first learn the Yīn side of training, namely the theory and methods of Embryonic Breathing. With this tool, he can manipulate the situation and balance the body's Yīn and Yáng easily and effectively.
3. **Build up Qì only as much as necessary.** Traditionally a student would build up Qì to a highly abundant level, encountering the attendant dangers. Before he has accumulated too much Qì, he should learn to circulate it. In this way, there is not enough Qì to cause the problem of "entering the fire" (Zǒuhuǒ, 走火).
4. **Use the mind to circulate before the Qì storage reaches a harmful level.** Traditionally one accumulated abundant Qì, then learned to circulate it. If we reverse this procedure, before a student's Qì has reached a harmful level, he can already lead it smoothly. That is like teaching a student driver with a small car. Only when he has become a skilled driver is a bigger and more powerful car provided. The disadvantage of this is that weaker Qì takes longer to overcome blockages and widen its path, like opening a blocked water pipe with less water.

5. **First practice Small Small Circulation.** Using Small Small Circulation (Xiǎo Xiǎozhōutiān, 小小周天) can help beginners to avoid danger, especially at the tailbone area, while learning to circulate Qì in coordination with the breathing, abdomen, and perineum.
6. **Carefully select the Qì turning points to avoid the problem of Qì stagnation.** Before completing the whole Small Circulation, first train the correct turning points where Qì can be returned to the Lower Dāntián. If the turning points are wrong, Qì stagnation can occur, as can "entering the fire'. These turning points were kept secret in the past. I have modified them, and believe these are safer than the traditional points used in the past. Once you understand the theory, you can modify the training path without causing any problem.

5-3. Small Circulation and Qì network (Xiǎozhōutiān Yǔ Jīngluòxué, 小周天與經絡學)

Qì Network

1. **Diaphragm** (Héng Gé Mó, 橫膈膜, Junction of Upper and Lower Level Qì)
   A. The diaphragm is a good electric conductor sandwiched between fasciae, which are poor conductors. This area acts as a battery to store Fire Qì (Huǒqì, 火氣), and is called the Middle Dāntián (Zhōng Dāntián, 中丹田).
   B. It divides the body into upper and lower bodies, in terms of Qì. The chest area above it is where the External Qì (Wàiqì, 外氣, oxygen and carbon dioxide) is exchanged. The diaphragm pumps the air in and out. The stomach and abdomen below the diaphragm constitute the biobattery where Internal Qì (Nèiqì, 內氣, bioelectricity) is stored. This Lower Dāntián (Xià Dāntián, 下丹田) produces Qì and stores it. The abdomen is the Qì pump, while the Huìyīn (Co-1, 會陰, perineum) is the controlling gate which regulates its flow.
   C. External Qì (air) and internal Qì (bioelectricity) are closely related to one other. Oxygen (air) and bioelectricity are proportional to each other. When oxygen supply is more abundant, more glucose will be converted into Qì to manifest as physical action, heat, and light.
   D. When too much Qì accumulates at the Middle Dāntián, the heartbeat will be faster and the breathing heavier, disturbing the Emotional Mind.

2. **Jīng** (Primary Qì channels, 經)

A. There are twelve primary Qì channels, six Yīn and six Yáng. They act as rivers which follow the limbs and distribute Qì throughout the body. Three Yáng (large intestines, Triple Burner, and small intestines) and three Yīn (lungs, pericardium and heart) channels connect six internal organs with the upper extremities. Another three Yáng (stomach, bladder, and gall bladder) and three Yīn (spleen, kidneys, and liver) channels connect the other six internal organs with the lower extremities. When Qì circulation stagnates in these rivers, sickness is initiated.

B. The heart, lungs, and pericardium coexist and are isolated from the other organs by the diaphragm. These three Yīn organs are closely related and harmonize with each other. For example, when the heart beats faster, the breathing is faster. When the breathing is slower, the heartbeat slows. The pericardium acts as a cooler for the heart which, like a car engine, needs a radiator to maintain its function. These three Yīn organs are connected to the thumb (lungs), middle finger (pericardium), and pinky (heart) and to three Yáng organs, namely the large intestine (index finger), triple burner (middle finger), and small intestine (pinky).

3. **Luò** (Secondary Qì channels, 絡)

A. There are millions of secondary channels, called Luò, branching out like streams from the primary channels and distributing Qì throughout the body. They are like capillaries in the blood system. They branch out from the primary channels, circulating Qì laterally.

B. Luò connect the primary channels to the skin surface and bone marrow, and to the organs. When more Qì is led out through the Luò from the primary Qì channels (Jīng), the Guardian Qì (Wèiqì, 衛氣) is strengthened, Qì manifests more externally, so the body becomes warmer. When more Qì is led in through Luò from the primary Qì channels, the Marrow Qì (Suǐqì, 髓氣) is enhanced. More Qì is stored internally and physical manifestation is weakened, so you feel chilly.

C. When exhalation is longer than inhalation, more Qì is led out and manifested. When inhalation is longer than exhalation, more Qì is led in and stored. With the sounds of Hā (哈) and Hēng (哼), manifestation and storage are more effective.

4. **Mài** (Vessels, 脈)
   Vessels (Mài, 脈) are like reservoirs which regulate Qì in the Twelve Primary Channels. One of the oldest Chinese medical books, *Nànjīng* (難經), said, "Mài includes strange meridians eight vessels, which do not belong to the Twelve Meridians."[1] Lǐ, Shí-Zhēn (李時珍) also explains in his book, *The Study of Strange Meridians and Eight Vessels* (*Qíjīng Bāmài Kǎo,* 奇經八脈考), "Strange meridians include eight vessels which are not restrained like twelve meridians. There is no matching and coordination on the surface or internally, so they are called strange."[2]
   Chinese medicine recognizes the importance of the Conception and Governing Vessels (任脈・督脈) used in acupuncture practice. That is why, together with the Twelve Primary Qì Channels (Shíèrjīng, 十二經), they are commonly called Fourteen Channels (Shísìjīng, 十四經) in Chinese acupuncture. Due to limited understanding of the other six vessels, acupuncture usually does not manipulate them. In the book *The Study of Practical Chinese Medical Qìgōng* (實用中醫氣功學), it says, "Governing Vessel originates from Huìyīn, Qì moves up the back of the body, and is the total governor of the Yáng vessels. Therefore, it is called the ocean of the Yáng vessel. Conception Vessel begins from Huìyīn, (Qì) circulates along the abdomen up the front of the body and is responsible for all Yīn vessels. Therefore, it is called ocean of the Yīn vessels. If one circulates Qì smoothly in these two, then hundreds of vessels all transport. Qì circulates through the body without hindrance or stagnation. The Dào of longevity depends on this."[3,4]

How do these two vessels control the Qì status of the whole body? Let us conclude this from available documents.

Conception Vessel—Ocean of Yīn Vessels (Rènmài, 任脈) (陰脈之海) (Figure 5-1)[4,5]

1. This vessel circulates right at the center of the chest and abdomen to meet three Yīn primary Qì channels of the feet (liver, spleen, and kidneys) at Zhōngjí (Co-3, 中極) and Guānyuán (Co-4, 關元) cavities. It joins Yáng Línking Vessel (Yángwéimài, 陽維脈) at Tiāntū (Co-22, 天突) and Liánquán (Co-23, 廉泉) cavities, and connects with Thrusting Vessel (Chōngmài, 衝脈) at Yīnjiāo (Co-7, 陰交).
2. The three Yīn primary Qì channels of the feet join the three Yīn primary Qì channels of the hands (heart, lungs, and pericardium). Through this network, the Conception Vessel regulates all six Yīn channels.

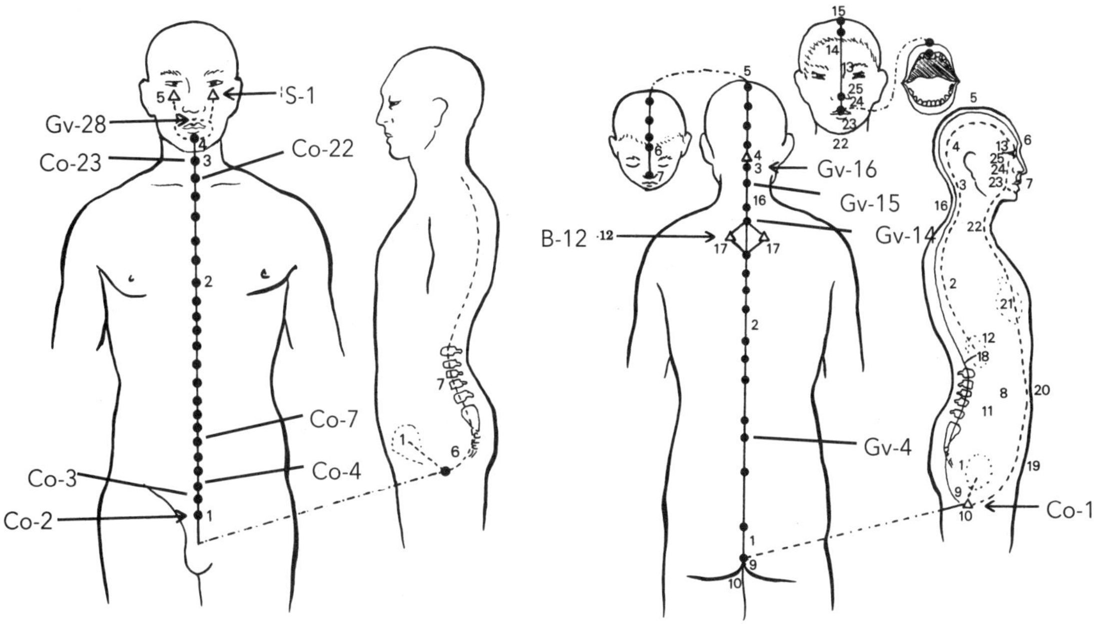

Figure 5-1. Conception Vessel (Rènmài)- Ocean of Yīn Vessels

Figure 5-2. Governing Vessel (Dūmài)–Ocean of Yáng Vessels

Governing Vessel—Ocean of Yáng Vessels (Dūmài, 督脈) (陽脈之海) (Figure 5-2)[4,6]

1. This vessel circulates right at the center of the back. It meets several times with the six Yáng primary Qì channels of the hands and feet. The most central place is Dàzhuī (Gv-14, 大椎) cavity. All three Yáng channels of the hands and feet meet here.
2. The Girdle Vessel (Dàimài, 帶脈) begins below the hypochondrium at the level of the 2nd lumbar vertebra connecting to Mìngmén (Gv-4, 命門), and encircles the waist like a girdle or belt. Yáng Línking Vessel (Yángwéimài, 陽維脈) also connects to the Governing Vessel (Dūmài, 督脈) at Fēngfǔ (Gv-16, 風府) and Yǎmén (Gv-15, 啞門). In this way, the Governing Vessel governs the function of the Yáng vessels.

Mài and Internal Elixir Meditation

How important are the vessels to Internal Elixir (Nèidān, 內丹) practice? Lǐ, Shí-Zhēn (李時珍, 1518–1593 CE) explains this in his book, *The Study of Strange Meridians and Eight Vessels* (*Qíjīng Bāmài Kǎo*, 奇經八脈考): "The Eight Vessels introduced in all existing books are too brief and not understood in detail. So for those doctors who do not know them, it is harder to explore the origin of sickness. For those immortal family (Qìgōng practitioners for enlightenment) who do not know them, it is hard to install the furnace and tripod (position spirit and Qì). Shi-Zhen is not wise, so refers to all available discussions and gathers information here, so those immortal family and doctors can use it. If those doctors know these Eight Vessels, then the major contents of Twelve Primary Qì Channels and fifteen secondary Qì channels can be understood. If those immortal researchers know these Eight Vessels, then the marvelousness of ascending and descending, tiger and dragon, and the hidden profound detail of Xuánpìn can be obtained."[7] Xuánpìn (玄牝) is what is called Tàijí (Grand Ultimate, 太極) in the *Yìjīng* (*Book of Changes*). This Tàijí is the Dào (道) of lives in the great nature. Therefore, Xuánpìn can be called the root of creation, variation, bearing, and raising of millions of lives. It is the mother of millions of objects of heaven and earth, another name for Dào.

Finally, I summarize the key points of the Eight Vessels.

1. **Conception Vessel** (Rènmài, 任脈)
   a. A Yīn vessel which balances the Qì status of the Yáng Governing Vessel.
   b. Responsible for regulating Qì in the six Yīn primary channels. When Qì is abundant, it circulates smoothly in the six Yīn primary Qì channels.
   c. With the Yáng Governing Vessel, it completes the Small Circulation. When Qì circulates smoothly in Small Circulation, the physical body can be conditioned and health improved. Small Circulation is the Fire Path (Huǒlù, 火路) of Internal Elixir (Nèidān, 內丹) practice. Qì circulates strongly in the Fire Path during the daytime.

2. **Governing Vessel** (Dūmài, 督脈)
   a. A Yáng vessel which balances the Qì status of the Yīn Conception Vessel.
   b. Governs and regulates the Qì in the six primary Yáng Qì channels. When Qì is abundant in this vessel, it circulates smoothly in the six primary Yáng Qì channels.
   c. With the Yīn Conception Vessel, it completes the Small Circulation.

3. **Thrusting Vessel** (Chōngmài, 衝脈)
   a. The main section of the Thrusting Vessel is the spinal cord, which connects the brain (Upper Dāntián) with the second brain (Real Lower Dāntián), constituting the central Qì system. Upper and lower brains are the two poles of this system.

b. Qì circulates strongly at night, and the brain obtains its energetic nourishment at this time. Due to abundant Qì supply at night, hormone production is enhanced, and the pituitary and pineal glands, adrenals, testicles, and ovaries function fully.

c. This path is responsible for spiritual growth, while the Small Circulation accounts for physical life. So circulating Qì in the Thrusting Vessel (Water Path) is for spiritual cultivation (Marrow/Brain Washing), while circulating it in the Small Circulation (Fire Path) is for physical conditioning (Muscle/Tendon Changing).

d. Among the Eight Vessels, this vessel is classified as extreme Yīn and balances the Girdle Vessel which is classified as extreme Yáng. When Qì accumulates here, the body is calm, and the marrow and brain obtain nourishment (marrow washing).

e. This central energy line gives a feeling of being centered.

4. **Girdle Vessel** (Dàimài, 帶脈)

a. This vessel's Qì circulates strongly whenever you are standing up. This gives a feeling of physical and mental balance, from which you find your center. This vessel is classified as extreme Yáng and balances the Thrusting Vessel. One provides balance, while the other provides a centered feeling. Thus, though there are two vessels, they function as one.

b. The Qì circulating in this vessel is responsible for the body's Guardian Qì (Wèiqì, 衛氣). When this Qì expands abundantly, you are more balanced and the immune system functions well.

c. How much the Guardian Qì can expand depends on the amount of Qì stored in the Real Lower Dāntián. The more Qì stored in the Real Lower Dāntián, the more healthy, balanced, and centered you are.

5. **Yīn Heel Vessel** (Yīnqiāomài, 陰蹺脈) and Yīn Línking Vessel (Yīnwéimài, 陰維脈)

a. These two vessels connect at the Huìyīn (Co-1) (會陰) with the Conception and Thrusting Vessels. At the bottom, they connect to the concave area of the feet. When sexual energy is strong, the Qì stored in these two vessels is strong, manifesting as the strength of the legs. When sexual energy is depleted, the legs are weak.

b. These two vessels balance the Qì status of the Yáng Heel and Yáng Línking Vessels. While the Yīn vessels store the Qì, the Yáng vessels manifest it.

6. **Yáng Heel Vessel** (Yángqiāomài, 陽蹻脈) and Yáng Línking Vessel (Yángwéimài, 陽維脈)
   a. These two vessels balance the Qì status of the Yīn Heel and Yīn Línking Vessels. While the Yīn vessels store Qì, the Yáng vessels manifest it. When the Qì is strong, the lower part of the body will be strong.
   b. These two Yáng vessels balance the above two Yīn vessels. Though physically they are two, in function they are one.

Zǐ and Wǔ Major Qì Flow (Zǐwǔ Líúzhù, 子午流注)

To understand the Qì network, recognize that the body is alive and the Qì circulation in it is affected by nature. This relationship with the cycles of nature is called Zǐwǔ Líúzhù (子午流注), which you need to follow to circulate Qì efficiently.

Zǐ (子) is the period between 11 pm and 1 am, and Wǔ (午) is the period between 11 am and 1 pm Líú (流) means flow, and Zhù (注) means tendency. So Zǐwǔ Líúzhù (子午流注) means "the major Qì flow tendency which follows the time changes."

The *Inner Classic* (*Nèijīng*, 內經) calls this the correspondence of heaven and man.[8] The major Qì flows of the Twelve Primary Qì Channels differ from each other. Qì flowing in the Conception and Governing Vessels (Fire Path) is also affected by the natural cycle. As it circulates, the Qì level in one part of the path is always higher than elsewhere. This area of stronger Qì moves around the path regularly, completing a cycle every twenty-four hours. It is this area of higher Qì potential which keeps the Qì flowing. Just as water only flows from a higher to a lower level, Qì only moves from a place of higher potential to one of lower potential.

Great Collection of Golden Elixir (Jīndān Dàchéng Jí, 金丹大成集) said, "Zǐ and Wǔ are the middle points of heaven and earth. In heaven, they are the sun and the moon; in humans, they are the heart and kidneys; in time, they are Zǐ (子, midnight) and Wǔ (午, noon); in the Eight Trigrams, they are Kǎn (Water, 坎) and Lí (Fire, 離); in orientation, they are the south and the north."[9] Also, Dr. Yáng, Jì-Zhōu (楊繼洲, 1522–1620 CE) explained in his book, The *Complete Book of Acupuncture and Moxibustion* (Zhēnjiǔ Dàchéng, 針灸大成), "Conception and Governing Vessels of a human body, back and front are analogous to nature's Zǐ-Wǔ (midnight-noon, 子午). If analogous to south and north, they can be divided and combined. When divided, Yīn and Yáng are not disordered, and when combined, they coordinate seamlessly with each other. One is two and two is one."[10] In the Small Circulation Fire Path, Qì circulates more strongly in the Conception Vessel (Rènmài, 任脈) than in the Governing Vessel (Dūmài, 督脈) during daytime, while it circulates more strongly in the Governing Vessel at night. It seems they are two vessels, but in function they are one, since they belong to the same circuit.

Lǐ, Shí-Zhēn (李時珍, 1518–1593 CE) discussed this in *The Study of Strange Meridians and Eight Vessels* (*Qíjīng Bāmài Kǎo*, 奇經八脈考): "Conception and Governing

Vessels are the body's Zǐ-Wǔ (子午). It is the Dào of ascending and descending of Yánghuǒ (陽火) and Yīnfú (陰符), used by the Elixir Family (Dānjiā, 丹家, Qìgōng society). It is the key place of Kǎn and Lí."[11] Yánghuǒ (Yáng fire, 陽火) means the way to increase the body's fire to make it more Yáng. Yīnfú (Yīn magic water, 陰符) is the way to enhance the body's water, making its Yáng more Yīn. Fú (符) is the magic water (Fúshuǐ, 符水) for curing disease.

In the Fire Path, the major Qì flow at noon is at the Middle Dāntián (Zhōng Dāntián, 中丹田). It moves down to the Lower Dāntián between 2 and 4 pm It goes down to Huìyīn (Co-1, 會陰) at sunset and moves to the back in the evening, reaching the top of the Bǎihuì (Gv-20, 百會) at midnight. At sunrise, the Qì is in the face, and by noon, it has reached the Middle Dāntián to complete the cycle. This cycle is used by martial artists for vital cavity strikes (Diǎnxuè, 點穴) (Figure 5-3).

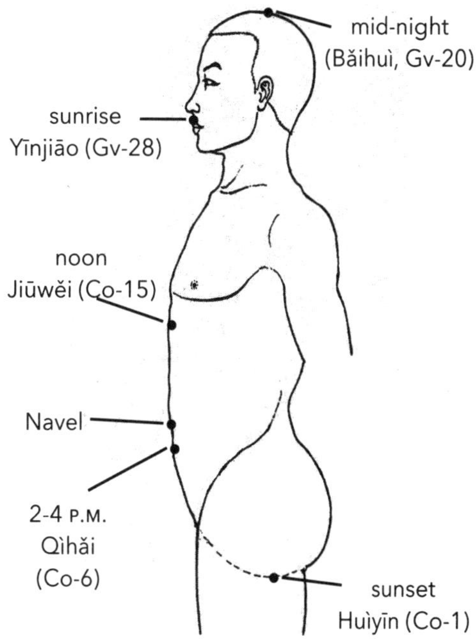

Figure 5-3. Natural Qì Circulation in the Fire Path

Cavities Related to Meditation 靜坐有關之穴道

Let us summarize the important cavities used in Small Circulation practice, so it will be easier to follow the discussion in the rest of the book.

1. **Shàng Dāntián** (Upper Elixir Field, 上丹田)
   The whole brain is regarded as the Upper Dāntián. Brain cells are highly conductive and can store and consume a lot of electricity. The space between the two hemispheres of the brain is called the Spiritual Valley (Shéngǔ, 神谷) where the Valley Spirit (Gǔshén, 谷神) resides. At the bottom center of the valley, where the pituitary and pineal glands are situated, is the Mud Pill Palace (Níwángōng, 泥丸宮). The brain is responsible for conscious thought, while this space without any brain cells is related to your subconscious mind. It is where you connect with nature since birth. While your conscious mind is in the false human matrix, your subconscious mind is free and truthful.
   Bǎihuì (Gv-20, 百會) at the crown and Yìntáng (M-NH-3, 印堂, third eye) are the two gates where your spirit communicates with the natural energy and spirit. Though Bǎihuì is open, Yìntáng has been sealed in humans for a long time.

2. **Zhōng Dāntián** (Middle Elixir Field, 中丹田)

   There are different opinions about the location of the Middle Dāntián. Some documents believe Shānzhōng (Co-17, 膻中) is the Middle Dāntián since behind it is the thymus gland, related to your heart (Emotional Mind). Others claim the heart itself is the Middle Dāntián since it relates to your Emotional Mind and stores Post-birth Fire Qì. Still others believe that Jiūwěi (Co-15, 鳩尾, Wide Pigeon's Tail, lower sternum) is where it is located (Figure 5-4).

   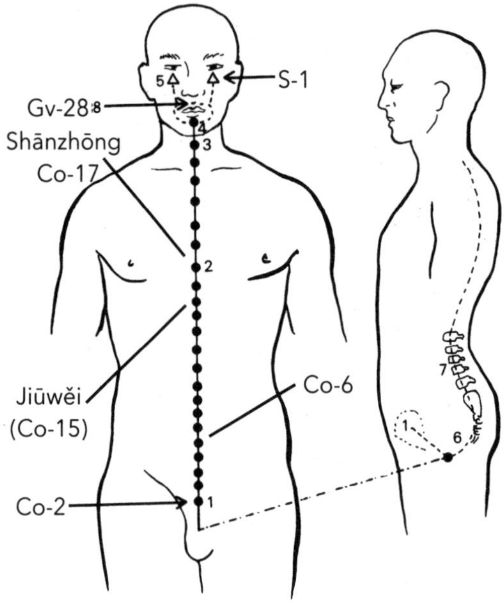

   Figure 5-4. Shānzhōng (Co-17) and Jiūwěi (Co-15)

   Looking at the body's structure, we see the diaphragm, a good electric conductor, sandwiched between fasciae (poor conductors) on both sides. This is like a battery, able to store charge to an abundant level. It is between the lungs where air is exchanged and the stomach where food is converted, so Post-birth Qì can be stored to a high level. Qì stored in this area also affects the Emotional Mind.

3. **Jiǎ Xiàdāntián** (False Lower Elixir Field, 假下丹田)

   The False Lower Dāntián is located about two inches below the navel in the abdominal area. This is Qìhǎi (Ocean of Qì, Co-6, 氣海) in Chinese medicine (Figure 5-5). Daoists call it Dānlú (Elixir Furnace, 丹爐). These names indicate that this area can produce Qì (grow elixir) as abundantly as the ocean.

   When you move your abdomen up and down through Abdominal Breathing, you produce Qì. This movement is called Qǐhuǒ (起火), which means to "start the fire." Two ways of breathing build up the fire and store Qì. One is Normal Abdominal Breathing (Zhèng Fùhūxī, 正腹呼吸), the other Reverse Abdominal Breathing (Fǎn, Nì Fùhūxī, 反・逆腹呼吸). Abdominal Breathing is also called Returning to Childhood Breathing (Fǎntóng Hūxī, 返童呼吸) or Post-Heaven Breathing (Xiāntiān Hūxī, 先天呼吸). A fetus uses this pumping movement to suck in nutrition and oxygen from its mother through the umbilical cord. Most small children retain this habit of abdominal movement. These two ways of breathing have been discussed in section 4-3 and will be scientifically analyzed in the next section.

4. **Zhēn Xiàdāntián** (Real Lower Elixir Field, 真下丹田)
Daoists regard the regular Lower Dāntián at the abdomen as the false one. The real one is inside the body under the stomach, in front of the kidneys (Nèishèn, 內腎), and above the External Kidneys (Wàishèn, 外腎, testicles). The Real Lower Dāntián is the Large and Small Intestines where the second brain or biobattery is located, as understood by scientists today (Figure 5-5). Daoists regard the regular Lower Dāntián as false because when Qì accumulates there, it automatically enters the Conception Vessel and disperses into the Twelve Primary Qì Channels. So, though it generates Qì and stores it to some degree, it cannot reach an abundant level. Though Qì stored at the False Lower Dāntián is beneficial for health, it is not enough for spiritual enlightenment. The Real Lower Dāntián is the lower pole of the central energy line, connected with the brain (Upper Dāntián) through the spinal cord (Thrusting Vessel). To have enough Qì to nourish the brain for spiritual enlightenment, first condition your biobattery and store Qì there to an abundant level.

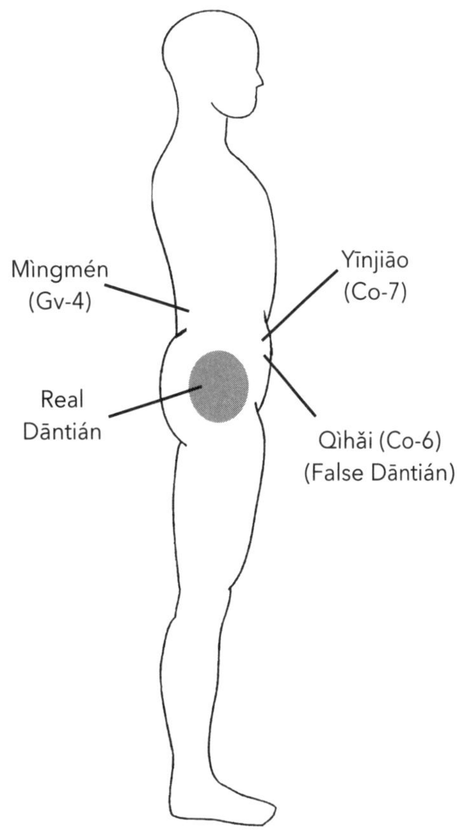

Figure 5-5. Real and False Lower Dāntián

The document Observing Vessels (Màiwàng, 脈望) says, "(Real) Dāntián is the root of life. This is why Daoists who meditate for spiritual cultivation and Buddhists who meditate for Buddhahood all gather real Qì (Original Qì) under the navel. There is a Spiritual Turtle (Shénguī, 神龜) in the Dāntián which inhales and exhales this Real Qì (Zhēnqì, 真氣). This respiration is not breathing through the mouth and nose, which are only the doors for respiration. Dāntián is the origin of Qì and the place for those holy men to begin their cultivation. This is the place where they keep and store the Real Oneness (Zhēnyī), so it is called Embryonic Breathing."[12]

Zhēnyī (真一) means Real One or True Singularity, namely the central Qì system constituted by the Two Poles. The Yáng pole at the Real Lower Dāntián provides the quantity of Qì, and the Yīn pole at the Upper Dāntián controls the quality of its manifestation as life (spirit). Physically there are Two Poles, but in function there is only one, since they are the Yīn and Yáng of the same thing. If you keep your mind in this Real One or True Singularity, you raise your Spirit of Vitality (Jīngshén, 精神) and establish abundant Qì storage.

5. **Huángtíng** (Yellow Yard, 黃庭)

Huángtíng (黃庭) can imply various places in the body. Líáng, Qiū-Zi (梁丘子) interpreted Huángtíng in Classic of Huángtíng's Internal Scene (Huángtíng Nèijǐng Jīng, 黃庭內景經): "Yellow (Huang), is the middle (color) of colors. Yard (Ting) is the center of a square. Externally, it means the center of heaven (Tiānzhōng, 天中), the center of a man (Rénzhōng, 人中), and the center of the earth (Dìzhōng, 地中). Internally, it means the center of the brain (Nǎozhōng, 腦中), the center of the heart (Xīnzhōng, 心中), and the center of the spleen (Pízhōng, 脾中)."[13] So Huángtíng can imply the center of many things.

Shí, Hé-Yáng (石和陽) interpreted Huángtíng in *Classic of Huángtíng's External Scene* (*Huángtíng Wàijǐng Jīng*, 黃庭外景經): "Above Mìngmén, there are two esoteric marvelous apertures, left is Xuán (玄) and right is Pìn (two internal kidneys, 牝). There is an empty place between named Huángtíng."[14]

The document *Secret Recording of Nourishing Life* (*Yǎngshēng Mìlù. Jīndān Wèndá,* 養生秘錄・金丹問答) said, "Where exactly is Huángtíng? Above the bladder, under the spleen, in front of the kidneys, left of the liver, and right of the lungs."[15] So Huángtíng is the center of where the internal organs are located (i.e., center of gravity).

Huángtíng is also called *Yùhuánxuè* (*Jade Ring Cavity,* 玉環穴), the name first used in the *Illustration of Brass Acupuncture and Moxibustion* (*Tóngrén Yúxuè Zhēnjiǔ Tú*, 銅人俞穴針灸圖) by Dr. Wáng, Wéi-Yī (王唯一). The Daoist book Wánglù Shíyú (王錄識餘) said, "In the Illustration of Brass Acupuncture and Moxibustion it was recorded that within the body's cavities of viscera and bowels, there is a Jade Ring (Yùhuán), but I do not know what the Jade Ring is." Later, Zhāng, Zǐ-Yáng (張紫陽) described the place the immortals use to form the elixir: "The heart is on top, the kidneys are underneath, the spleen is to the left, and the liver is to the right. The life door (Shēngmén, 生門, navel) is in front, the closed door is to the rear, they are connected like a ring, white like cotton, an inch in diameter. It encompasses the Essence and the refinement of the whole body. It is opposite the navel and is the root of life. This is the Jade Ring."[16] "The life door is in the front means the Qì door is open in front, and closed to the rear. This concept was also confirmed in the document Muscle/Tendon Changing Classic; Appendix (Yìjīnjīng·Fùlù, 易筋經・附錄).[17] Mìhù (密戶) means Concealed Door (Mìngmén, Gv-4, 命門) located between L2 and L3 vertebrae (Figure 5-6). Some believe Huángtíng is actually the second brain, the Real Lower Dāntián (Zhēn Xiàdāntián, 真下丹田) or biobattery of the body. This place is the center of gravity which stores abundant Qì or bioelectricity.

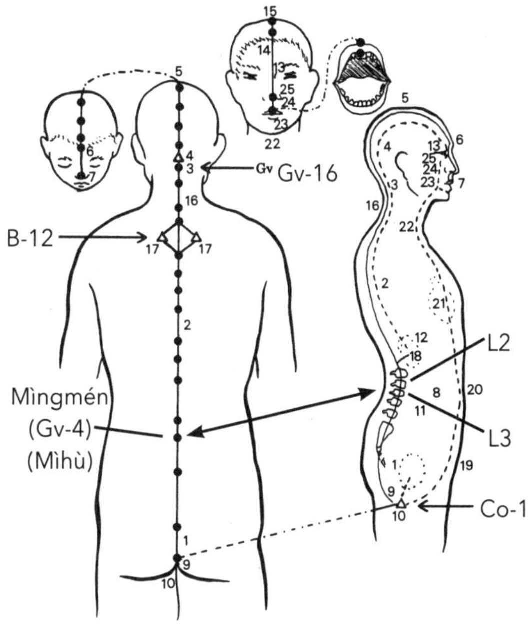

Figure 5-6. Mìhù (Mìngmén, Gv-4)

Other documents claim Huángtíng to be between the kidneys, while others place it under the heart. I believe Huángtíng means the place above the Real Lower Dāntián, behind the navel, and in front of the kidneys. In Daoist spiritual enlightenment practice, this is where Kǎn and Lí interact. Water Qì is stored at the Real Lower Dāntián while Fire Qì is accumulated at the Middle Dāntián. Water and Fire Qì interact at Huángtíng, to conceive the Spiritual Embryo.

6. **Bǎihuì** (Gv-20, 百會, Hundred Meetings)

   Bǎihuì is located on top of the head and is where the whole body's Qì gathers (hundred meetings). This is the most Yáng part of the body, just as Huìyīn (Co-1, 會陰, perineum) is the most Yīn part of the body. Through the Thrusting Vessel, these two cavities connect to each other (Figure 5-7). When Qì manifests at Bǎihuì, the spirit (Shén, 神) can be raised high and the body's Qì governed efficiently by the mind.

   Bǎihuì is the gate where the spirit exits and enters. Through it, the spirit leaves the body and enters to return to its residence, the Mud Pill Palace (Níwángōng, 泥丸宮).

7. **Yìntáng** (M-NH-3, 印堂, Sealed Hall)

   Yìntáng (M-NH-3, 印堂) cavity, as it is called in Chinese medicine, is called Tiānyǎn or Tiānmù (天眼・天目, Heaven Eye) in Daoist society, and the "third eye" in the West (Figure 5-8). It is called Heaven Eye because when it is open, you can communicate with the Qì and spirit of heaven. You can communicate telepathically with other living beings. You are enlightened, knowing many

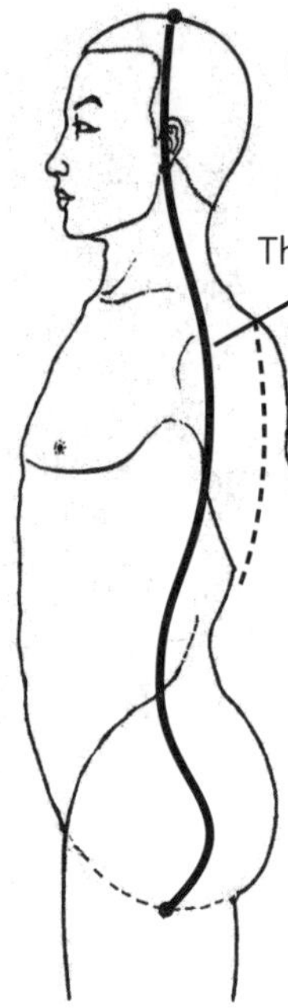

Figure 5-7. Bǎihuì (Gv-20) and Huìyīn (Co-1) connected by Thrusting Vessel

natural secrets and seeing true reality. This is a paired cavity with Qiángjiān (Gv-18, 強間). These two cavities are located at the end of the Spiritual Valley (Shéngǔ, 神谷).

8. **Yínjiāo** (Gv-28, 齦交, Gum Junction) (Figure 5-8)
   This is the last cavity in the Governing Vessel (Dūmài, 督脈), and it connects with the Conception Vessel (Rènmài, 任脈). Yīnjiāo cavity is the junction or bridge connecting the Yīn Conception and Yáng Governing vessels.
9. **Rénzhōng** (Gv-26, 人中, Philtrum) or Shuǐgōu (水溝, Water Ditch) (Figure 5-8)
   This cavity under the nose is also called Shuǐgōu (水溝, water ditch). It is a matching cavity with Nǎohù (Gv-17, 腦戶, Brain's Household) at the top of the neck. It connects with the conscious mind, and when one is unconscious, pressing this cavity can awaken you.
10. **Tiāntū** (Co-22, 天突, Heaven's Prominence) (Figure 5-8)
    Tiāntū is at the bottom of the throat. When attacked, breathing capability can be affected. Its Qì corresponds with that of Dàzhuī (Gv-14, 大椎) on the back.
11. **Jiūwěi** (Co-15, 鳩尾, Wide Pigeon's Tail or Xīnkǎn (心坎, Heart Pit) (Figure 5-9)
    Jiūwěi is at the bottom of the sternum. It is connected with the heart and with Língtái (Gv-10, 靈臺), its paired cavity on the back. When these two cavities are struck at noon time, heart attack can occur. Jiūwěi is called Xīnkǎn (心坎) in Chinese martial arts society.
12. **Zhōngwǎn** (Co-12, 中脘, Middle Cavity, Solar Plexus) (Figure 5-9)
    Zhōngwǎn is at the solar plexus and is called "center" in Qìgōng society. Behind it is the Huángtíng (黃庭) cavity. Through Yīn and Yáng interaction of Fire and Water Qì at Huángtíng, the Spiritual Embryo is conceived.
    This cavity is one of the vital cavities in martial arts society. When struck

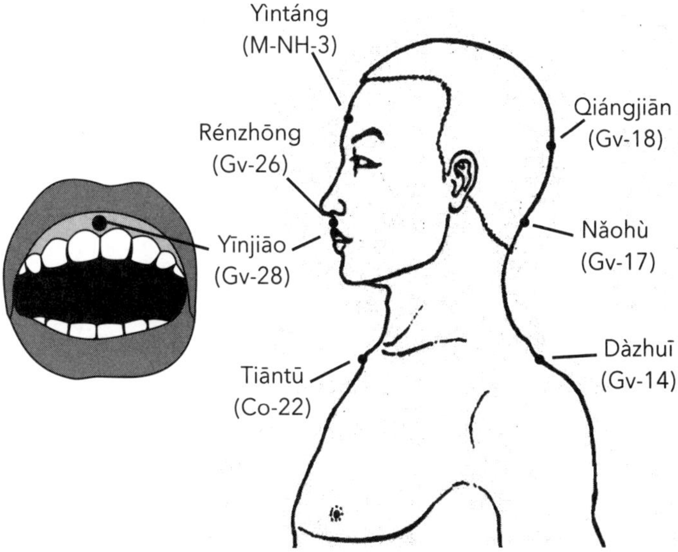

Figure 5-8. Yìntáng (M-NH-3), Qiangjian (Gv-18), Yínjiāo (Gv-28), Rénzhōng (Gv-26), Nǎohù (Gv-17), Tiāntū (Co-22), and Dàzhuī (Gv-14)

upward with force, heart attack can occur. When struck straight forward, nausea can occur. When struck downward, the lungs can be sealed and breathing prevented.

13. **Abdomen Yīnjiāo** (Co-7, 陰交, Yīn Junction) (Figure 5-9)
    This should not be confused with Yínjiāo (Gv-28) at the mouth. This cavity is the junction of the Yīn Conception Vessel and Yīn Thrusting Vessel. It connects to the Real Lower Dāntián and allows Qì to enter and exit from the human biobattery. It is a paired cavity with Mìngmén (Gv-4, 命門, Life's Door) located between L2 and L3 vertebrae.
14. **Qìhǎi** (Co-6, 氣海, Sea of Qì) (Figure 5-9)
    Qìhǎi is about two inches below the navel and regarded as the False Lower Dāntián in Daoist society. It is also called Elixir Furnace (Dānlú, 丹爐), since it produces Qì. When moved up and down, fat (food essence) is converted into Qì.

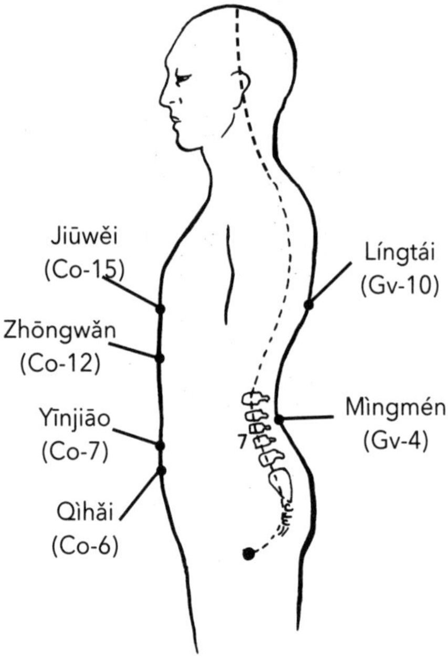

Figure 5-9. Jiūwěi (Co-15), Língtái (Gv-10), Zhōngwǎn (Co-12), Abdomen Yínjiāo (Co-7), Mìngmén (Gv-4), and Qìhǎi (Co-6)

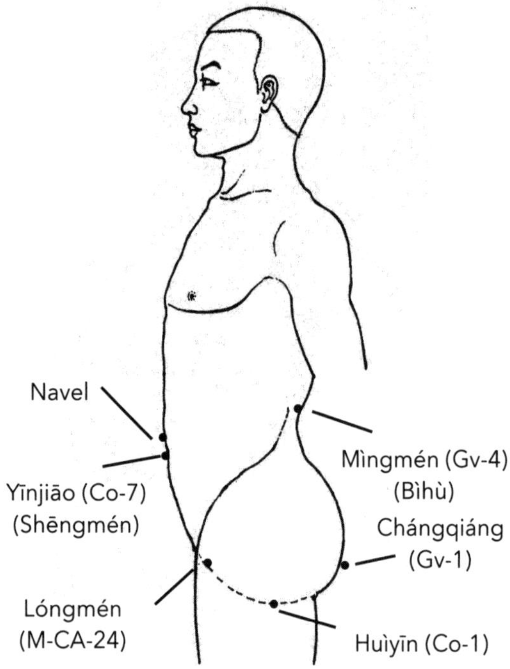

Figure 5-10. Lóngmén (M-CA-24), Chángqiáng (Gv-1), Huìyīn (Co-1)

15. **Lóngmén** (M-CA-24, 龍門, Dragon's Gate) or Xiàyīn (Low Yīn, 下陰) (Figure 5-10)
    The groin area is called Lóngmén. It is also called Xiàyīn (Low Yīn, 下陰) since the Qì here is Yīn. It and Chángqiáng (Gv-1, 長強, Long Strength; or Wěilǘ, 尾閭, Coccyx) are considered to be a pair of corresponding Qì cavities.
16. **Huìyīn** (Co-1, 會陰, perineum) (Figure 5-10)
    Huìyīn means to Meet Yīn, since it connects the four main Yīn vessels, Conception, Thrusting, Yīn-Heel, and Yīn-Línking Vessels. It is regarded as a secret gate (Qiàomén, 竅門) in Internal Elixir Qìgōng. When opened (pushed out), Qì stored in the body can be released, and when closed (held up), Qì can be retained and stored. This gate is the pump of the body's inner Qì, which controls Qì storage and manifestation. This cavity and Bǎihuì (Gv-20, 百會, Hundred Meetings) are corresponding paired gates in the body's central Qì system.

17. **Chángqiáng** (Gv-1, 長強, Long Strength) or Wěilǘ (Coccyx, 尾閭) (Figure 5-10)
    Chángqiáng is the first gate obstructing the path of Small Circulation meditation. The Qì passage is narrow here due to the structure of the area. Since there is little conductive muscle or tendon here, the passage of this area becomes narrower as one gets older. To widen this gate is the first task of Small Circulation. This is the first dangerous gate. When one does not know the correct way to lead Qì past it, the Qì can flow into the legs instead, damaging the nerves.

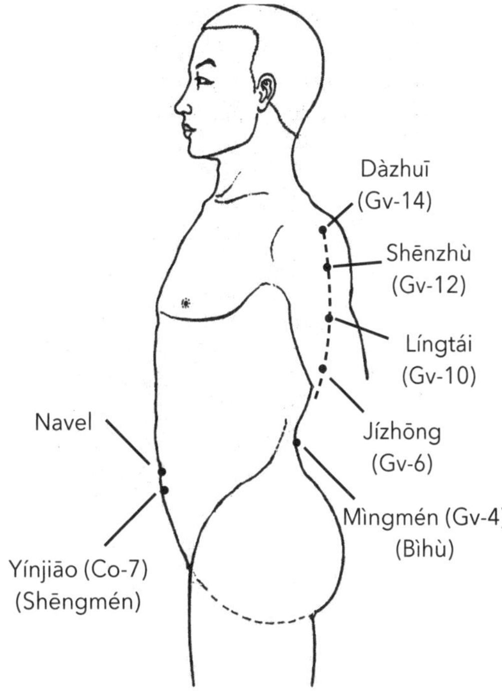

Figure 5-11. Mìngmén (Gv-4), Yīnjiāo (Co-7), Jízhōng (Gv-6), Língtái (Gv-10), Shēnzhù (Gv-12), and Dàzhuī (Gv-14)

18. **Mìngmén** (Gv-4, 命門, Life Door) (Figure 5-11)
    Mìngmén means Life Door, connected to the Real Lower Dāntián. It should not be confused with Gv-10 behind the back, called Língtái (靈臺) in medical society but Mìngmén by martial arts society.
    Mìngmén is a corresponding cavity with Yīnjiāo (Co-7, 陰交) at the abdominal area. Qì stored at the Real Lower Dāntián can be led either from Yīnjiāo or from Mìngmén to enter the Small Circulation orbit.
19. **Jízhōng** (Gv-6, 脊中, Mid-spine) (Figure 5-11)
    Jízhōng is located at the middle of the spine. It is a Qì turning point for beginners in Small Circulation practice.
20. **Língtái** (Gv-10, 靈臺, Spiritual Platform) or Jiájí (Squeeze the spine, 夾脊) or Mìngmén (Life Door, 命門) (Figure 5-11)
    Língtái is a Chinese medical name. Due to its location between the shoulder blades, it is called Jiájí (squeeze the spine) in Daoist society. It is often called Mìngmén (Life Door) in martial arts society, because when it is struck at the right time, the heart can be shocked.
    Língtái is the second dangerous gate or obstacle in Small Circulation meditation. There is no anatomic structure to cause Qì stagnation, but it is connected to the heart. When excess Qì is led there, it can go to the heart and make it

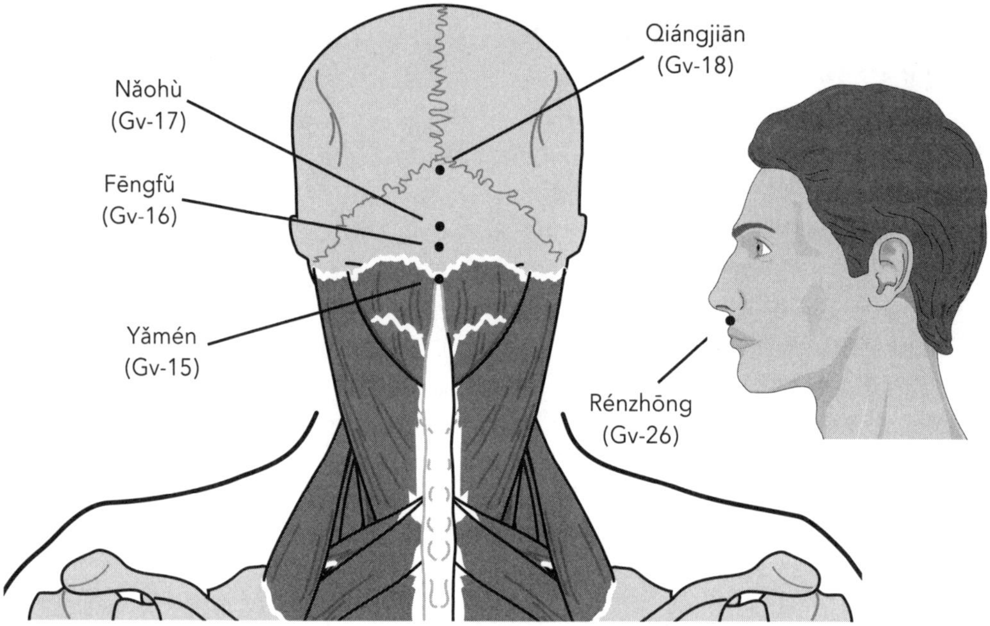

Figure 5-12. Yǎmén (Gv-15), Fengfu (Gv-16), Rénzhōng (Gv-26), Nǎohù (Gv-17), and Qiángjiān (Gv-18)

too Yáng, causing faster heartbeat. This may induce one to pay attention to the heart and thus lead more Qì there, precipitating a heart attack. So it is a dangerous cavity. When you practice, beware of it. If the heartbeat increases, simply ignore it and continue leading Qì up the spine.

21. **Shēnzhù** (Gv-12, 身柱, Body Pillar) and Dàzhuī (Gv-14, 大椎, Big Vertebra) (Figure 5-11)
    Both Shēnzhù and Dàzhuī cavities can be used as turning points, because they join the path of the spine with that of the arms. Any Qì stagnation can be removed easily.
22. **Yǎmén** (Gv-15, 啞門, Door of Muteness) (Figure 5-12)
    Yǎmén is at the rear center of the neck. Neck movement easily removes stagnant Qì in this area, so it can also be used as a Qì turning point.
23. **Fēngfǔ** (Gv-16, 風府, Wind Dwelling) (Figure 5-12)
    Fēngfǔ is a paired cavity with Rénzhōng (Gv-26, 人中) and is located exactly opposite it. It is a major cavity for treatment of stiff neck, numbness of the limbs, common cold, headache, stroke, and mental illness.

24. **Nǎohù** (Gv-17, 腦戶, Brain's Household) or Yùzhěn (Jade Pillow, 玉枕) (Figure 5-12)
    Nǎohù is about one inch above Fēngfǔ, also called Jade Pillow (Yùzhěn, 玉枕) by Daoist society. It is the Third Gate of Small Circulation practice. When abundant Qì reaches this cavity, excess Qì may enter and cause brain damage, so one needs caution here. We discuss the Three Gates (Sānguān, 三關) in more detail later.
25. **Qiángjiān** (Gv-18, 強間, Between Strength) (Figure 5-12)
    Qiángjiān is opposite the Heaven Eye (Tiānyǎn, 天眼, third eye). These two are corresponding cavities, although Nǎohù (Gv-17, 腦戶) is also often considered a paired cavity of the Third Eye.

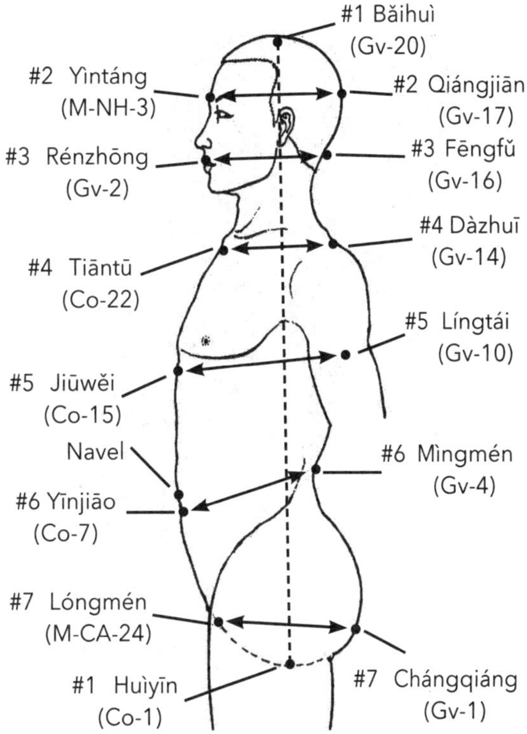

Figure 5-13. Seven Pairs of Corresponding Qì Gates

Seven Pairs of Corresponding Qì Gates

The human body has seven major pairs of corresponding Qì gates from which its Qì structure is constituted: 1. Huìyīn (Co-1, 會陰) and Bǎihuì (Gv-20, 百會); 2. Yìntáng (M-HN-3, 印堂) and Qiángjiān (Gv-17, 強間) [or Nǎohù (Gv-18, 腦戶)]; 3. Rénzhōng (Gv-26, 人中) and Fēngfǔ (Gv-16, 風府); 4. Tiāntū (Co-22, 天突) and Dàzhuī (Gv-14, 大椎); 5. Jiūwěi (Co-15, 鳩尾) and Língtái (Gv-10, 靈臺); 6. Yīnjiāo (Co-7, 陰交) and Mìngmén (Gv-4, 命門); and 7. Lóngmén (M-CA-24, 龍門) [or Xiàyīn (下陰)] and Chángqiáng (Gv-1, 長強) [or Wěilǘ (尾閭)]. Among these seven, two pairs are the most important: Huìyīn (Yīn) and Bǎihuì (Yáng), and Yīnjiāo (Yīn) and Mìngmén (Yáng). Huìyīn is connected to Bǎihuì through the Thrusting Vessel ,which establishes the central balance of Qì distribution in the body. Yīnjiāo is also connected to Mìngmén through the Thrusting Vessel and joins the Conception Vessel in front and the Governing Vessel behind, providing front and rear Qì balance to the body. These four are the main Qì gates (Figure 5-13).

Tiāntū controls vocal vibrations and generates the sounds of Hēng (Yīn, 哼) and Hā (Yáng, 哈) for manifestation of Qì. It is a gate of expression, and its energy is balanced with Yìntáng, where the spirit resides. When spirit is high in Yìntáng, the energy manifested is strong, and alertness and awareness are high. Jiūwěi and Língtái connect to the heart (Emotional Mind) and offer strong driving force to raise up the spirit. These four minor gates control manifestation of Qì in the body. So the Eight Gates are defined.

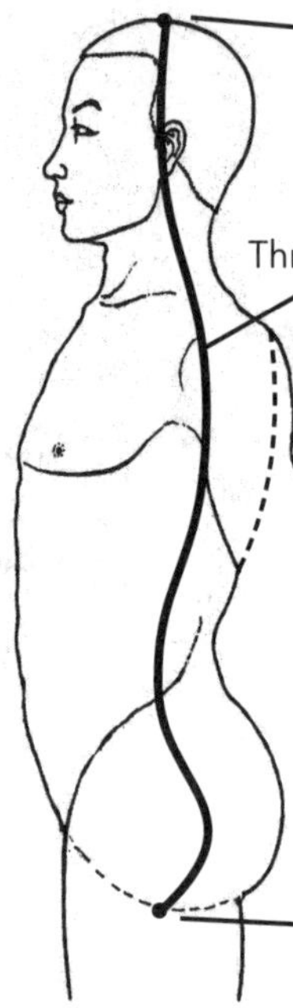

Figure 5-14. Qì Circulates in Thrusting Vessel and Bone Marrow at Night

5-4. Theory of Small Circulation Meditation (Xiǎozhōutiān Zhī Lǐlùn, 小周天之理論)

In this section, I propose a theory of Small Circulation practice from both Eastern and Western understanding. If any ancient practice has survived thousands of years with its function and effectiveness verified, it must be correct. Then we should be able to interpret it in terms of modern scientific logic. Ancient theory and practice should be consistent with modern scientific interpretation, otherwise either theory or practice needs to be modified. I propose to demonstrate this connection and offer a new theoretical concept of this practice.

General Concepts

1. From Chinese medicine and Qìgōng, we understand that the major Qì flow in the daytime is in the Conception and Governing Vessels, while at night it is in the Thrusting Vessel. The Conception Vessel regulates Qì circulation in the six primary Yīn channels, while the Governing Vessel regulates the six primary Yáng channels. These Twelve Primary Qì Channels (Shíèrjīng, 十二經) distribute Qì throughout the body via millions of secondary Qì channels (Luò, 絡). During the day, when there is physical activity, Qì circulates strongly in these two vessels. Exhalation is longer than inhalation, and Guardian Qì (Wèiqì, 衛氣) expands. At night, your body relaxes and rests. Inhalation is longer than exhalation, leading Qì into the Thrusting Vessel and the bone marrow (Figure 5-14). The brain and glands are nourished with Qì, while hormone production increases. We conclude that Qì in the Small Circulation path nourishes the body (Muscle/Tendon Changing), while that in the Thrusting Vessel promotes longevity and spiritual cultivation (Marrow/Brain Washing).

2. Qì is stronger in the Conception Vessel during the day and in the Governing Vessel at night. During the daytime, the natural world around you is Yáng, so Yīn Qì in the Conception Vessel balances this external Yáng. At night, the external environment is Yīn, and Qì in the Yáng Governing Vessel balances the natural Yīn (Figure 5-15).
3. There are three major obstacles to Qì circulation in the Small Circulation orbit, all located in the Governing Vessel. There is no obstacle in the Conception Vessel.
4. The Conception and Governing Vessels are constructed from many different layers of tendon and fascia (Figure 5-16). Since the conductivity of tendons is higher than that of the surrounding muscles, we can assume that Qì circulation at this center line is more abundant than in the surrounding areas. Many layers of tendon (good conductor) and fascia (poor conductor) are sandwiched at these two vessels like a battery, able to store Qì to an abundant level. We assume electrical conductivity of tendons is higher than that of muscles, for the following reasons:
   a. The cross-section area of a tendon connected to a muscle is much smaller than that of the muscle itself. Since both are insulated by fascia (a poor conductor), and the same current passes through both areas, the current must flow faster through the tendon than through the muscle. So the electric conductivity of tendons is higher than that of muscles (Figure 5-17).
   b. Tendon is stronger than muscle, so its Qì must circulate stronger than in muscle.
   c. After physical exercise, tendons are colder than muscles. More Qì is trapped in the muscle and manifested as heat, which means the muscle has more resistance.

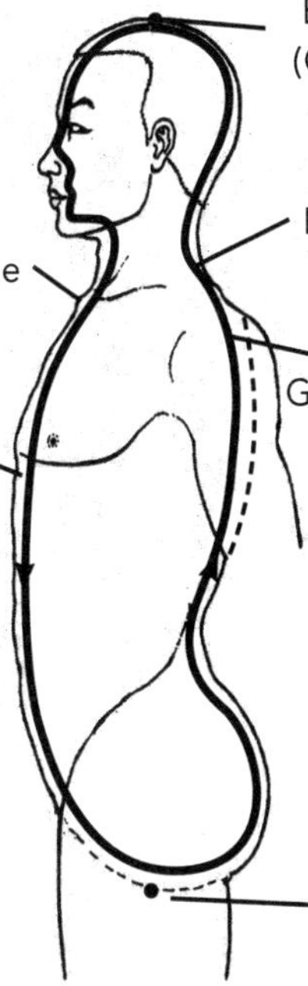

Figure 5-15. Qì is Stronger in the Conception Vessel during the Day and in the Governing Vessel at Night

These conclusions are derived from logical analysis, but require verification with modern scientific equipment.

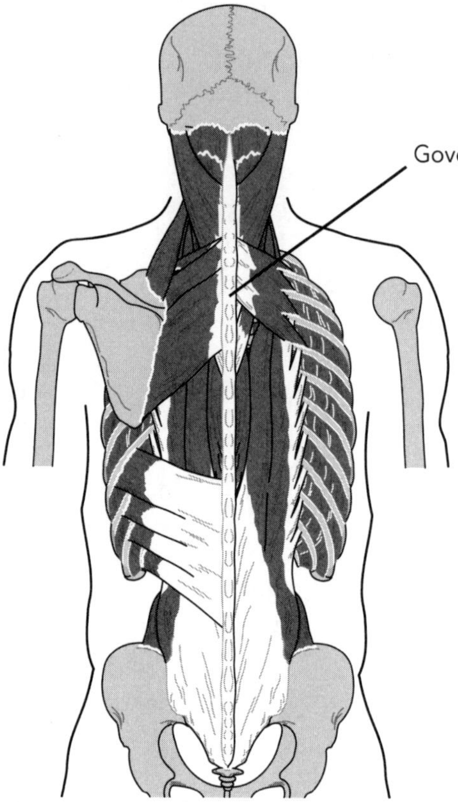

Figure 5-16. Conception and Governing Vessels are Constructed from Many Different Layers of Tendon and Fascia

Producing Qì (Shēngqì, 生氣)

Let us summarize the methods of producing and increasing Qì in the body.

1. **From metabolism of food and air.** The biochemical reaction is:

$$\text{glucose} + 6O_2 \longrightarrow 6CO_2 + 6H_2O$$

$$\Delta G^{o'} = -686 \text{ Kcal (energy content)}$$

From digestion of food and inhalation of oxygen, energy is generated. Different foods produce different quantity and quality of Qì, and herbs especially are used to manipulate the Qì status of the body. This is called Fire Qì (Huǒqì, 火氣) or Post-Heaven Qì (Hòutiānqì, 後天氣).

2. **From abdominal exercise.** The Lower Elixir Field (Xià Dāntián, 下丹田), called Qì Ocean (Qìhǎi, Co-6, 氣海) by Chinese medicine, is at the front of the abdomen a few inches below the navel. Qì is generated here as abundantly as the ocean. This center is also called Furnace Tripod (Dǐnglú, 鼎爐) or Elixir Furnace (Dānlú, 丹爐), but is said to be a False Dāntián (Jiǎ Dāntián, 假丹田) by Daoists. Even though it produces Qì, it cannot store it to an abundant level.

   The up-and-down movements of "back to childhood breathing" facilitate the biochemical reaction that converts stored fat into Qì. This is called Water Qì (Shuǐqì, 水氣), Pre-Heaven Qì (Xiāntiānqì, 先天氣), or Original Qì (Yuánqì, 元氣). It is pure and clean like water to calm you physically and mentally. Fat is the essence of food which has been processed, purified, and stored in the body. Fat has a high caloric content and can be converted efficiently into energy.

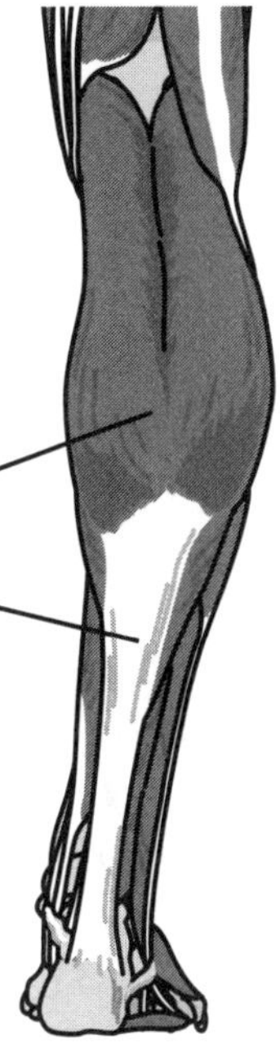

Figure 5-17. Electric Conductivity of Tendons is Higher Than That of Muscles

   Water Qì is also called Pre-Heaven Qì or Original Qì because your Qì is converted from your Original Essence (Yuánjīng, 元精), i.e., hormones. In my view, however, since hormones act as catalysts in the body's biochemical reactions, they cannot be converted into Qì. All they do is facilitate the process of converting fat into Qì.

   How is Qì generated at the Lower Dāntián? The abdomen has six layers of muscle and fascia. A lot of fat is stored in the layers of fascia. When you move your abdomen up and down, your mind controls contraction and relaxation of the muscles. This causes food essence to be converted to Qì through biochemical reaction. When those places where fat is stored are exercised, the fat gradually turns into energy and disappears, so it is reasonable to assume the same happens when we move the abdomen.

   Since muscles are good conductors while fasciae are poor conductors, this area can act like a battery to store the Qì. All animals store fat (food essence) to survive in nature. In this way, extra food is stored for when there is none available. The largest storage place is the abdomen. Qì is converted and stored more abundantly here than any other place in the body and distributed efficiently to the body through the Conception and Governing Vessels. Abdominal movement is coordinated with breathing in Qìgōng practice. This is called "Starting the Fire" (Qǐhuǒ, 起火), and there are two ways of doing so. One is Normal Abdominal Breathing (Zhèng Fùhūxī, 正腹呼吸) and the other Reversed Abdominal Breathing (Fǎn, Nì Fùhūxī, 反、逆腹呼吸). According to the intensity of Qì production, the practice is classified as Martial Fire (Wǔhuǒ, 武火), or Scholar Fire (Wénhuǒ, 文火). Rapid breathing quickly generates Martial Fire Qì to an abundant level, which is used to energize the body for battle, or for Wàidān Qìgōng practice. It is hard to store this Qì in the Real Lower Dāntián. If you intend to store Qì internally, breathe softly and slenderly, then lead it to the Real Lower Dāntián and store it there. This is called Scholar Fire (Wénhuǒ, 文火) Breathing.

3. **From massaging the abdominal area.** In Muscle/Tendon Changing, massage used in conjunction with herbs converts the fat into Qì, as described in *Qìgōng—The Secret of Youth*.

Storing Qì to an Abundant Level (Xùqì, 蓄氣)

Having produced extra Qì at the False Lower Dāntián, lead it inward and store it at the Real Lower Dāntián. When it is left at the False Lower Dāntián on the Conception Vessel, it is distributed through the Small Circulation path to the Twelve Primary Qì Channels. This improves strength and health, but it is then not available to nourish the brain for enlightenment. Remember, each brain cell requires up to twelve times more Qì than other cells. To achieve enlightenment, along with mental conditioning, you need to lead considerable Qì to the brain from storage at the Real Lower Dāntián. My book, *Qìgōng Meditation—Embryonic Breathing* discusses this in detail. Here, I will summarize key theories and training methods.

1. **Condition the Lower Dāntián to store abundant Qì.** Conditioning is achieved through massage and physical stimulation (pounding and beating) of the stomach and abdominal area (Huángtíng, 黃庭). This converts fat into Qì and reduces fat between the layers of muscle, allowing your "battery" to store a charge far stronger than that of other people. The most important factor is conditioning the nervous system in this area to raise its pain threshold. Qì cannot generally be stored abundantly because it causes pain and tension when storage reaches its threshold of tolerance, leading the Qì to disperse. Conditioning increases the tolerance of the nerves, allowing Qì storage to increase.

2. **Increase the efficiency of conversion from fat to Qì.** This depends on the hormones (Original Essense) to regulate the metabolism. Hormones act as catalysts for the biochemical reaction that converts food into Qì, and when they are adequate, the reaction proceeds smoothly.
   There are three major glands surrounding the abdominal area (Huángtíng), namely the adrenals at the back, pancreas in front, and testicles or ovaries at the bottom. To increase their production of hormones, supply them with extra Qì through massage.
   There are two ways to massage the adrenals located on top of the kidneys. One is through alternating pressure on the lower back. The other is to massage the kidneys directly. When you reach a high level of practice, you can lead Qì directly to the kidneys using the mind.
   Massage the pancreas through abdominal exercise and massage. In the past, Qìgōng practitioners seldom used the mind to lead Qì to the pancreas, because they did not recognize its capability of producing Original Essence.
   Testicles and ovaries are massaged directly, or the focused mind leads Qì there with the assistance of correct breathing. Qì is also led there by tensing and relaxing the Huìyīn (Co-1, 會陰, perineum).
3. **Store Qì to an abundant level at the Real Lower Dāntián to reach spiritual enlightenment.** Embryonic Breathing (Tāixí, 胎息) is the way to achieve this. Locate the two Poles of the body, Mud Pill Palace and Real Lower Dāntián, and focus your mind there. Focus at the Mud Pill Palace so your mind is calm, centered and focused, and the spirit raised. Focus at the Real Lower Dāntián to conserve Qì and lead it back to its residence.
   Once you synchronize these two centers, the strength of the central Qì system is firmly established. Next, bring your mind to the Huángtíng, where spirit and Qì are united, returning your being to the beginning of life. This is called Unification of Mother (Qì) and Son (Spirit), namely Mǔzǐ Xiāngshǒu (母子相守), or Wújí Breathing (Wújí Hūxī, 無極呼吸).

Circulating Qì (Xíngqì, 行氣)

There are two main reasons to practice Small Circulation. One is to accumulate abundant Qì in the Conception and Governing Vessels, and the other is to circulate it smoothly in these vessels to regulate Qì in the Twelve Primary Qì Channels. Qì already circulates naturally in these two vessels, otherwise you would have encountered some physical problem. But this circulation becomes stagnant as we age, and the path of circulation becomes narrow. Small Circulation widens this path so Qì can circulate smoothly and abundantly again. There are three places, called Three Gates (Sānguān, 三關), where the path is especially narrow, causing Qì circulation to stagnate. The aim of practice is to open and widen these three gates, a process called "Pass Through Three Gates" (Tōngsānguān, 通三關).

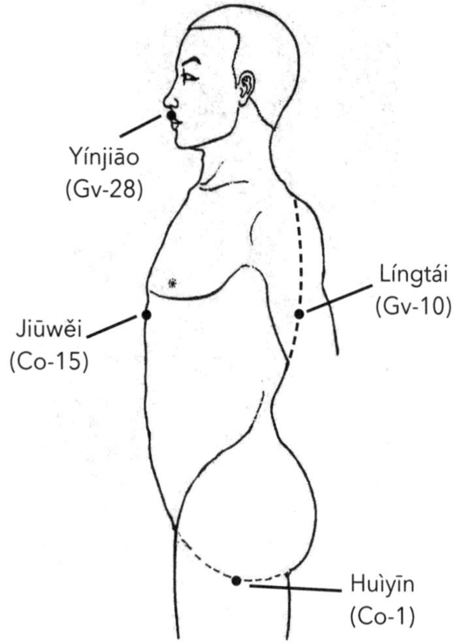

Figure 5-18. Huìyīn (Co-1), Yínjiāo (Gv-28), Jiūwěi (Co-15), and Língtái (Gv-10)

We now describe natural Small Circulation, the theory of opening the gates, and the traditional and modified methods of Small Circulation practice. Since the Three Gates are so important, we will discuss them separately in the next section.

1. **Natural Qì Circulation in the Small Circulation Orbit.** "Internal Qì circulation in the Governing Vessel is from the bottom to the top. It connects at Yínjiāo (Gv-28, 齦交, Gum Junction) with the Conception Vessel and circulates down the Conception Vessel, becoming cyclic circulation. The junctions of the Governing and Conception Vessels, at the top and bottom, are called Upper Magpie Bridge (Shàng Quèqiáo, 上鵲橋) and Lower Magpie Bridge (Xià Quèqiáo, 下鵲橋)."[18,19] Qì circulates from top to bottom in front of the body, and from bottom to top in the back. The two vessels are joined at the Magpie Bridges. They are Huìyīn (Co-1, 會陰) and Yínjiāo (Gv-28, 齦交), which control Qì in Small Circulation practice (Figure 5-18).
   The major Qì flow in these two vessels is determined by the time of day and thus controlled by the sun. At midnight (11 pm to 1 am) Qì accumulates at Bǎihuì, connected with its corresponding gate, Huìyīn, so Huìyīn can also be classified as midnight. At dawn, depending on the season, the major Qì flow is at the mouth (Yínjiāo). Since external Qì is changing from Yīn (night) to Yáng (day), internal Qì circulation also changes from Yáng (Governing Vessel) to Yīn (Conception Vessel). At noon, the major Qì flow is at Jiūwěi (Co-15, 鳩尾) and its corresponding gate Língtái (Gv-10, 靈台) at the back. If these cavities are attacked at noon, a heart attack can be triggered. At dusk, the major Qì flow is at Huìyīn, where Qì circulation is changing from Yīn to Yáng, while

external Qì is changing from Yáng to Yīn. The correlation between Qì flow and the time of day was kept top secret in Chinese martial arts society, since serious injury can follow an attack on these cavities.

2. **Theory of Opening the Gates.** As you age, the Qì channels gradually block, choking the flow of Qì. Age spots, wrinkles, pain, numbness, and organ malfunctions develop, made worse by lack of exercise. As the channels get narrower, the Qì circulation slows, narrowing them still further. In Qìgōng we widen the path of Qì circulation in the Conception and Governing Vessels. Qì stagnation is more serious at cavities like Chángqiáng and Nǎohù. The path is widened through abundant Qì circulation, just as when a river is blocked with garbage, abundant water can flush it away and restore the flow. Small Circulation practice accumulates abundant Qì and uses the mind to circulate it. The Conception and Governing Vessels control Qì circulation in the Twelve Primary Qì Channels, spreading Qì to the whole body, so once Small Circulation is accomplished, the body becomes strong and healthy.
3. **Traditional Method and Modified Method.** In traditional practice, the master would teach his student to produce extra Qì in the Lower Dāntián through abdominal breathing. After a long time, about ten years of practice, this area would be conditioned and plenty of Qì stored. Only then would the master teach his trusted student to lead the Qì. The main goal, besides increasing the quantity of Qì circulating in the Conception and Governing Vessels, would be to widen the Three Gates so Qì could circulate smoothly. Qì was stored to an abundant level first, to be able to restore Qì flow and widen the path. However, this may cause injury if it enters the wrong path, causing shock to the nervous system and affecting normal function. To avoid the danger of injury, I have modified the ancient training procedures, through twenty years of teaching experience, in three major ways. I teach students Embryonic Breathing first, rather than Abdominal Breathing. This is the root of Internal Elixir practice. In the past, Embryonic Breathing was not practiced for Small Circulation, due to the secrecy surrounding it. It was hidden in Buddhist and Daoist monasteries for spiritual enlightenment practice. Having mastered Embryonic Breathing, you can manipulate Qì even if it is very strong. Second, I reverse the order of traditional teaching. When a student has some Qì, I teach him to circulate it immediately. There is no danger since the Qì is not strong enough to cause harm. Having learned to circulate it, he spends the rest of his life accumulating Qì and gradually widening the path. Naturally, this revised method takes longer to achieve. Third, to prevent danger caused from passing the first gate at Wěilǘ (尾閭;

Chángqiáng, Gv-1, 長強), I teach circulating Qì in a smaller orbit called Small Small Circulation (Xiǎo Xiǎozhōutiān, 小小周天). The student leads the Qì to Huìyīn, passes Wěilǘ and re-enters the Real Lower Dāntián through Mìngmén (Gv-4, 命門) to complete this Small Small Orbit. Only then is he taught regular Small Circulation.

Practicing Theory and Keys

If you grasp the theory, you can achieve the goal more quickly. You should study the book *Qìgōng Meditation—Embryonic Breathing*. The theory and practice of Embryonic Breathing is the essential root of Internal Elixir Qìgōng.

1. **The Body Is the Battlefield** (Tiáoshēn, 調身).
   The body is like a battlefield, and Qì is like soldiers engaged in battle against sickness and aging. For religious Qìgōng, Qì generates crucial power to reopen the Third Eye. Qìgōng practice aims to increase the quantity of Qì and improve the quality of its manifestation. So arrange the battlefield in your favor.
   Regulating the Body (Tiáoshēn, 調身) means keeping the torso upright, neck relaxed, joints opened, and legs crossed comfortably, as you strive for extreme relaxation of the whole body. This reduces to a minimum the resistance to Qì flow, allowing it to circulate smoothly and abundantly. Blood flows smoothly too, carrying oxygen, water, nutrients, and Qì throughout the body. The body's metabolism is effective, so damage to the body can be repaired and the aging process slowed.
   Most important of all, your mind becomes peaceful and calm so it can focus on leading the Qì. This is called Harmonious Balance of Body and Mind (Shēnxīn Pínghéng, 身心平衡).
2. **Breathing as Strategy** (Tiáoxí, 調息)
   Breathing is the strategy in Qìgōng practice. When you breathe correctly, Qì circulates smoothly, and when it is awkward, Qì stagnates. The keys to regulating the breath are: A. Calm and silent (Jìng, 靜), B. Slender (Xì, 細), C. Deep (Shēn, 深), D. Long (Cháng, 長), E. Continuous (Yōu, 悠), F. Uniform (Yún, 勻), G. Slow (Huǎn, 緩), and H. Soft (Mián, 綿). Once you reach this stage, oxygen and carbon dioxide exchange smoothly and the metabolism is healthy. Your mind is calm and peaceful and the body relaxed. This is called Mutual Dependence of the Xīn and Breathing (Xīnxí Xiāngyī, 心息相依). Xīn is the Emotional Mind which makes you excited, confused, or distracts you from leading the Qì.

3. **Mind Is the General** (Tiáoxīn, 調心)
   Mind is the general in charge of the battlefield (body), strategies (breathing), and soldiers (Qì). If the general's mind is calm and clear, he controls the situation effectively. If it is confused and scattered, his control will be weak and shallow.
   The mind generates EMF so Qì can be directed. When this mind is confused and weak, the Qì is poorly led. A highly concentrated mind can be achieved in a drowsy, semi-hypnotic state. Your conscious mind is there, yet not there. Entering the Herbal Mirror (Rùyàojìng, 入藥鏡) describes this state, "The state of trance, remote and profound. Body and mind are naturally comfortable, as though drunk and like an idiot. Muscles and skin are refreshed and transparent. Its beauty is hidden within."[20] Lǐ, Shí-Zhēn (李時珍) describes this state in his book, The Study of Strange Meridians and Eight Vessels (Qíjīng Bāmài Kǎo, 奇經八脈考): "Dusky (tranced) and silent, like a drunk and like an idiot."[21]
   To reach this state, your Wisdom Mind (Yì) governs your Emotional Mind (Xīn). Once emotion is calm, use Yì to lead your Qì.
4. **Spirit Is the Soldiers' Morale** (Tiáoshén, 調神)
   The spirit of practice is more important than the mind, Qì, or body. Spirit is invisible but controls the morale of the army. When morale is high, orders are executed effectively. When your spirit is down, your immune system is weak and you easily get sick. Raise up the spirit with a firm mind and strong will. Keep your motivation to practice high at all times, and govern Xīn with Yi. Be decisive, with confusion reduced to a minimum. Keeping spirit at a high level, you harmonize Spirit and Qì (Shénqì Xiànghé, 神氣相合), so Qì is led effectively.
5. **Huìyīn is the Pump, and the Abdomen is the Bellows.**
   The Huìyīn cavity is the crucial valve controlling Qì in the four Yīn vessels. When it is pushed out, the stored Qì is released, and when it is held up, the valve is closed, holding Qì in and conserving it. So the Huìyīn pumps Internal Qì (Nèiqì, 內氣) and governs the manifestation or preservation of the body's Qì. Controlling Huìyīn in your practice makes a significant difference. Traditionally this was one tricky place which the master would keep secret until the student was trustworthy.
6. **Tongue Is the Bridge of Yīn and Yáng.**
   The tongue is the bridge or switch which connects the Yīn Conception and Yáng Governing Vessels, necessary so Qì can circulate smoothly between the two vessels. Your tongue should touch your palate whenever you practice Qìgōng.

5-5. Three Gates (Sānguān, 三關)

If one does not follow the correct method, practicing Internal Elixir Qìgōng can be very dangerous. There are two dangers to be faced. One is Zǒuhuǒ (走火), which means "Walk into the Fire." Qì enters into the wrong path, which may cause physical and mental damage. The other is Rùmó (入魔), which means "Enter the Demon," or being bewitched. The mind enters the state of illusion or imagination during meditation.

Each organ or part of the body has its own Qì threshold. When Qì becomes deficient or exceeds this threshold, damage can occur. For example, if too much Qì enters the heart, it can cause heart attack.

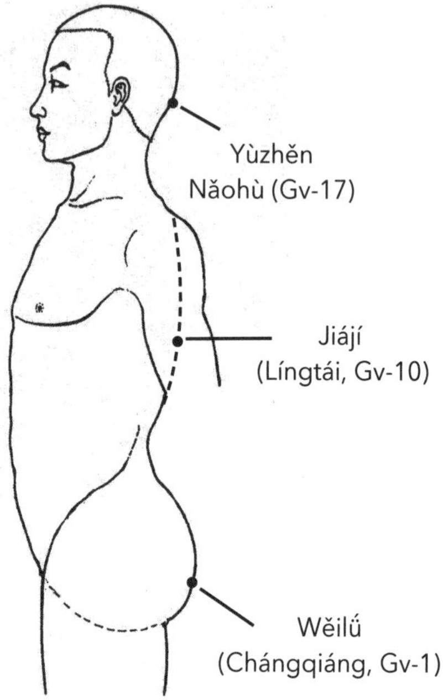

Figure 5-19. Three Gates (San Guan): Yùzhěn, Jiájí, and Wěilǘ

When you meditate, you accumulate abundant Qì at your Lower Dāntián and then circulate it. If your mind directs this Qì and keeps it in the Small Circulation orbit, there will be no problem. But if it strays from this path and enters the wrong one, damage can follow. So your mind plays a key role when you meditate.

In the meditative state, your body is extremely relaxed and your mind calm and clear, so you are vulnerable to energy disturbances around you. These disturbances can cause illusion, which can lead your mind astray, as when a cold breeze makes you feel you are in the presence of a ghost.

There are three gates (Sānguān, 三關) which can cause one to Walk into the Fire and Enter the Demon: Yùzhěn (玉枕), Jiájí (夾脊), and Wěilǘ (尾閭). *The Collection of Great Achievements in Golden Elixir* (*Jīndān Dàchéng Jí*, 金丹大成集) said, "Behind the brain is Yùzhěn Guan. Jiájí is called Lùlúguān, while the junction of water and fire is called Wěilǘ Guan."(Figure 5-19)[22] Yùzhěn means "jade pillow." In ancient times, rich people would thread small pieces of jade together to make a pillow. Yùzhěn is a Daoist term, known in acupuncture as Nǎohù. Jiájí means "squeeze the spine," the center of the spine between the shoulder blades. Jiájí is also called Lùlúguān (Windlass Gate, 轆轤關) because it is at the center where the shoulders turn, like a windlass. It is also called Mìngmén (Life Door, 命門) by martial artists, since it is connected to the heart and can cause death when struck. In acupuncture it is called Língtái (Gv-10, 靈臺, Spiritual Platform). Wěilǘ (tailbone) is called Chángqiáng (Gv-1, 長強, Long Strength) in acupuncture, but in Qìgōng society has always been conflated with Huìyīn (Co-1, 會陰, perineum). It is the junction where Qì enters either the water or fire path.

First Gate: Wěilǘ (尾閭), Chángqiáng (Gv-1, 長強)

The Wěilǘ cavity is also called Xūwēi (Endangered Cavity, 虛危穴). It has many names, due to its importance in Internal Elixir cultivation. *The Complete Book of Principal Contents of Human Life and Temperament* (*Xìngmìng Guīzhǐ Quánshū*, 性命圭旨全書) lists them:[23]

- Tiānrén Héfā Zhījī (天人合發之機): The pivotal place for unification of heaven and man
- Zǐmǔ Fēntāi Zhīlù (子母分胎之路): The path of separation of son (embryo) and mother
- Rèn Dū Jiējiāo Zhīchù (任督接交之處): The junction of Conception and Governing Vessels
- Yīn Yáng Biànhuà Zhīxiāng (陰陽變化之鄉): The village (location) of variations of Yīn and Yáng
- Jiǔlíng Tiěgǔ (九靈鐵鼓): The iron drum of nine spirits (meaning unknown)
- Sānzú Jīnchán (三足金蟾): Golden toad with three legs (meaning unknown)
- Tàixuánguān (太玄關): Grand mysterious gate
- Cángjīndòu (藏金斗): Hidden golden dipper (meaning unknown)
- Wěilǘ Xuè (尾閭穴): Tailbone cavity
- Shēngsǐ Xuè (生死穴): Cavity of life and death
- Cháotiānlǐng (朝天岭): Approach remote heaven
- Qìhǎimén (氣海門): The gate to the Qì ocean
- Cáoxīlù (曹溪路): Cao Xi road (meaning unknown)
- Sānchàkǒu (三岔口): The junction of three paths
- Píngyì Xuè (平易穴): Peace and easy cavity (meaning unknown)
- Xiánchí (咸池): Pond of wholeness
- Yīnduān (陰端): Yīn extremity
- Jìnmén (禁門): Forbidden gate
- Huìyīn (會陰): Meet Yīn
- Gǔdào (穀道): Grain path
- Lónghǔ Xuè (龍虎穴): Cavity of dragon and tiger (Yīn and Yáng)
- Sānchàgǔ (三岔骨): Junction bone of three paths
- Héchēlù (河車路): The path of river car (transporting Qì)
- Shàngtiāntī (上天梯): The ladder to heaven (enlightenment)

Much attention has been focused on this cavity in Chinese Qìgōng history. *The Complete Book of Principal Contents of Human Life and Temperament* (*Xìngmìng Guīzhǐ Quánshū*, 性命圭旨全書) said, "It is because this cavity is where Jīng (essence) and Qì are gathered and dispersed, where water and fire begin, where Yīn and Yáng vary, where the substantial (body) and insubstantial (spirit) enter and leave, where son and mother separate." "This cavity is the center between the Conception and Governing Vessels. Upward, it communicates with Tiāngǔ (Spiritual Valley), and downward, it reaches Yǒngquán." "This cavity has the strongest influence (on life), it is the key of one's life and death. So the immortals called it the hole of life and death." The book Cāntóngqì (參同契) said, "This is where to establish and to firm the spiritual cultivation, the place to retain the storage, and the controlling gate of Qì." Yellow Yard Classic (Huángtíngjīng, 黃庭經) said, "This is where to seal and close the life door so the jade (precious life) can be protected. This is also where to seal the path of sperm, so you may live long."[24]

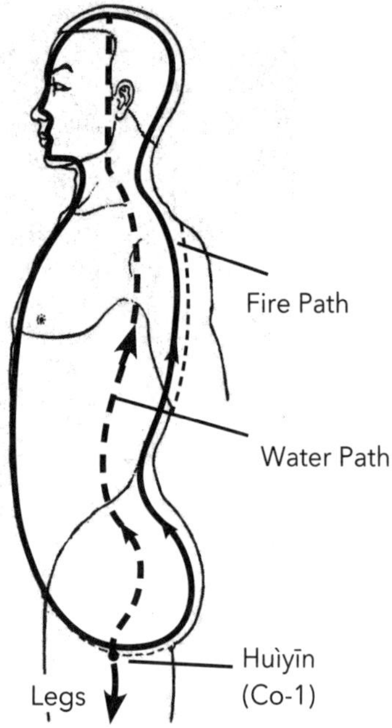

Figure 5-20. Huìyīn (Co-1) is the Junction of Fire Path, Wind Path, and Legs

The documents are not clear on where exactly the cavity is, whether it refers to the tailbone (Wěilǘ, 尾閭), or to the Huìyīn. The anus is also sometimes considered to be the place and is commonly called Gǔdào (穀道), or grain path.

If we analyze the anatomy and the historical background, the confusion disappears. Almost everyone in those days was illiterate and had difficulty understanding special medical terminology such as Huìyīn. Since the muscles of the anus area are connected with the perineum, it was easier to write anus instead of Huìyīn. Through contraction and relaxation of the perineum, Qì can be regulated. If the anus is gently held up, the perineum tightens and seals the Qì gate. When it is gently pushed out, the perineum relaxes, and the Qì gate opens.

Also recognize that Huìyīn is the key cavity where Qì divides into three paths, Fire Path (Huǒlù, 火路) through the Governing Vessel, Water Path (Shuǐlù, 水路) through the Thrusting Vessel, and also down to the bottom of the feet through the Yīn Heel Vessels (Yīnqiāomài, 陰蹺脈) and Yīn Línking Vessels (Yīnwéimài, 陰維脈) (Figure 5-20). When Qì circulates abundantly in the Fire Path, then the Twelve Primary Qì Channels (Shíèrjīng, 十二經) will also be full.

If Qì is led up strongly through the Water Path, the brain is nourished and energized. This is the key to Marrow/Brain Washing for spiritual enlightenment. Huìyīn also regulates Qì flow from the sexual organ to the legs, so when sexual energy is strong, the legs are strong.

Qì enters the Fire or Water paths through the tricky gate at Wěilǘ (tailbone, Chángqiáng, 長強). Contracting and relaxing the Huìyīn muscles pumps Qì through Wěilǘ into the Fire Path or the Water Path. In the beginning, Qì will tend to flow down to the legs instead, because the Qì paths to the legs are wide open.

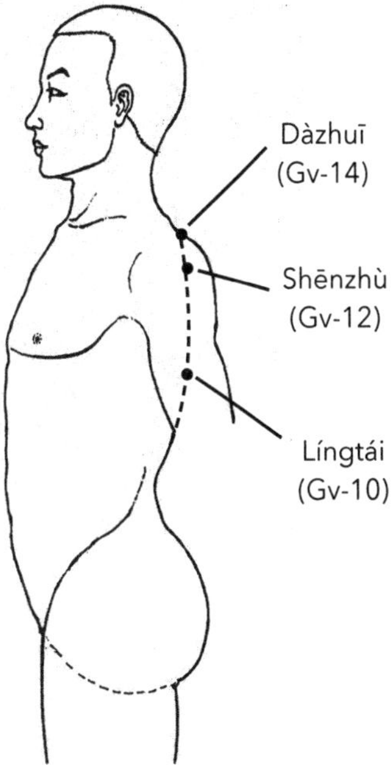

Figure 5-21. Língtái (Gv-10), Dàzhuī (Gv-14), and Shēnzhù (Gv-12)

This is not a problem if the Qì is weak, but abundant Qì can be dangerous if you don't lead it into the correct path. When abundant Qì encounters its first obstacle at the Wěilǘ gate, it may instead rush down to the legs and damage the nervous system there. This is called "Walking into the Fire" (Zǒuhuǒ, 走火), well-known as the first danger of practice, which can paralyze the legs. When you meditate, it is important to sit with crossed legs to block the Qì flow to the legs. If too much Qì nevertheless rushes there during meditation, first try to lead it back to the Lower Dāntián. Then hit the legs to stimulate them, leading Qì from deep inside to dissipate at the skin.

Second Gate: Jiájí (夾脊), Lùlú (轆轤), Língtái (Gv-10, 靈臺)

This gate is not narrow and can be passed easily, but is dangerous because abundant Qì there can enter the heart, causing palpitations. A beginner may be distracted by this, focusing on the heart and triggering a heart attack.

In practice, simply ignore this cavity. If you sense Qì flow to the heart, focus on the Dàzhuī (Gv-14, 大椎) or Shēnzhù (Gv-12, 身柱) cavities and lead the Qì there instead (Figure 5-21). With practice you get used to it and find that as long as your mind is calm and clear, there is no problem leading Qì past this cavity.

Third Gate: Yùzhěn (Jade Pillow, 玉枕), Nǎohù (Gv-17, 腦戶)

This is at the base of the skull and is dangerous due to its physical structure. There is a thin layer of muscle between the skull and the skin. The Qì path suddenly narrows as the neck tendons end. When abundant Qì accumulates here, some of it can enter the brain

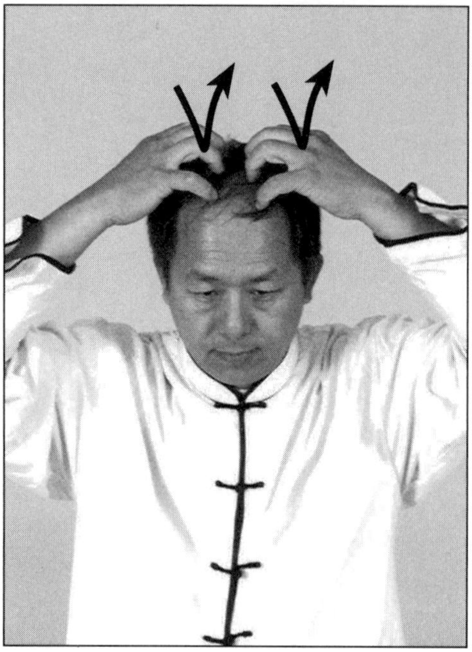

Figure 5-22

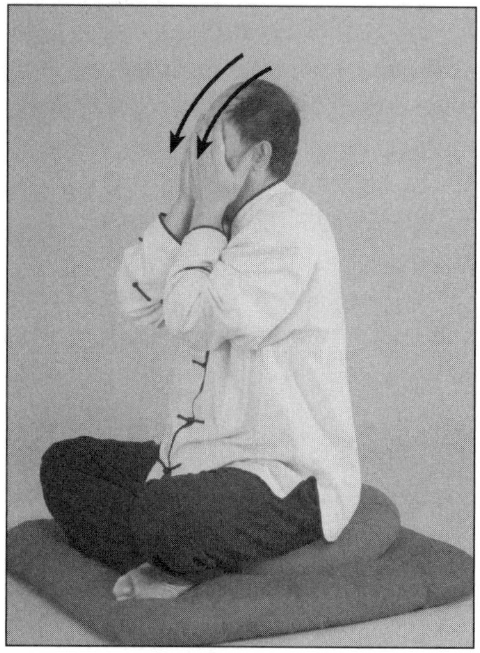

Figure 5-23

through Nǎohù, which can excite the nervous system in the brain, damage its function, or even cause mental disorder.

Be careful when you lead Qì past this cavity. Various sensations are generated. Pay attention to Bǎihuì, and Qì will go there. If some Qì enters the brain through Nǎohù, first lead it back to the Lower Dāntián. Tap the head with your fingertips to lead Qì to the surface (Figure 5-22), then brush it forward and down the Fire Path with your palms (Figure 5-23).

Having opened and widened these three gates, you complete the Small Circulation path. As you continue your practice, you accumulate more abundant Qì circulating in this Fire Path. The more abundant it is, the better your health and the stronger your foundation for Muscle/Tendon Changing practice.

5-6. Different Paths for Small Circulation (Xiǎozhōutiān Zhī Bùtóng Tújìng, 小周天之不同途徑)

By examining the body's Qì network and physical structure, we can conclude a few possible paths for Small Circulation. Due to lack of information and personal experience, I will only discuss those paths I am familiar with.

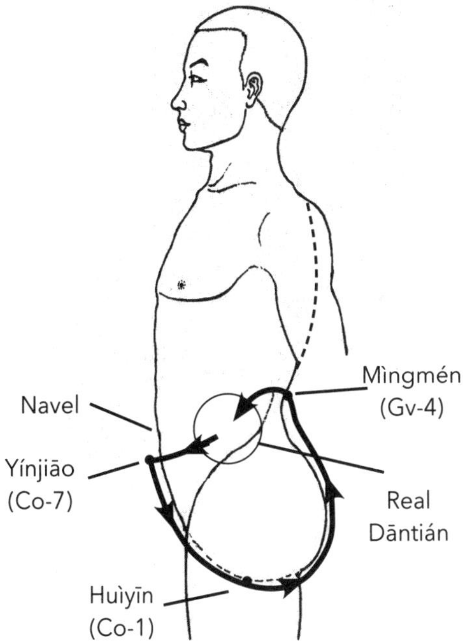

Figure 5-24. Small Small Circulation

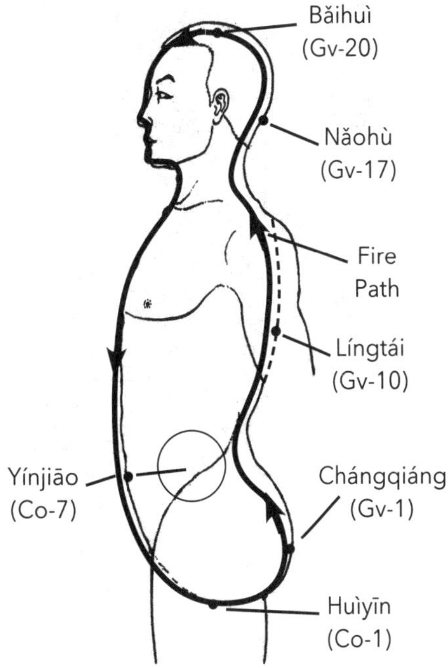

Figure 5-25. Fire Path

1. **Small Small Circulation** (Foundation, Xiǎo Xiǎozhōutiān, 小小周天-根基)
   This path is very safe, and much easier for beginners learning to pass the first gate at Wěilǘ. Practice this path first until you can lead the Qì smoothly, before continuing the Fire Path practice.
   Lead the Qì down from the Real Lower Dāntián, through Yīnjiāo, down to Huìyīn, up past Chángqiáng, and finally enter Mìngmén to reach the Qì residence at the Real Lower Dāntián (Figure 5-24). This is described in detail in Chapter 8.
2. **Fire Path** (Regular Path, Huǒlù, 火路, Shùnxíng, 順行)
   Fire Path is the regular path that follows natural Qì circulation and is the one most commonly practiced. It is often called Large Returning Elixir (Dàhuándān, 大還丹). Returning Elixir Secret (還丹訣) said, "Keep the body upright and sit correctly, transport Qì from Wěilǘ, with one breath pass through Sānguān (Three Gates) up to Níwán, harmonize with the spiritual water (saliva) and descend back to Dāntián. This is Large Returning Elixir (Dàhuándān). From kidneys to liver, from liver to heart, from heart to spleen, to lungs, and then repeat. Finally end at the Dāntián. This is called Small Returning Elixir (Xiǎohuándān, 小還丹)."[25]

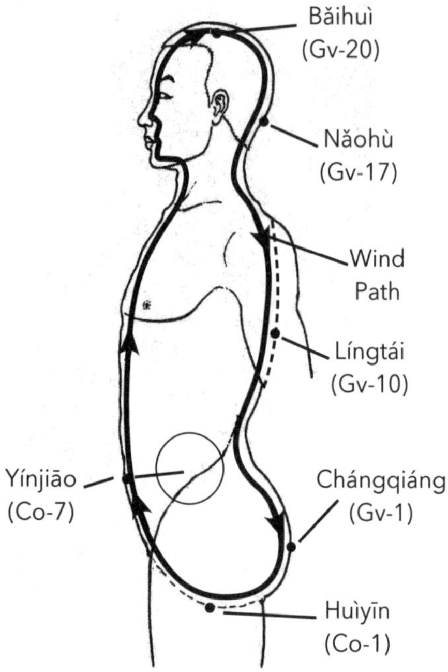

Figure 5-26. Wind Path

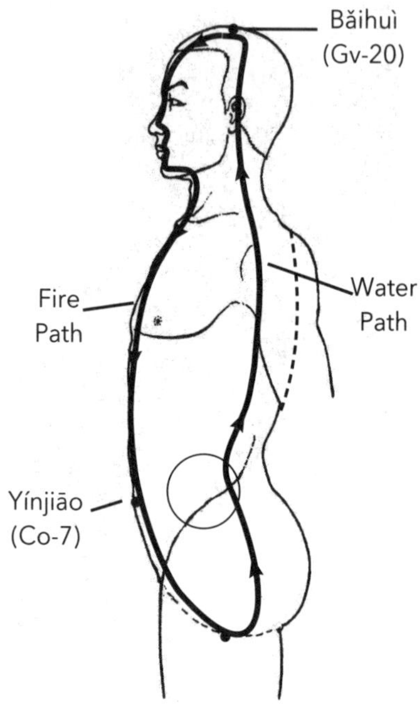

Figure 5-27. Combination of Water Path and Front Fire Path.

In this path, you lead Qì from the Real Lower Dāntián, passing Yīnjiāo, Huìyīn, Chángqiáng, Língtái, Nǎohù, and Bǎihuì, then down through the Conception Vessel back to Yīnjiāo and the Real Lower Dāntián (Figure 5-25). This is also described in detail in Chapter 8.

3. **Wind Path** (Reversed Regular Path, Fēnglù, 風路, Nìxíng, 逆行)
   Wind Path is the reverse of the natural path, so it generates resistance (wind) (Figure 5-26). Its purpose is to slow down Qì circulation in the fire path. Lead Qì up the front, down the back, then back to the Real Lower Dāntián.
4. **Combination of Water Path and Front Fire Path**
   Qì is led up the Thrusting Vessel (Water Path) to Bǎihuì, then down the Conception Vessel back to the Real Lower Dāntián (Figure 5-27). This can be done by those with abundant Qì at the Real Lower Dāntián and who are able to lead it up to nourish the brain. You may feel Qì moving by itself in the Thrusting Vessel, as all paths are already open to some extent. What you practice is to build abundant Qì, to circulate and to nourish.

5. **Combination of Back Fire Path and Reverse Water Path**
   This path brings Fire Qì down through the Thrusting Vessel. Qì follows the Fire Path up to Bǎihuì, and then goes down through the Thrusting Vessel back to the Real Lower Dāntián (Figure 5-28). When the Qì is led up the Thrusting Vessel, the Shén is raised up and Qì activity increases. But when the Qì is led down the Thrusting Vessel, it returns to its residence. Physical and mental activities gradually cease. Once you complete the Fire Path, try this path, which is relatively safe and very efficient in bringing down your Fire Qì.

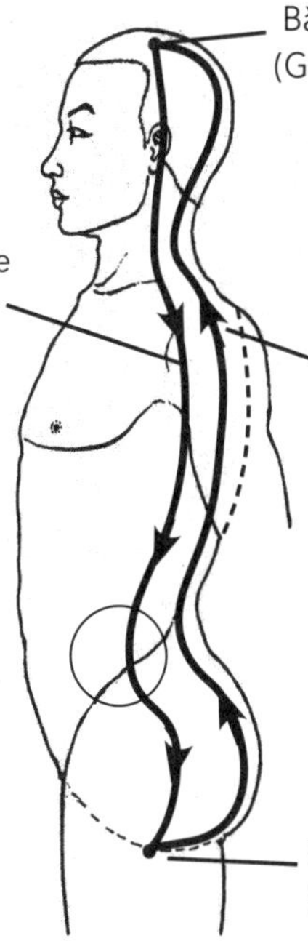

Figure 5-28. Combination of Back Fire Path and Reverse Water Path.

6. **Back Fire Path—Dàzhuī— Tiāntū —Front Fire Path**
   This path is little known and seldom practiced. Qì is led up the Fire Path to Dàzhuī (Gv-14, 大椎), then forward to Tiāntū (Co-22, 天突). It then goes down the Conception Vessel to Yīnjiāo, returning to the Real Lower Dāntián (Figure 5-29).
7. **Back Fire Path—Dàzhuī—Reverse Water Path**
   To avoid Qì going to the wrong path in the head, some practitioners use this path to cool down the fire, instead of path number 5. Qì is led up the Fire Path to Dàzhuī, forward to the Thrusting Vessel, then down to the Real Lower Dāntián (Figure 5-30).

There is no path which enters the Jiájí cavity and then goes forward. This would lead extra Qì to the heart, and would be extremely dangerous.

All paths are already open to some extent. Too much stagnation or blockage would have made you sick already. You aim to increase the level of Qì circulating there, to smooth its flow and to widen the path. Follow five basic steps: 1. Train yourself (Liànjǐ, 煉己), 2. Modulate the herbs (Tiáoyào, 調藥), 3. Produce the herbs (Chǎnyào, 產藥), 4. Pick the herbs (Cǎiyào, 采藥), and 5. Refine the herbs (Liányào, 煉藥). That means to regulate your Emotional Mind and cultivate your temperament. Be patient and study the method of cultivation. After that, use this calm mind to regulate your breathing and Qì flow. You accumulate abundant Qì through Abdominal and Embryonic Breathing,

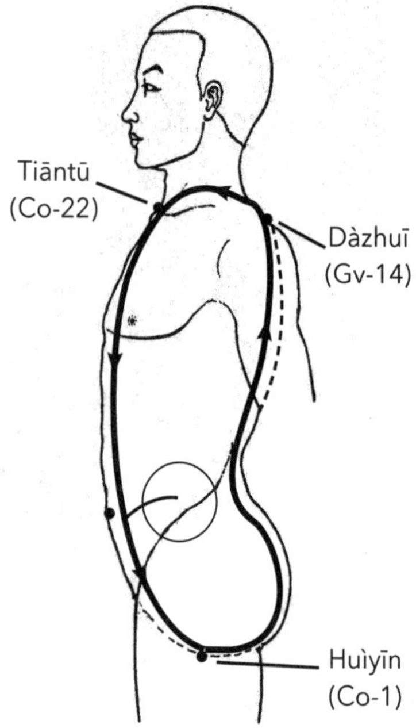

Figure 5-29. Back Fire Path–Dàzhuī–Tiāntū–Front Fire Path.

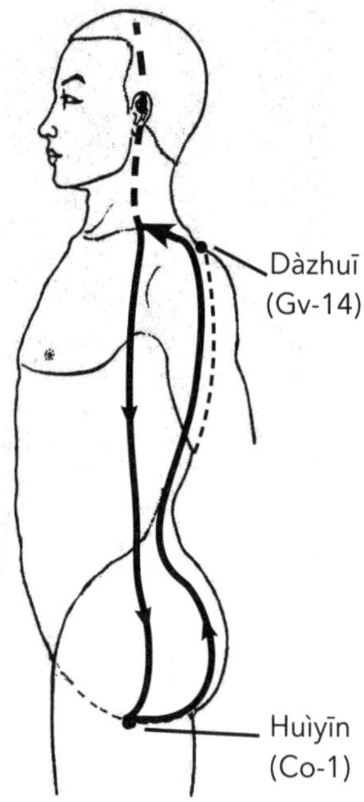

Figure 5-30. Back Fire Path–Dàzhuī–Reverse Water Path.

then use it for Muscle/Tendon Changing and Marrow/Brain Washing. Constantly refine your breathing, build up your Qì, and circulate it for the rest of your life.

Once your mind can lead the Qì efficiently, you can lead it any way you like in your body. "Transport Qì as though through a pearl with a nine-curved hole, it will reach even the tiniest place."[26]

5-7. Táng Dynasty Internal Elixir Meditation Illustration (Tángdài Nèidān Jìngzuò Nèijǐngtú, 唐代內丹靜坐內景圖)

This was painted during the Táng Dynasty (618–907 CE, 唐代) and revealed to secular society by a Daoist, Sùyún (素雲). Internal Elixir cultivation (Nèidān, 內丹) is specified very clearly even though it was still in its early stages. Internal Elixir for longevity and enlightenment was brought to China from India by Dámó during the Liáng Dynasty (502–557 CE, 梁朝). His two classics, *Yìjīnjīng* (*Muscle/Tendon Changing,* 易筋經) and *Xǐsuǐjīng* (*Marrow/Brain Washing,* 洗髓經) have strongly influenced Chinese Qìgōng society.

This illustration was revealed more than a thousand years ago. Even though disagreements and discrepancies crept in later, the main structure and contents remain accurate today. Keep a few things in mind:

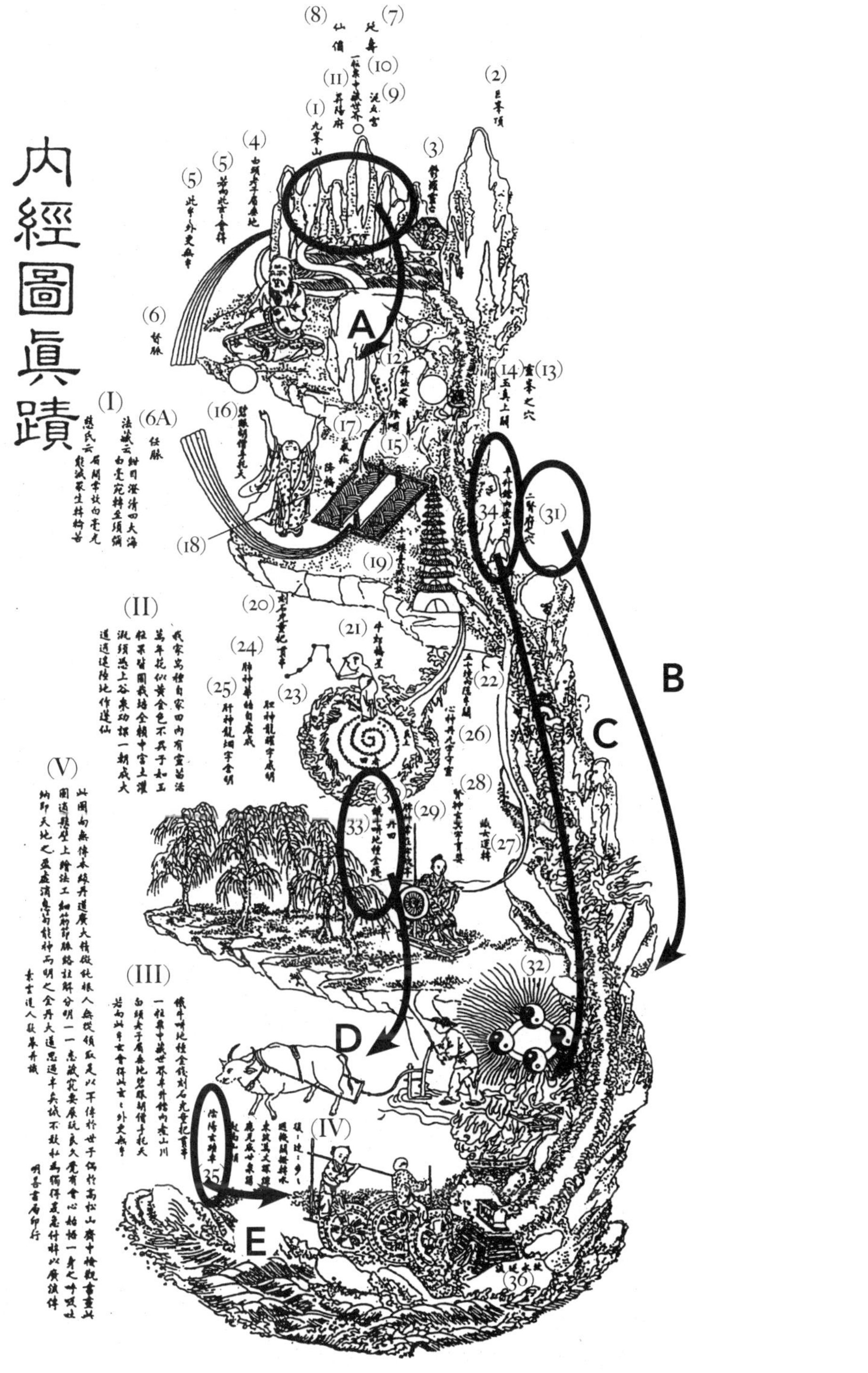

Figure 5-31. Corrections of Tang Dynasty Internal Elixir Meditation Illustration

1. Always question what you see and read. Think, and challenge the source. Then you will see much more clearly. If you simply believe, you can easily be led astray.
2. This illustration can be interpreted in various ways, so refer to all of them, and depend on your own thinking, experience, and judgment.
3. At least five functions were deliberately misplaced in the illustration (Figure 5-31): A. The Mud Pill Palace, which refers to the pituitary and pineal glands, is located at the top of the head. It should be at the center of the head behind the eyes. B. The right-hand column of characters behind the throat should be at the kidneys behind the spine, where the lady is weaving. C. The left-hand column of characters behind the throat refers to the small boiler under the Real Lower Dāntián, where the four Yīn-Yáng symbols are located. D. The column of Chinese characters under the heart should be placed above the Iron Bull cultivating the land, which symbolizes cultivating Qì in the Dāntián. E. The column of Chinese characters below the bull's head should be placed near the water wheels.
4. The following interpretations derive from my current understanding, which may change in the future, and should not be taken at face value (Figure 5-31).

(I)
Fǎzàng said:
Use the Buddhist heart (mind) and viewpoint to understand the four great oceans (world). Then your spirit will reach the fullness of virtue gradually and softly.

法藏云：
紺目澄清四大海
白毫宛轉至須彌

Gàn (紺) means Buddhist temple, and implies using the Buddhist heart to make judgment. Mù (目) means eyes, and implies viewing and observing. Báiháo (白毫) means many tiny white beams, and implies the spiritual light emitted from the head (the third eye). Wǎnzhuǎn (宛轉) means soft, gradual, and gentle. Xūmí (須彌) is the Daoist term for the spiritual being in the fullness of human virtue.

As long as you have a Buddha heart, you will have a neutral and clear point of view to judge whatever you see. You will be able to cultivate your temperament in the fullness of human virtue.

Císhì said:
Once the space between the eyebrows (third eye) can emit tiny white beams frequently, it can help seculars to eradicate the suffering of reincarnation.

慈氏云：
眉間常放白毫光
能滅眾生轉輪苦

Continuously cultivate your spirit to open the third eye located between the eyebrows to achieve enlightenment. Countless tiny beams of spiritual white light will emit from this place. You reach the first stage of Buddhahood and are able to solve secular emotional suffering, which arises from recurrent reincarnation.

(II)
I am engrossed in cultivating my own land in my family (body). There is a spiritual seed in it which can live ten thousand years (longevity).
Its flower is like yellow gold without different color (precious), and its fruits are like jade granules all around.
To plant and cultivate, rely on the Earth in the Central Palace, and to irrigate it, depend on the spring in the Upper Valley.
When the achievement of reaching the great Dào has been completed through practice, you become an immortal who lives leisurely without worry in this land.

我家耑種自家田
內有靈苗活萬年
花似黃金色不異
子如玉粒果皆圓
栽培全賴中宮土
灌溉須憑上谷泉
功課一朝成大道
逍遙陸地作蓬仙

The spirit is like a seed, precious as gold. Cultivate it correctly, so it allows you to live long. When cultivated and bearing fruit, it makes your spirit full. To cultivate it, rely on two things. First, build up elixir Qì at the Central Palace (Zhōnggōng, 中宮), the

Huángtíng (黄庭) or the Real Lower Dāntián. Also cultivate the spirit residing in the Spiritual Valley (Shéngǔ, 神谷). The holy Spiritual Embryo conceived at the Huángtíng establishes the seed of spiritual enlightenment. The quantity of Qì at the Real Lower Dāntián provides healthy physical life. The spirit at the Upper Dāntián governs the quality of Qì which manifests as life.

Having cultivated these two, unify them at the Real Lower Dāntián. This is called the unification and harmonization of Shén and Qì (Shénqì Xiànghé, 神氣相合). This is the goal of Embryonic Breathing. Water Qì at the Real Lower Dāntián is led up to interact with Fire Qì descending from the Middle Dāntián to conceive the Spiritual Embryo at the Huángtíng. This is the first step to reaching spiritual enlightenment. Having reached enlightenment, you live as an immortal in this secular world.

(III)
Iron Bull tills the land to plant the golden coins.
The stone-carving child threads them (golden coins) together.

鐵牛耕地種金錢 (33)

刻石兒童把貫串 (20)

The False Lower Dāntián is where the elixir land is plowed and the precious golden coins (Qì) grown. To build up Qì (start the fire) through Abdominal Breathing (Fùhūxī, 腹呼吸), you must be patient and persistent like the stubborn Iron Bull. (The Chinese characters were misplaced, and should be near the bull.)

To store abundant Qì (thread coins together), you need a childlike, innocent heart, free from emotional bondage. The child at the heart area (Middle Dāntián area) means the innocent and pure mind. Stone carving is hard work demanding patience, as needed to store Qì to an abundant level.

A single grain of rice can conceal the world,
A half-liter boiler can heat the mountains and the rivers.

一粒米中藏世界(10)

半升鐺內煮山川 (34)

A single grain of rice is very small. It refers to the Mud Pill Palace (Níwángōng, 泥丸宮) where the Shén resides. Keep your spirit there without being distracted by secular Xīn, then you can use this Shén to govern your life. The physical body is heaven and earth (Tiāndì, 天地), country (Guó, 國), world (Shìjiè, 世界), or mountains and rivers (Shan Chuan, 山川). Qì is called the people, and spirit is called the king.

The tiny boiler at the Lower Dāntián produces enough Qì to supply the mountains and rivers (physical body). Abundant Qì at the Lower Dāntián will supply the whole body's needs. Maintain your Shén at its residence to govern the quality of Qì manifestation, which means the quality of life. (The Chinese characters behind the throat were misplaced and should be under the four Yīn-Yáng symbols.)

The eyebrows of the white-headed old man reach to the ground.
The foreign monk with the blue eyes holds up heaven with his hands.

白頭老子眉垂地 (4)

碧眼胡僧手托天 (16)

The long eyebrows and white hair imply very old age and mean immortality can be reached through cultivation. Hands holding up heaven means the tongue is touching the palate of the mouth. This technique originated from Dámó (達摩), also known as Bodhidharma, who had been a prince in southern India. From the Mahayana school of Buddhism, he was considered to have been a bodhisattva, an enlightened being who renounced nirvana to save others. From fragmentary historical records, it is believed he was born about 483 CE. He arrived in Canton in 527 CE during the reign of the Wèi Xiàomíng emperor (魏孝明帝, 516–528 CE) or the Liáng Wǔ emperor (梁武帝, 502–557 CE).

If one comprehends the knack of this mystery,
then beyond it, there is no more mystery.

若向此鄉玄會得 (5)

此玄玄外更無鄉 (5)

These are the secrets of spiritual cultivation. Grasp them, then there is nothing more to be understood.

(IV)
Repeatedly and continuously, step by step repeat the cycle.
The pump turns the water and makes it flow to the East.
When the bottom of a deep lake of ten thousand fathoms can be seen,
then the sweet spring will emerge from the end of the southern mountains.

復復連連步步週
機關撥轉水東流
萬丈深潭應見底
甘泉湧起南山頭

Huìyīn is the secret cavity which controls manifestation of the body's Yīn and Yáng. From this area, you lead Qì in the Fire Path. Your body is strong and healthy, manifesting Qì into physical form.

However, if you lead the Qì up through the Thrusting Vessel, you enter the Water Path, which calms the body and raises the spirit.

The boy and girl represent Yīn and Yáng, manifesting through continuously pumping the water wheel (Huìyīn). Yīn manifests the Water Path, while Yáng manifests the Fire Path.

There was said to be an island called Pénglái Xiāndǎo (蓬萊仙島), in the eastern ocean, where the immortals lived. Through cultivation, you can attain immortality.

Your mind must be clear and calm like a very deep lake, through which the bottom can be seen clearly. This means you are not in emotional bondage, and your spirit is free and pure.

Once your mind is calm and peaceful and the spirit clear and focused, then saliva (sweet spring) is generated in the mouth, to the south of the head.

九峰山 (1)

Nine-peaked mountain. The top of the head is commonly referred to as the peak of a mountain or of heaven. Nine-peaked mountains means the brain in the top half of the head. Brain is also called Jiǔgōng (九宮), which means "Nine Palaces."

巨峰頂 (2)

Top of giant peak. The brain at the back of the head right behind Bǎihuì.

鬱羅靈臺 (3)

Obscure spiritual platform. Bǎihuì is where spirit leaves and enters its residence.

督脈 (6)

Governing Vessel. One of four Yáng vessels regulating the Qì status of the six primary Yáng channels.

任脈 (6A)

Conception Vessel. One of four Yīn vessels regulating the Qì status of the six primary Yīn channels.

延壽 (7)

Extending life. Embryonic Breathing (Tāixí, 胎息) condenses the spirit at the Mud Pill Palace (Níwángōng, 泥丸宮), where growth hormone and melatonin are produced in the pituitary and pineal glands. This is the key to longevity and immortality. (Mud Pill Palace is misplaced and should be at the center of the head.)

仙儷(8)

Immortal realm. The same as 7 above.

泥丸宮 (9)

Mud Pill Palace. Center of the head where pituitary and pineal glands are situated. Considered the Yīn center (Yīnhé, 陰核) of the Yáng Shén's (陽神) manifestation, and the residence of Original Shén (Yuánshén, 元神). Condensing the spirit here through Embryonic Breathing produces hormones, the secret of longevity. When this center is firmed and under control, manifestation of Yáng can be elevated to a magnificent level without inducing chaos. (These Chinese characters were misplaced, and should be at the center of the head.)

昇陽府 (11)

Uprising Yáng residence. Same as Mud Pill Palace above.

昇法之源 (12)

The origin of natural rule in spiritual raising. Same as Mud Pill Palace above.

靈峰之穴 (13)

Cavity of spiritual peak. Called Jade Pillow (Yùzhěn, 玉枕) by Daoists or Nǎohù (Gv-17, 腦戶) by Chinese medicine. The Qì at this cavity balances that at the Tiānyǎn (天眼, third eye), called Yìntáng (M-NH-3, 印堂) by Chinese medicine. Through the Qì balance of this gate, the third eye can be opened. This is the third gate needing to be opened in Small Circulation meditation. It is very precious in training, like jade. Because it helps open the third eye to reach the truth, it is a true gate.

玉真上關 (14)

Jade true upper gate. Another name for Jade Pillow, see 13 above.

飡咽 (15)

Food swallowing. The entrance of food into the body. When saliva is correctly swallowed with a sound Ń (嗯), health is maintained and significant progress made in meditation.

氣疾 (17)

Qì urgency. This Qì is Kōngqì (空氣, air). In meditation you regulate your breathing to be slender, soft, smooth, and natural. Without first calming body and mind, the mouth will be dry and breathing urgent. Calm the body and mind through correct breathing, then saliva will be generated.

降橋 (18)

Descending bridge. Under this bridge, saliva (heavenly water, Tiānchíshuǐ, 天池水) is generated. If swallowed correctly, Qì descends and strengthens the Yīn, assisting physical and mental calm during meditation.

十二樓臺藏秘訣 (19)

In the twelve-storied pagoda, secrets are hidden. Twelve-storied pagoda is the throat. Sounds express emotions, controlling the body's Qì. For example, a "Hā" (哈) sound on exhalation raises the spirit and leads Qì outward, strengthening Guardian Qì (Wèiqì, 衛氣). A "Hēng" (哼) sound on inhalation calms the spirit, leading Qì inward and nourishing Marrow Qì (Suǐqì, 髓氣).

This sentence can also be interpreted to mean that through asking, you will learn all hidden secrets of practice.

牛郎橋星 (21)

Cowherd bridge stars. The bridge joins Cowherd (Niúláng, 牛郎) and Weaving Lady (Zhīnǚ, 織女), so the baby embryo can be conceived. This bridge is the Xīn (heart). The mind brings Yīn and Yáng together so they can interact.

五十境內隱鄉關 (22)

In the fifty realms, the mysterious gateways are concealed. Fifty realms are the vertebrae, within which the spinal cord (Thrusting Vessel) is concealed. "Mysterious gateways" refers to the Water Path (Shuǐlù, 水路), circulating in the Thrusting Vessel. Water Path meditation is crucial to Brain Washing (Xǐsuǐ, 洗髓) for spiritual enlightenment. Its secrets have been concealed in Buddhist and Daoist monasteries for more than fifteen centuries.

膽神龍曜字威明 (23)

Gall bladder spirit, Lóngyào, means majestic and bright. The spirit of the gall bladder is called Lóngyào (龍曜). It is also associated with the liver. When it manifests, the eyes are bright and majestic. The gall bladder (Yáng organ) is the paired organ of the liver (Yīn organ).

肺神華皓自虛成 (24)

Lung spirit, Huáhào, is completed from emptiness. The spirit of the lungs is called Huáhào (華皓). It is associated with the nose, which takes in air (emptiness) and fills the lungs with life.

肝神龍煙字含明 (25)

Líver spirit, Lóngyān, contains brightness. The spirit of the liver, called Lóngyān (龍煙), is associated with the eyes. When the liver is healthy, the eyes are bright and sharp.

心神丹元字守靈 (26)

Heart spirit, Dānyuán, contains and maintains the Líng. The spirit of the heart is called Dānyuán (丹元). It contains the Líng (靈) and maintains its activities.

織女運轉 (27)

Weaving lady circulates and turns the wheel. This is the Huángtíng (黃庭) cavity where the Spiritual Embryo is conceived. The lady is preparing for the baby's birth.

腎神玄冥字育嬰 (28)

Kidney spirit, Xuánmíng (玄冥), contains nourishment for the baby. It nourishes the production of sperm. The kidneys are called Internal Kidneys (Nèishèn, 內腎), while the testicles are called External Kidneys (Wàishèn, 外腎). They are related to each other in function, responsible for reproduction and nourishment of new life.

脾神常在宇魂亭 (29)

Spleen spirit, Chángzài, is concealed in the soul pavilion. The spleen spirit, Chángzài (常在), is related to the soul.

中丹田 (30)

Middle Dāntián. The diaphragm, under the heart.

二腎府之穴 (31)

Cavities of two kidney residences. These two cavities are also called Shènshū (B-23, 腎俞, Kidney's Hollow). Through them, the kidney Qì enters and leaves at the back. (The descriptive characters should be behind the kidneys, not the throat.)

正丹田 (32)

Real Lower Dāntián. Second brain or biobattery where abundant Qì is accumulated in Qìgōng practice. This maintains physical strength and health. From here, Qì is led up through the Thrusting Vessel (Chōngmài, 衝脈) to nourish the brain, open the third eye, and attain spiritual enlightenment.

陰陽玄踏車 (35)

Stepping car (water pump) of Yīn-Yáng mystery. Water pump or water wheel, which implies the Huìyīn. Through control of the Huìyīn cavity, you can lead Qì to the Fire Path (Huǒlù, 火路, Yáng) or the Water Path (Shuǐlù, 水路, Yīn). This method of controlling the body's Yīn and Yáng was kept secret in the past. (Chinese characters should be placed closer to the water pump.)

坎水逆流 (36)

Kǎn water flows in the reverse direction. Kǎn (坎) represents water in the Eight Trigrams. Kǎn water (Kǎnshuǐ, 坎水) refers to the Qì circulating in the body. Through the pumping action of the Huìyīn, Kǎn water is led up to nourish the brain.

(V)
"This illustration has never before been passed down to others, because this Elixir Dào (Dào of refining elixir, 丹道) is so wide and refined. Those not wise enough will not be able to gain (the key), so it is rarely seen in this world. By accident, I found this illustration and writing in Gāosōng Mountain (high pine mountain, 高松山). It was hanging on the wall. The skills of this drawing are very refined, and the tendons, joints, vessels, and Qì channels are clearly indicated and interpreted. Every one conceals the important key in detail. I looked and pondered it for a long time, and feel I have comprehended some meaning within. Consequently, I started to realize deeply that the uttering and taking (Tǔnà, 吐納) of the whole body is just like the substantial and insubstantial of heaven and earth. If one can enlighten it and comprehend it clearly, then more than half of the achievement of reaching Great Dào of Golden Elixir (Jīndān Dàdào, 金丹大道) will have been achieved already. I dare not keep this secret to myself and thus publish it enthusiastically so it can be spread to the public."

— Copied and discerned by Sùyún Daoist

此圖向無傳本，緣丹道廣大精微，鈍根人無從領取，是以罕傳於世。子偶於高松山齋中檢觀書畫。此圖適懸壁上，繪法工細，筋、節、脈、絡註解分明。一一悉藏竅要，展玩良久，覺有會心。始悟一身之呼吸吐納，即天地之盈虛消息。苟能神而明之，金丹大道，思過半矣！誠不敢私為獨得，爰急付梓，以廣流傳。

素雲道人敬摹并識

References

1. 《難經・二十七難》：〝脈有奇經八脈者，不拘于十二經。〞

2. 李時珍《奇經八脈考》：〝奇經凡八脈，不拘制于十二正經，無表里配合，故謂之奇。〞

3. 《實用氣功學》：〝督脈起於會陰，循背而行于身之后，為陽脈之總督，故曰陽脈之海。任脈起於會陰，循腹而行于身之前，為陰脈之承任，故曰陰脈之海。〞〝人能通此兩脈，則百脈皆通，自然周身流轉，無有停壅之患，而長生久視之道斷在此矣。〞

4. *The Study of Practical Chinese Medical Qìgōng* (實用中醫氣功學), by Mǎ, Jì-Rén (馬濟人), 上海科學技術出版社, Shànghǎi, China, 1992.

5. 任脈：一・它循行于胸腹之正中，并在中極、關元穴與足三陰經交會，在天突、廉泉穴與陰維脈交會，在陰交穴與衝脈交會。二・足三陰經上接手三陰經。這樣任脈就可以溝通手、足三陰經的全部六條陰經了。

6. 督脈（總督諸陽）：一・它循行于背部之正中，其脈氣多次與十二正經的手、足的全部六條陽經相交會。最集中的地點是大椎穴，手足三陽經都在這裡左右相會。二・帶脈出于第二腰椎繞腰一轉，陽維脈與督脈也交會在風府、啞門，這樣督脈就起著統率的作用了。

7. 李時珍《奇經八脈考》：〝八脈散在群書者，略而不悉。醫不知此，罔探病機；仙家不知此，難安爐鼎。時珍不敏，參考諸說，萃集于左，所以備學仙、醫者筌蹄之用云。〞〝是故醫而知乎八脈，則十二經、十五絡之大旨得矣；仙而知乎八脈，則虎龍升降、玄牝幽微之竅妙得矣。〞

8. 《內經》：〝天人相應。〞

9. 《金丹大成集》：〝子午乃天地之中也，在天為日、月，在人為心、腎，在時為子、午，在卦為坎、離，在位為南、北。〞

10. 楊繼洲在《針灸大成》：〝人身之任督，以背腹言，天地之子午；以南北言，可以分，可以合者也。分之以見陰陽不雜，合之以見渾淪之無間，一而二，二而一也。〞

11. 李時珍在《奇經八脈考》：〝任督兩脈，乃身之子午也，乃丹家陽火陰符升降之道，坎水離火交媾之鄉。〞

12. 《脈望》：〝丹田，性命之本。道士思神，比丘坐禪，皆聚真氣于臍下，良由此也。丹田內有神龜，呼吸真氣，非口鼻之呼吸也。口鼻只是呼吸之門戶，丹田為氣之本源，聖人下手之處，收藏真一所居，故曰胎息。〞

13. 《黃庭內景經・梁丘子注》：〝黃者，中之色也；庭者，四方之中也。外指事即天中，人中，地中；內指事即腦中，心中，脾中。〞

14. 《黃庭外景經・石和陽注》：〝命門之上，有玄關二竅，左玄右牝，中虛一處，名曰黃庭。〞

15. 《養生秘錄・金丹問答》：〝黃庭正在何處？答曰：在膀胱之上，脾之下，腎之前，肝之左，肺之右也。〞

16. 王錄識餘云：〝銅人針灸圖，載臟腑一身俞穴有玉環，余不知玉環是何物。〞張紫陽玉清金華祕文，論神仙結丹處曰：〝心上腎下，脾左肝右，生門在前，密戶居後，其連如環，其白如棉，方圓徑寸，密裹一身之精粹，此即玉環。〞

17. 《易筋經・附錄》：〝神仙結丹處。曰：心下腎上脾左肝右，生門在前，密戶居后，

其連如環，其白如綿，方圓徑寸，包裹一身之精粹。・・・其處與臍相對。人之命脈根蒂也。〞

18. 〝督脈的內氣循行上向是自下而上，但至上唇齦交穴與任脈交接后，內氣則沿任脈上而下。成循環周流的情況。督脈與任脈上下交接處，分別稱為上鵲橋與下鵲橋。〞

19. *The Study of Practical Chinese Medical Qìgōng* (實用中醫氣功學), by Mǎ, Jì-Rén (馬濟人), 上海科學技術出版社, Shànghǎi, China, p. 682, 1992.

20. 《入藥鏡》：〝恍恍惚惚，杳杳冥冥，自然身心如暢，如醉如痴，肌膚爽透，美在其中。〞

21. 《奇經八脈考》：〝昏昏默默，如醉如痴。〞

22. 《金丹大成集》：〝腦後曰玉枕關，夾脊曰轆轤關，水火之際曰尾閭關。〞

23. 據《性命圭旨全書・采藥歸壺圖》所列：天人合發之機；子母分胎之路；任督接交之處；陰陽變化之鄉；九靈鐵鼓；三足金蟾；太玄關；藏金斗；尾閭穴；生死穴；朝天岭；氣海門；曹溪路；三岔口；平易穴；咸池；陰端；禁門；會陰；穀道；龍虎穴；三岔骨；河車路；上天梯等。

24. 《性命圭旨全書・天人合發采藥歸壺》：〝蓋精氣聚散常在此處，水火發端也在此處，陰陽變化也在此處，有無出入也在此處，子母分胎也在此處。〞〝其穴言于任督二脈中間，上通天谷，下達湧泉。〞又〝此穴干涉最大，系人生死岸頭。故仙家名為生死窟。《參同契》云：筑固靈株者此也。拘畜禁門者此也。《黃庭經》云：閉塞命門保玉都者此也。閉子精路可長活者，此也。〞

25. 《還丹訣》：〝端身正坐，運氣自尾閭起，一撞三關至泥丸。合而神水下降，復還丹田。曰大還丹。自腎轉肝，自肝傳心，自心傳脾，傳肺，周而復始，再至丹田，曰小還丹。〞

26. 行氣如九曲珠，無微不到。

Chapter 6

Embryonic Breathing

6-1. Introduction (Jièshào, 介紹)

More than a hundred ancient documents which discuss Embryonic Breathing (Tāixí, 胎息), were written by experienced Qìgōng masters in different historical periods. Embryonic Breathing is one of the very few subjects discussed seriously and in depth. Why has this subject been regarded as so important to Nèidān (內丹, Internal Elixir) Qìgōng practitioners?

In the previous chapter, we discussed the body's circulatory network of bioelectricity, or Qì. For this Qì to circulate smoothly, we must first concern ourselves with the biobattery, the energy supply source of this network. For longevity we need a strong and healthy body, and an efficient Qì system. When this Qì system performs efficiently, we can not only maintain physical health, but also lead extra Qì up the spinal cord (Chōngmài, 衝脈) to nourish the brain, which enhances the spirit of vitality. The method of using Qì to strengthen the body is called Muscle/Tendon Changing Qìgōng (Yìjīngōng, 易筋功), while using it to nourish the marrow and brain for enlightenment is called Marrow/Brain Washing Qìgōng (Xǐsuǐgōng, 洗髓功).

In realizing these benefits, we need to condition the biobattery, the Real Lower Dāntián, to produce Qì and store it abundantly. Embryonic Breathing is the method for this, developed through thousands of years of experience.

Embryonic Breathing is also called Cavity Breathing (Xuèwèi Hūxī, 穴位呼吸) or Dāntián Breathing (Dāntián Hūxī, 丹田呼吸). I call it No Extremity Breathing (Wújí Hūxī, 無極呼吸) or Second Brain Breathing. It is also called Wújí Breathing because its final goal is the Wújí state, where you focus only at the center of your Real Lower Dāntián (Zhēn Xiàdāntián, 真下丹田).

The purposes of Embryonic Breathing are:

1. **To calm the body and mind.** The first goal is to establish the mind in a state of extreme calm, in the Real Lower Dāntián. Then Qì is not led away from the center and consumed. The brain is not agitated nor the body excited, and Qì can be accumulated in abundance. *Dào Dé Jīng*, Chapter 16 (道德經・

十六章) said, "Approach the nothingness (emptiness) to its extremity, and maintain calmness with sincerity..."[1] This implies extreme calm of the body and mind. Your conscious mind gradually disappears, and the subconscious mind connected to the spirit awakens.

2. **To condition the Real Lower Dāntián (biobattery) and improve the storage capacity of Qì.** To increase Qì storage capacity higher than ordinary people, the Real Lower Dāntián must be conditioned. Refer to *Qìgōng—The Secret of Youth.*
3. **To accumulate abundant Qì in the Real Lower Dāntián.** This process charges the biobattery to an abundant level and facilitates the Qìgōng practice of Muscle/Tendon Changing and Marrow/Brain Washing.
4. **To stimulate production of hormones (Original Essence) in the adrenals, testicles or ovaries, and pancreas.** Hormones catalyze the body's biochemical reactions. Abundant healthy hormones keep the body's metabolism and Qì production smooth and healthy. Establishing healthy hormone levels is the key to longevity.
5. **To make the body strong and healthy through Muscle/Tendon Changing.** When abundant Qì accumulates in the Real Lower Dāntián, that in the Eight Vessels (Bāmài, 八脈) and Twelve Primary Qì Channels (Shíèrjīng, 十二經) will also flow strongly. This is crucial to maintaining physical health.
6. **For longevity and enlightenment, through Marrow/Brain Washing.** When abundant Qì is led into the bone marrow, the production of blood cells proceeds smoothly. This is vital in slowing down the aging process, because blood cells are the main carriers of oxygen and nutrition. Also, when abundant Qì is led up through the spinal cord to nourish the brain, the spirit of vitality is raised and the third eye can open. This is the achievement of Buddhahood or enlightenment.

6-2. Theory of Embryonic Breathing (Tāixí Lǐlùn Zhī Jiǎnjiè, 胎息理論之簡介)

Since so many documents are available, we cannot include them all in this book. Here we briefly discuss the concepts and methods of Embryonic Breathing, as they relate to spiritual cultivation. Again, for a more detailed discussion, refer to the book, *Qìgōng Meditation—Embryonic Breathing.*

Definition of Embryonic Breathing (Tāixí Zhī Dìngyì, 胎息之定義). According to the ancient documents, there are two definitions of Embryonic Breathing. One is to locate the spiritual center and the Qì center, then unite Shén and Qì at the Real Lower

Dāntián. These two centers are the two poles of the energy body. Bring the Shén down to unite with the Qì at the Real Lower Dāntián, which is the Qì center (Figure 6-1). Thus you return to the Wújí state, the origin of life. You are returning to the Real Lower Dāntián where you were conceived as a fetus. In this Wújí state, you return your being to nature.

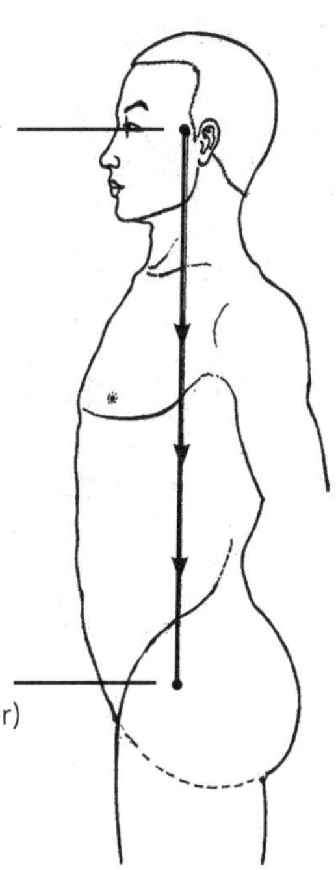

Figure 6-1. Unification of Shén and Qì at the Wújí Center

The earliest document in which this concept of Embryonic Breathing was propounded is Lǎozi's *Dào Dé Jīng*. Chapter 16 says, "Approach the nothingness (emptiness) to its extremity, and maintain calmness with sincerity. Millions of objects (lives) in action allow me to observe their cyclic repetition. Though there are so many objects, each individual must repeatedly return to its root (origin). When it returns to the root, it means calmness. When it is calmed, it means repetition of a life. When the life repeats, it means constant natural cycle."[2] From this document we see the purpose of Embryonic Breathing in tracing back the root of our lives, and understanding the cyclic repetition of nature. That means returning our spiritual being to the Wújí state (No Extremity, neutral state, 無極) of human life and thus reaching the origin of our spiritual nature.

Regulate Shén through cultivating the mind to an empty, neutral state. Shén finds its center and stays at its residence. Without this, we remain locked in the human emotional matrix. The mind cannot see the origin of the spirit, nor can we lead Qì to its residence (Real Lower Dāntián) and keep it there. The very beginning of Embryonic Breathing is searching for the spiritual origin in the center of the brain (Upper Dāntián) and the origin of Qì at the center of physical gravity, the Real Lower Dāntián.

To regulate Shén, Chapter 6 of *Dào Dé Jīng* said, "The Valley Spirit (Gǔshén, 谷神) does not die, then it is called Xuánpìn (玄牝). The door (key) to reach this Xuánpìn is the root of heaven and earth (nature). It is very soft and continuous as though it existed. When used, it will not be exhausted."[3] Shén is called Valley Spirit (Gǔshén, 谷神) because it resides in the Spiritual Valley (Shéngǔ, 神谷), the space between the two hemispheres of the brain. Xuánpìn (玄牝) means the marvelous and mysterious Dào, the mother of creation of millions of objects. The goal of regulating the Shén is to keep it at the Spiritual Valley, its residence.

Breathe softly, slenderly, and deeply like a newborn baby. Chapter 10 of *Dào Dé Jīng* said, "When bearing and managing the Pò (Vital Spirit, 魄) and embracing the state of oneness (Bàoyī, 抱一), can it be not separate? When concentrating Qì to reach softness, can it be soft as a baby? When cleansing the thought to reach purity, can it be without flaw?"[4] Língjiànzi Dǎoyǐn Zǐwǔ Recording (靈劍子導引子午記注) said, "What is Embryonic Breathing? It is a method of Embracing Oneness (Bàoyī, 抱一) and keeping it in the neutral state."[5]

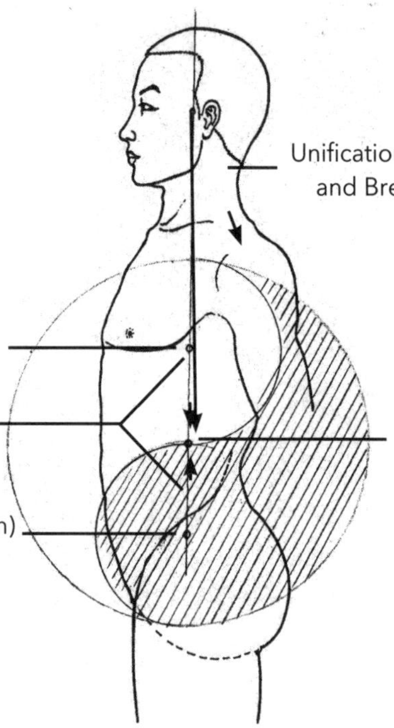

Figure 6-2. Conceiving the Spiritual Embryo

Embryonic Breathing means to regulate the mind and Shén to their most calm and concentrated state, and to accumulate abundant Qì at the Real Lower Dāntián, then unite the Shén and Qì to return the being to its origin. Embryonic Breathing has always been very important in Chinese Qìgōng practice, being the method of storing Qì in the Real Lower Dāntián. Through Embryonic Breathing you charge your biobattery to a high level. Then your vital energy is raised, the immune system is strengthened and the body reconditioned.

In Buddhist and Daoist tradition, Embryonic Breathing is defined as conceiving a Spiritual Embryo (Shéntāi, 神胎) at the Huángtíng cavity (黃庭). When it is ready, lead it up to the Upper Dāntián to be born (opening the third eye). To achieve this, first build up a high level of Water Qì (Shuǐqì, 水氣, Original Qì) at the Real Lower Dāntián. Lead it up, and lead Fire Qì (Huǒqì, 火氣, Post-Heaven Qì) down from the Middle Dāntián, so they meet at the Huángtíng (黃庭). This process is called Intercourse of Dragon and Tiger (Lónghǔ Jiāogòu, 龍虎交媾), the interaction of Yīn and Yáng, commonly called Kǎn and Lí (坎離). This results in the conception of life. Then you lead Shén down to meet this life, until a new Shén develops in the embryo. This process is called Mutual Dependence of Mother and Son (Mǔzǐ Xiāngyī, 母子相依). Mother means Qì and Son means Shén. From this process, a Spiritual Embryo is conceived (Figure 6-2).

When the Spiritual Embryo is ready, lead it up through Chōngmài to the brain. When the energy reaches a high level, the third eye (Tiānyǎn, 天眼) opens.

Theoretical Foundations of Embryonic Breathing 胎息之理論基礎. Here we review the role and function the Eight Vessels (Bāmài, 八脈) play in Qìgōng practice, especially in Nèidān (內丹) Qìgōng.

1. The Eight Vessels comprise four Yīn and four Yáng vessels which balance each other. These eight vessels comprise the major framework of the body's Qì network and regulate the Qì in the Twelve Primary Qì Channels (Shíèrjīng, 十二經).
2. They are Qì reservoirs that store Qì, but like Yīn and Yáng primary channels, the Yáng vessels manifest Qì, while the Yīn vessels preserve it.
3. The Conception Vessel (Rènmài, 任脈) in front is a Yīn vessel that balances the Yáng Governing Vessel. It regulates the Qì in the six primary Yīn channels (Qì rivers) while the Governing Vessel (Dūmài, 督脈) governs the Qì of the six primary Yáng channels. Since these Twelve Channels distribute Qì through the body, the two vessels control Qì distribution throughout the body.
4. The physical structure of the vessels is very likely constructed of various layers of tendon sandwiched between fasciae. Tendons are better conductors than muscles, while fasciae are insulators (poor conductors). This structure comprises a sort of battery to store Qì, which flows better in tendons than muscles. The Governing Vessel exhibits various layers of tendons attached at the center line of the spine, sandwiched by fasciae.
5. The Girdle Vessel (Dàimài, 帶脈) is extreme Yáng and counterbalances the Thrusting Vessel (Chōngmài, 衝脈) which is extreme Yīn. The Girdle Vessel's Qì expands horizontally, providing physical and mental balance, while the Thrusting Vessel centers your body and mind (Figure 6-3). These are the two most vital vessels of the Qì network. When Qì expands in the Girdle Vessel, Guardian Qì (Wèiqì, 衛氣) manifests strongly, as does the immune system. When Qì is abundant in the Thrusting Vessel, the central energy line is strong, and Shén is raised up. The glands along the central energy line—the pineal, pituitary, adrenals, and gonads—are nourished and their hormone production stimulated. Marrow Qì is also abundant, so healthy blood cells are produced. We will discuss this in more detail in the next book, Qìgōng Grand Circulation for Spiritual Enlightenment.

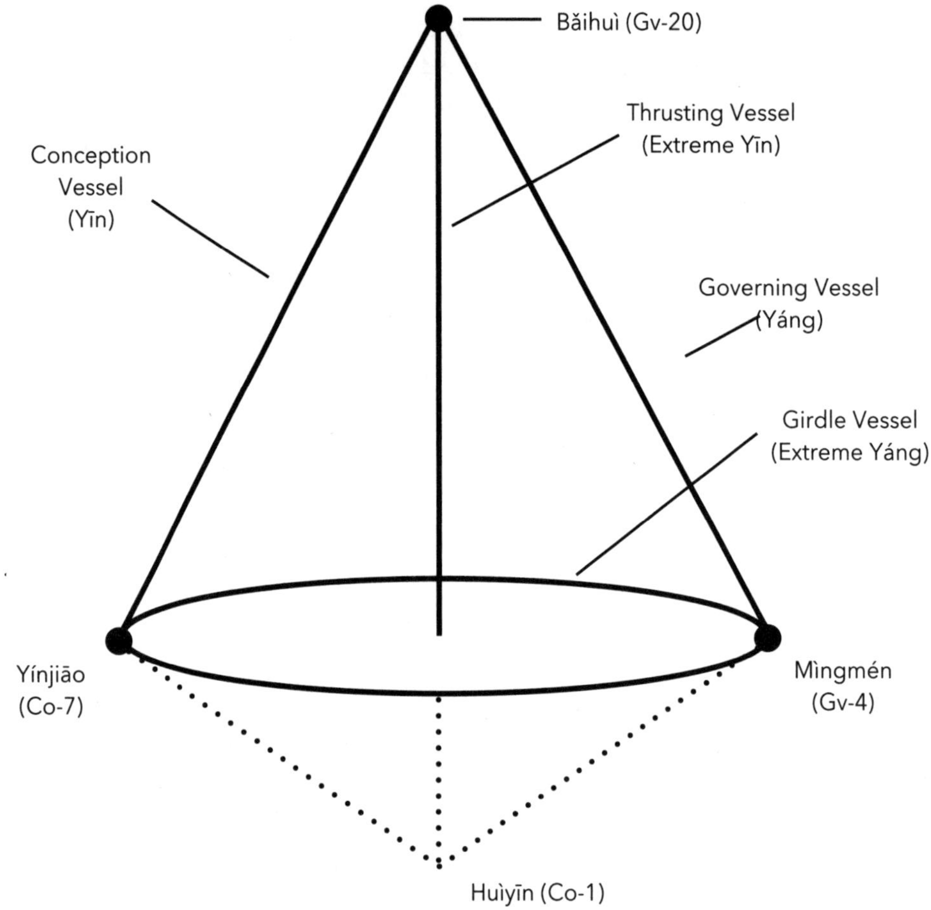

Figure 6-3. Thrusting Vessel and Governing Vessel

6. When you wake up in the morning, you start using your body. Your exhalation is longer than inhalation, since your mind is outside the body. Qì is led out to be manifested. The Conception and Governing Vessels regulate the Qì in the Twelve Primary Qì Channels, so it circulates aggressively in the Conception and Governing Vessels. But at night you sleep, with your body relaxed and your inhalation longer than exhalation. Qì is led inward to the central energy line, and Guardian Qì shrinks. Hormones are produced by the glands, and the brain obtains Qì nourishment. This promotes dreaming, as the brain cells readjust their energy.

   This is no different from the Qì cycle of a fish. During daytime, Qì circulates strongly along the upper and lower contours of the fish, so the fins and tail move aggressively. At night, this Qì circulation weakens and Qì is focused at the center line. Electromagnetic waves are emitted from the third eye of the fish, enabling it to swim without colliding with obstacles or other fish (Figure 6-4).[6]

During daytime, a tree's energy spreads up and out from the root, which is its biobattery, to exchange its Qì with that from the sun. At night, its Qì returns to its center and back down to the root (Figure 6-5). All living things are part of the Dào, which remains the same throughout nature. If you comprehend one clearly, you can interpret others easily.

7. The other four vessels exist in pairs. They are the Yīn Heel Vessel (Yīnqiāomài, 陰蹺脈), Yīn Línking Vessel (Yīnwéimài, 陰維脈), Yáng Heel Vessel (Yángqiāomài, 陽蹺脈)

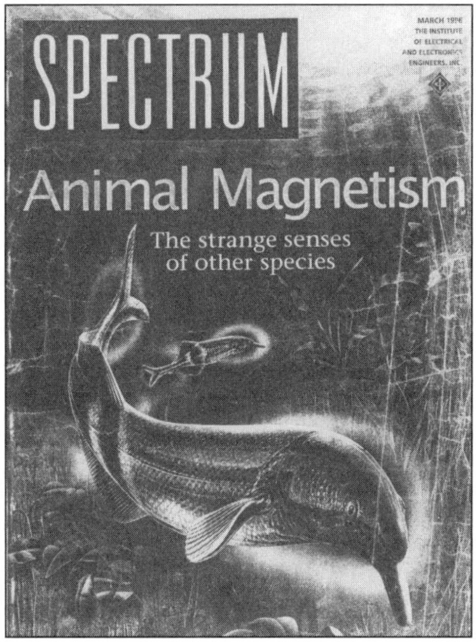

Figure 6-4. How Fish See Things in the Dark

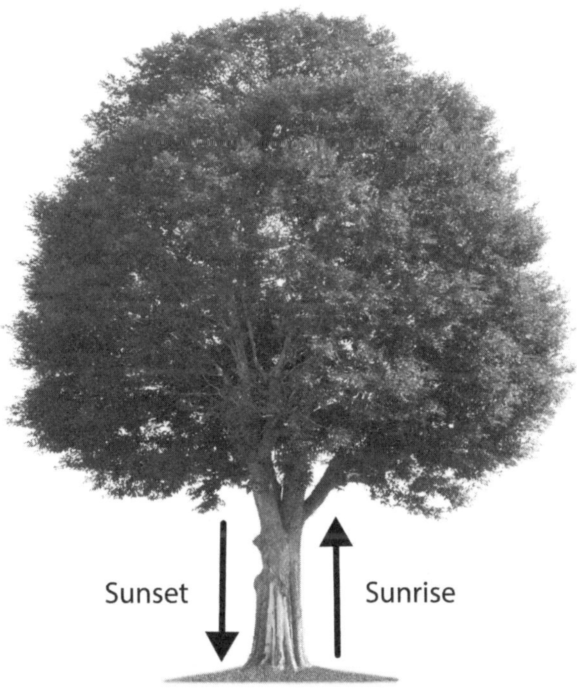

Figure 6-5. The Tree's Energy Moves Upward and Outward in the Daytime, and Moves Downward and Inward at Nighttime

(Photo by Shutterstock)

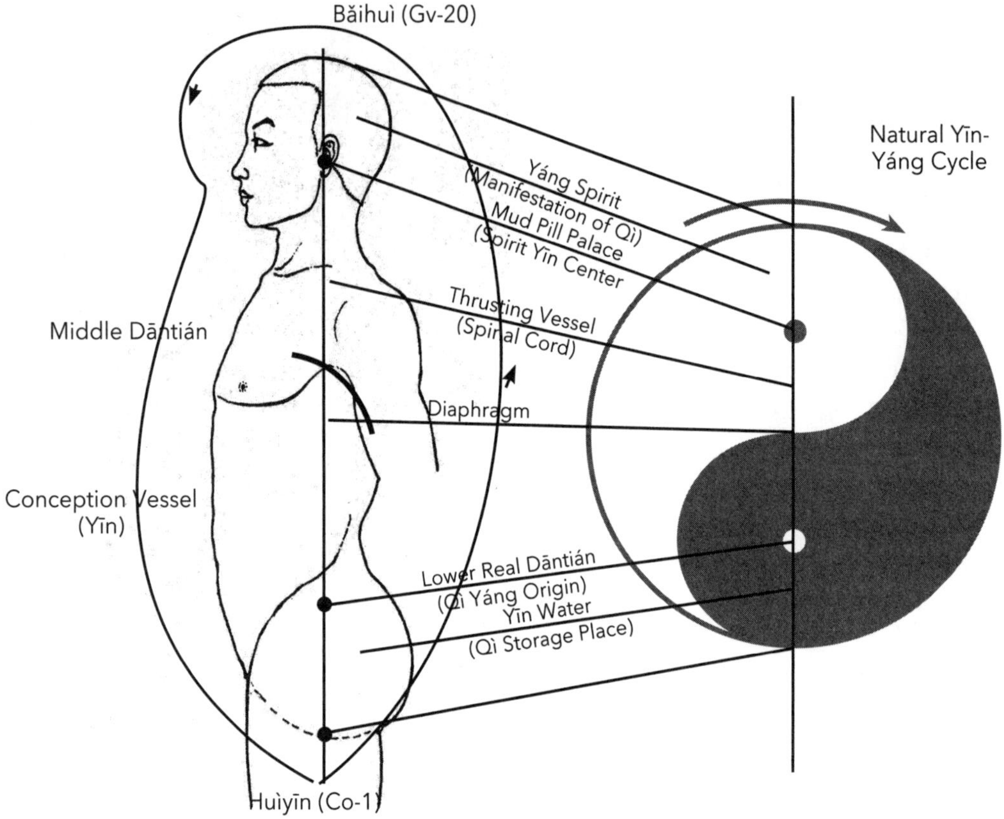

Figure 6-6. The Body's Yīn and Yáng, and the Two Polarity Centers

and Yáng Línking Vessel (Yángwéimài, 陽維脈). The two Yīn vessels connect at the Huìyīn, where they meet the other two Yīn vessels, the Conception and Thrusting Vessels. The perineum is called Huìyīn, the gate which connects all four Yīn vessels in the body. When this gate opens, Qì manifests, and when it closes, Qì is preserved. For example, when you are happy and excited, exhalation is longer than inhalation, and the body turns Yáng which leads excess Yáng to the internal organs, especially the heart. Then you automatically balance it by making a sound of "Hā" (哈) while pushing the perineum out. By contrast, when you are sad or scared, inhalation is longer than exhalation and you feel cold. To preserve Qì, you hold up the perineum automatically to close the gate. Using the perineum to control Qì in the body is one of the hidden keys in Qìgōng practice.

Illustration of the Body's Yīn and Yáng Poles (Rénshēn Yīny-Yáng Líǎngyí Jiě, 人身陰陽兩儀解). Here we compare the natural Tàijí Yīn-Yáng symbol with the body's Yīn-Yáng energy structure to discover the correspondences between them. Since one's body is part of nature, one should be able to interpret its Qì manifestation using the Yīn-Yáng symbol (Figure 6-6).

1. The direction of Qì circulation along the Conception and Governing Vessels is the opposite of the natural Yīn-Yáng cycle, so Yīn and Yáng in the body can be balanced by natural Yīn and Yáng.
2. Shén is considered Yáng, and the term Yángshén (Yáng Spirit, 陽神) is commonly used in Chinese Qìgōng documents. Shén is the general who controls the manifestation of Qì. When Shén is high, Qì is controlled and manifests effectively. Once you raise Shén to a high level, your vital force is enhanced. Normally, Shén is raised through the Bǎihuì, the place of extreme Yáng at the top of the Yīn-Yáng symbol. Bǎihuì means "hundred meetings," the meeting place of all the body's Qì. It is the pivotal point controlling all the body's energy, the most Yáng place in the body.
3. Huìyīn is the most Yīn place in the body. It is sometimes called Hǎidǐ (sea bottom, 海底), because Qì is similar to water, with the intestines as the ocean which stores it. While Qì remains here, the body is calm and peaceful, but when it is consumed through manifestation, mind and body are excited and Shén diverges. Keep calm by inhaling deeply and leading Qì down to the abdomen, then exhale while relaxing. In this way tension dissipates and blood pressure is lowered.
4. The body's Yīn and Yáng are connected by the Thrusting Vessel. The Spirit Yīn Center in the Mud Pill Palace controls, governs, and restrains the Yáng Shén's manifestation. If Shén stays here, it is focused and centered. To bring Shén to this Yīn center, first calm the mind, and avoid emotional disturbance and desire.
5. The Real Lower Dāntián produces Qì and stores it, supplying it to the body and brain. The Upper Dāntián controls the quality of Qì. With the Girdle Vessel (Extreme Yáng Vessel) and Thrusting Vessel (Extreme Yīn Vessel), it forms a spiritual cultivation triangle (Figure 6-7). The more Guardian Qì there is, the higher the Shén can be raised. The base of the triangle represents physical life, while the center line represents spiritual life.

Interaction of Yīn and Yáng (Intercourse of Dragon and Tiger) (Lónghǔ Jiāogòu, 龍虎交媾)

Keep your Shén and Qì at their centers to Embrace Oneness (Bàoyī, 抱一). These are two poles of the same life, which synchronize and correspond with each other. Physically they are two, but in function they are one. One is for physical life and the other for spiritual life, but they are indivisible.

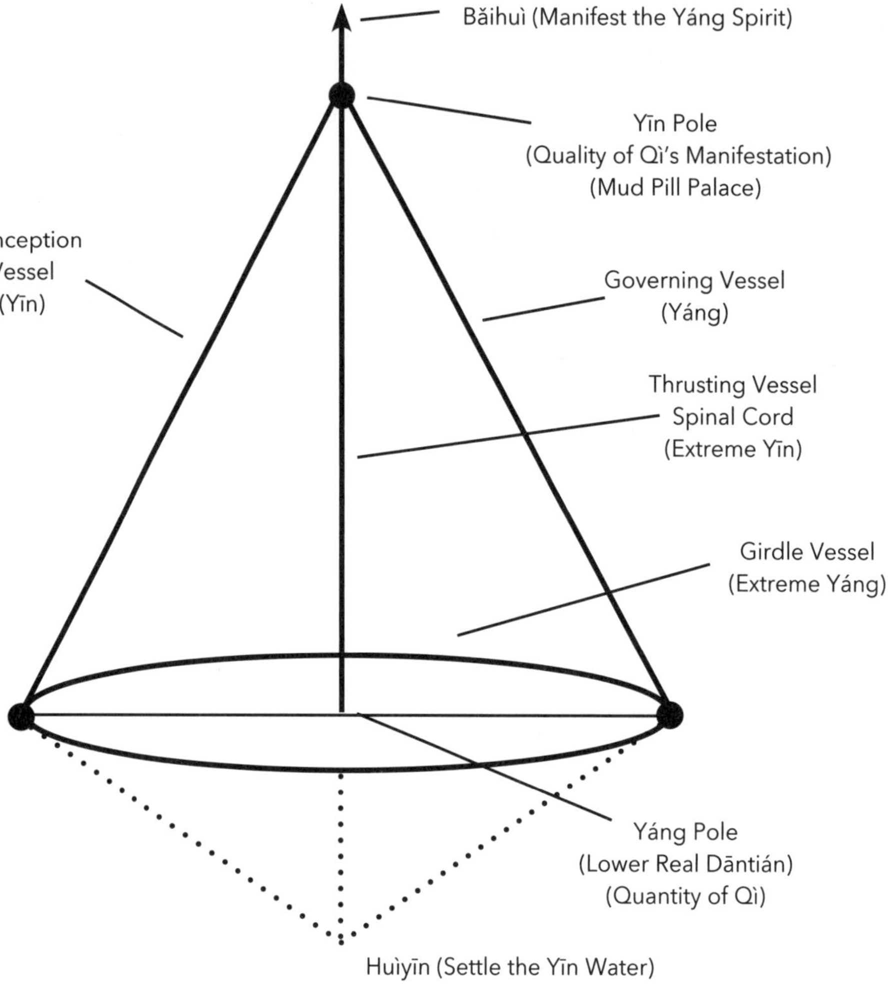

Figure 6-7. Spiritual Triangle

The first definition of Embryonic Breathing is to unite Shén and Qì at the Real Lower Dāntián, to return to the source of life. Here, life is initiated and developed. To many Daoists, the first goal of Embryonic Breathing is to find this center to unite Shén and Qì (Figure 6-8). Since the goal of this practice is to return to the Wújí center, I call this Wújí Breathing (Wújíxí, 無極息).

The second definition of Embryonic Breathing is to conceive a Spiritual Embryo (Shéntāi, 神胎) at the Huángtíng. Concentrate the Wisdom Mind (Yì, 意), lead Fire Qì down from the Middle Dāntián and Water Qì up from the Real Lower Dāntián to meet at Huángtíng (Figure 6-9). This interaction of Yīn and Yáng is called Intercourse of Dragon and Tiger (Lónghǔ Jiāogòu, 龍虎交媾), or Kǎn and Lí (坎離). Then you lead Shén down from the Upper Dāntián to unite with Qì and conceive the Spiritual Embryo.

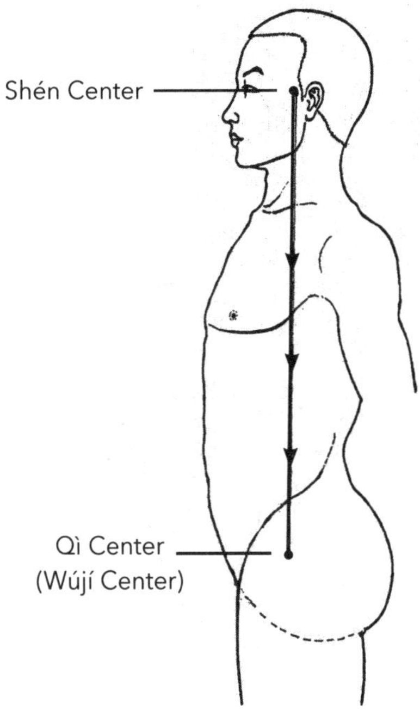

Figure 6-8. Unification of Shén and Qì at the Wújí Center

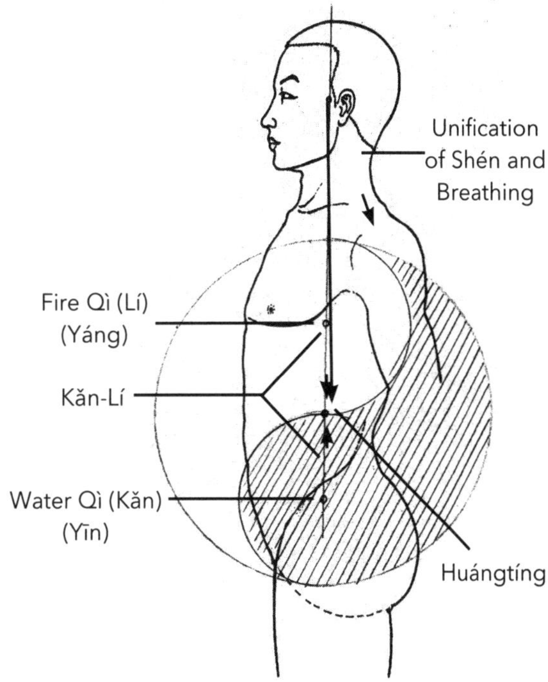

Figure 6-9. Conceiving the Spiritual Embryo

Summaries

1. *The Complete Book of Principal Contents of Human Life and Temperament, About Large and Small Tripod and Furnace*, (*Xìngmìng Guīzhǐ Quánshū, Dàxiǎo Dǐnglú Shuō*, 性命圭旨全書，大小鼎爐說) says, "Huángtíng (黃庭) is the tripod, Qìxuè (氣穴, Qì cavity) is the furnace. Huángtíng is just on top of Qìxuè, interconnected with numerous Luò (絡). It is the meeting place of hundreds of Qì vessels in the body. Original Qì (Yuánqì, 元氣) is dense between these two cavities and is called Small Tripod Furnace (Xiǎo Dǐnglú, 小鼎爐). If the Qián (brain, 乾) is the tripod and the Kūn (abdomen, 坤) is the furnace, then Níwán (Upper Dāntián, 泥丸) is the tripod and the Lower Dāntián is the furnace. This is called Big Tripod Furnace (Dà Dǐnglú, 大鼎爐)."[7] This document explains the large Yīn-Yáng and Small Yīn-Yáng symbols and how they relate to the body (Figures 6-10 and 6-11).
2. In the Small Tripod Furnace (Xiǎo Dǐnglú, 小鼎爐), you search for the Wújí state of Kǎn and Lí. Then the Spiritual Embryo (Shéntāi, 神胎) is conceived. Later, when it is mature, it is led up for cultivation of spiritual enlightenment.

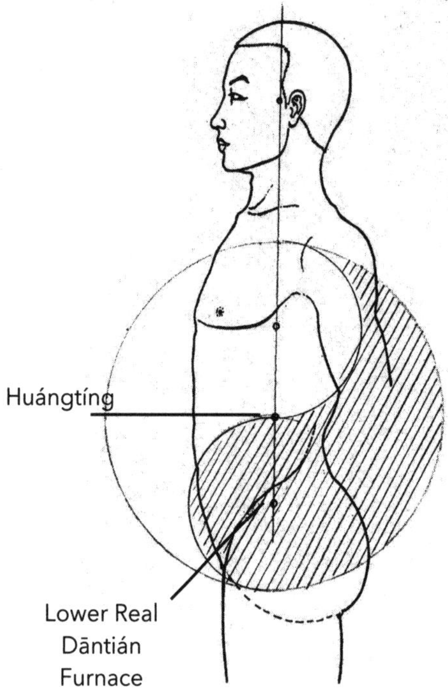

Figure 6-10. Small Tripod and Furnace

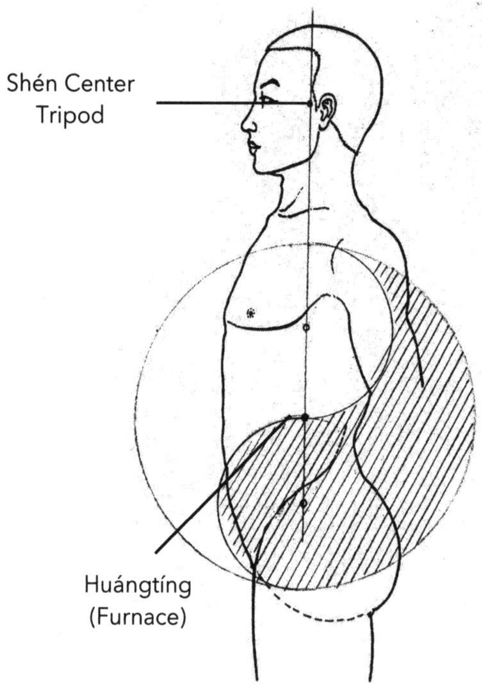

Figure 6-11. Large Tripod and Furnace

3. In the Big Tripod Furnace (Dà Dǐnglú, 大鼎爐), you look for the Wújí state of your original being, returning life to its very origin. Bring Shén down to the Real Lower Dāntián to unite with the Qì.

6-3. Methods of Embryonic Breathing (Tāixífǎ, 胎息法)

Here we discuss the practice of Embryonic Breathing. First, your mind must locate the Upper Dāntián and the Real Lower Dāntián. Next, you condense the spirit to a higher level of focus and produce more abundant Qì. Then lead the spirit and the Qì to their residences, and keep them there. Finally, you unite the spirit and the Qì at the Real Lower Dāntián.

We briefly discuss the method of the Qì's Kǎn and Lí and how to unite it with the Shén at the Huángtíng (黃庭) to conceive the Spiritual Embryo. The method of leading Qì up to nourish the brain and Shén will be discussed in the next book, *Qìgōng Grand Circulation for Spiritual Enlightenment*.

Times to Practice. The best times to practice are dawn, noon, dusk, and midnight, but this is not easy to achieve. I recommend dawn and right before you go to sleep. If your schedule allows you to take an afternoon nap, use this time to practice Embryonic

Breathing. Your body is most Yáng during early afternoon, and Embryonic Breathing stores the surplus Qì inside.

When your mind and body are very calm and relaxed, you may allow yourself to fall asleep. Embryonic Breathing is not the same as other Nèidān meditation in which you lead the Qì. In Nèidān you should not fall asleep, since Qì will enter the wrong path. However, in Embryonic Breathing your mind is not leading the Qì, so falling asleep will not cause any problem.

You should not be restricted to the suggested times. Once you have mastered Embryonic Breathing, you can practice anytime and anywhere.

Orientation of Practice. Embryonic Breathing takes advantage of natural Qì, the most significant being the Qì of the sun, moon, and earth. So orient your meditation accordingly. (Table 6-1) For a detailed exposition, refer to *The Root of Chinese Qìgōng*, by YMAA Publication Center.

Table 6-1. Meditation Orientation and Times

Timing	Purpose	Orientation	Natural Qì Source
Dawn	Nourishing	Face east	Sun
	Retreating*	Face west	Sun
Noon	To calm down	Any direction	——
Dusk	Prevent retreating	Face east	Sun
	Retreating	Face west	Sun
Night**	Nourishing	Face south	Earth's magnetic field
	Retreating	Face north	Earth's magnetic field

*Retreating means to remove some Qì from your body to make it more Yīn.

**To absorb Qì from the moon, meditate two to three days before full moon, facing the moon. Not recommended after full moon, since the moon then drains your Qì.

Recognize the Yīn Center of the Upper Dāntián and the Yáng Center of the Real Lower Dāntián

(Shàng Dāntián Yīnhéxīn Yǔ Xià Dāntián Yánghéxīn Zhī Rènshí, 上丹田陰核心與下丹田陽核心之認識, Xuèwèi Rèntóng, 穴位認同)

The first step is to recognize the Yīn center of the Upper Dāntián (Yīnshén, 陰神) and the Yáng center of the Real Lower Dāntián (Yángquán, 陽泉) (Figure 6-6). The only way to locate these two centers is through inner feeling.

The Upper Dāntián (Shàng Dāntián, 上丹田) is at the center of the Spiritual Valley (Shéngǔ, 神谷), where the pineal and pituitary glands are located. This is the Mud Pill Palace (Níwángōng, 泥丸宮), the central spiritual residence (Shénshì, 神室, Upper Dāntián). It lies where the line joining the tops of the ears meets the line joining the

Yìntáng (M-HN-3, 印堂) with the Qiángjiān (Gv-18, 強間). The Yīn Shén is at the center of the Dāntián, and has a different quality of feeling than the rest of the Dāntián itself. To recognize this point through feeling, be free of emotional disturbance and external attraction, so your mind is clear. Search for the place sincerely, and you will soon find it.

The Yángquán is the Yáng center of the Real Lower Dāntián (Zhēn Xiàdāntián, 真下丹田) where the large and small intestines are located, a couple of inches above the center of gravity. The whole digestive system constitutes the Real Lower Dāntián. If you can find its center, you can keep the Qì there, storing it to an abundant level. It is located behind Yīnjiāo (Co-7, 陰交) and in front of Shíqīzhūixià (M-BW-25, 十七椎下) below the 17th vertebra, at the center between these two cavities. Search for this point through feeling when you meditate, and you should find it in a short time.

Condensing Shén and Qì into Their Centers

(Regulating the mind, spirit, and Qì) (Tiáoxīn, 調心) (Tiáoshén, 調神) (Tiáoqì, 調氣)

Having located the Yīn center of the Upper Dāntián, you raise up the spirit and keep it there. Calm your Emotional Mind (Xīn, 心), cut off external distractions and the material attractions of desire and ambition. Concentrate your mind in raising your spirit, and condense it at the Yīn spiritual center. Whenever you encounter difficulties in this, simply focus on your breathing. Keep the inhalation soft, long, and slender. Exhale naturally and allow carbon dioxide to be released by itself. In this way you stabilize and calm your mind. Focus your spirit at the Yīn spiritual center. In this way the Yáng spirit (陽神), the manifestation of Qì by the spirit, is brought under control. On one hand you aim to raise your spirit to a high level, but on the other you need to bring it under the control of the Yīn spirit.

To condense Shén at this Yīn spiritual center, simply imagine your head as a ball, with the Mud Pill Palace (Níwángōng, 泥丸宮) as its center. Inhale deeply, softly, and slenderly, using Reverse Abdominal Breathing (Nì Fùhūxī, 逆腹呼吸) while holding up the Huìyīn gently. Imagine the ball shrinking and condensing inward to the Mud Pill Palace. When you exhale, relax, and allow the abdomen and Huìyīn to return to their normal state. You pay more attention to the inhalation, and the Yì of inhalation is strong, which leads Shén and Qì inward to condense at their centers.

Conditioning the Biobattery (Real Lower Dāntián)

(Zhēn Xiàdāntián Zhī Gǎiliáng, 真下丹田之改良)

To store abundant Qì at the Real Lower Dāntián, first condition it extensively to improve the storage capacity significantly. You cannot expect exceptional Qì capacity from an average biobattery.

The ancient classic of *Muscle/Tendon Changing and Marrow/Brain Washing Qìgōng* (*Yìjīnjīng; Xǐsuǐjīng*, 易筋經・洗髓經) describes the most efficient way of conditioning this biobattery (False and Real Lower Dāntiáns), namely through massage and stimulation. Massage gets rid of the fat hidden inside, so the circulation can be smooth, and stimulation conditions the nerves to store a significant amount of Qì there. The conditioning process is long and arduous, and you need a clear grasp of its theory. It is described in detail in the book *Qìgōng—The Secret of Youth.*

A. **Condition Your Nervous system**
Conditioning the biobattery requires stimulating the abdomen's nervous system, using abdominal breathing and massage. When enough energy is stored there, it agitates the nervous system, which at first may simply feel warm. After extensive stimulation, the nerves reach their tolerance threshold, and the muscles twitch and vibrate by themselves. No more Qì can be stored, but will simply disperse. It is best to start conditioning practice using massage. Appropriate methods are described in *Qìgōng—The Secret of Youth.*

B. **Improve the Quality of the Biobattery's Material Structure**
The higher the structural quality of the abdomen and bowels, the better the conditions for storing abundant Qì. There are two ways to reach this goal. One is through massage as described in the last section. The second is through pounding the area with special tools. The force reaches deeper and stimulates the whole system, qualitatively changing the area. Naturally you must be patient, using correct techniques to avoid injury.

C. **Reduce the Thickness of Fat (Insulators)**
To increase the charge of a battery, the insulator between the conductive area must be thin, but with high insulating capability. Fat and fasciae act as insulators in the body, sandwiched between good conductors (muscles). To store more Qì at the Real Lower Dāntián, you need to reduce the thickness of the fat and improve the insulating capacity of fasciae. This is achieved through massage and pounding, and also through abdominal exercises. Correct methods of exercise reduce the fat and condition the fasciae effectively.

Increase the Quantity of Qì (Qìliàng Zhī Jiāqiáng, 氣量之加強)

Having conditioned your biobattery, you need high quality Qì to store in it. There are three ways to increase the quantity of Qì in the body:

A. **Qì Furnaces**

About two inches below the navel is an area called Qìhǎi (Co-6, 氣海, Qì Ocean) in medical society. In Daoist society it is called Dānlú (丹爐) (Elixir Furnace) or Dāntián (Elixir Field), the place which produces Qì. Move the abdomen in Abdominal Breathing, facilitating the conversion of fat into Qì.

B. **Herbs**

Different diets affect the body's Qì differently, and Chinese medicine uses herbs extensively, some of which increase the body's Qì. Appropriate herbal prescriptions are listed in *Qìgōng—The Secret of Youth*, although some ingredients are difficult to find, not being in common use. I recommend consulting a qualified Chinese doctor, since these prescriptions have been passed down over fifteen hundred years, and their accuracy is in doubt. Be very cautious when you use them.

C. **Increase Hormone Production**

Hormones are called Original Essence (Yuánjīng, 元精) in Chinese Qìgōng. They act as catalysts to facilitate biochemical reactions in the body's metabolism. When hormones are abundant, Qì from biochemical reaction is enhanced. Hormone therapy can extend our lifespan significantly. Qìgōng practice targets the adrenals, the gonads, and the pituitary and pineal glands.

a. **Adrenals (Kidneys)**

Adrenal glands fit like small cups on top of the kidneys. Each is divided into two parts: the cortex or outer portion, and the medulla or central section. The cortex and medulla produce different hormones. The cortex, absolutely essential to life, secretes about thirty hormones and regulates several metabolic processes. The medulla produces the hormone epinephrine, commonly called adrenaline.

There are three ways to stimulate hormone production.

i. Massage. This includes circular rubbing and tapping the kidneys. Please refer to the YMAA book, *Qìgōng Massage*.

ii. Spinal Movement. Correct movement of the lower back and spine massages the kidneys, maintaining health and stimulating hormone production. Please refer to the YMAA book, Back Pain Relief.

iii. Deep Abdominal Breathing. This lowers the diaphragm and accesses the adrenal glands, enhancing hormone production.

b. **Testicles or Ovaries (Gonads)**

The testicles produce the male hormone testosterone, while the ovaries produce estrogen and progesterone. When these hormones are adequate, the life force is strong and activity is vigorous. There are two ways to stimulate production.

i. Massage. Traditional techniques for men are described in *Qìgōng—The Secret of Youth*. To massage the ovaries is more difficult, and the most common way is to circle and rub them gently with the palms.

ii. Testicle or Ovary Breathing. Lead the Qì to the sex glands, in coordination with abdominal breathing, to stimulate hormone production. Alternatively one may use imaginary sexual activity, but this can lead you into the domain of illusion and I do not recommend it.

c. **Pituitary and Pineal Glands**

These glands are located in the Mud Pill Palace (Níwángōng, 泥丸宮) where the spirit resides. This area can raise your spirit and increase your life span.

The pituitary gland produces growth hormone and stimulates, regulates, and coordinates the functions of the other endocrine glands. For this reason it is called the master gland. Scientists know little about the function of the pineal gland. It produces melatonin and is related to the body's time clock.

i. Massage. The Mud Pill Palace is connected to the sacrum through the spinal cord, and to the bottom of the feet through the two Yīn vessels (Yīn Heel and Yīn Línking Vessels, 陰蹻脈・陰維脈). When the sacrum or the bottoms of the feet are massaged, hormone production of the pituitary and pineal glands is stimulated.

ii. Brain Washing Qìgōng Practice. Lead the Qì up through the spinal cord to nourish the brain around the Mud Pill Palace, using Embryonic Breathing.

Store the Qì in Abundance—Embryonic Breathing (Cavity Breathing, Wújí Breathing) (Tāixí, 胎息)

These techniques enable you to produce more Qì. You need to store it in the Real Lower Dāntián, otherwise it flows out to be consumed in manifestation.

Keep your mind in the Real Lower Dāntián, then Qì will not be led away from its residence. Move the navel (Yīnjiāo) and the lower back at the same time. The navel is called Shēngmén (生門), the door of life. The lower back is called Bìhù (閉戶), the closed door, or Mìngmén (Gv-4, 命門) cavity between L2 and L3 (Figure 6-12). Through synchronized movement of the front and back, you can locate the Yáng water center easily. Your mind initially focuses on both front and back, but later, when you reach the stage of regulating without regulating, the mind will find the center. The Secret of Embracing Oneness and Containing Three (Bàoyī Hánsān Mìjué, 抱一函三秘訣) said, "Between the two kidneys is the root, called the elixir foundation of the ancestral herb."[8] This emphasizes the importance of the Mìngmén cavity, located between the two internal kidneys.

When you synchronize moving the two doors up and down, extra Qì is produced in both places. Also coordinate with movement of Huìyīn. Soon you feel Qì in the Girdle Vessel expanding and contracting (Figure 6-13).

These movements stimulate the glands and enhance production of insulin hormone in the Islets of Langerhans in the pancreas, DHEA (dehydroepiandrosterone) in the adrenal glands, and testosterone (male), or estrogen and progesterone (female), in the sex glands.

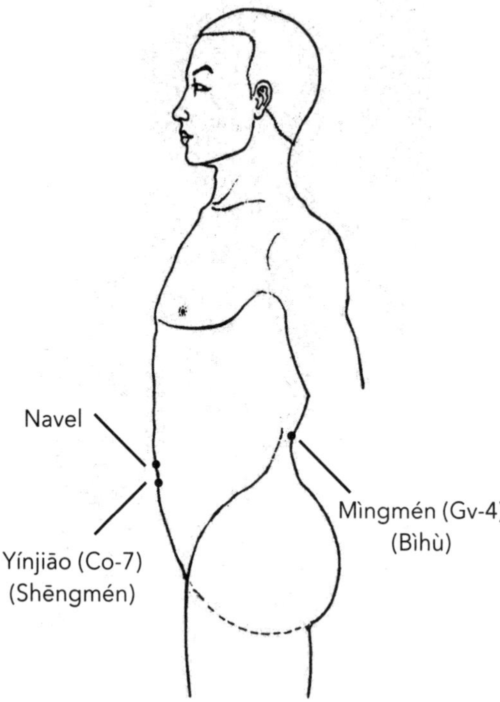

Figure 6-12. Shēngmén (the Door of Life) and Bìhù (the Closed Door)

In addition to focusing your mind at the Yáng center of the Real Lower Dāntián, also focus it at the Yīn center of the Upper Dāntián. These are the Two Poles of the central energy line, and they correspond and synchronize with each other. They are two aspects of the same thing and cannot be separated. Shén and Qì are like son and mother, which cannot be separated when you practice Embryonic Breathing.

When the mind concentrates at the Yīn center of the Upper Dāntián, production of melatonin (pineal gland) and growth hormone (pituitary gland) is also enhanced. These hormones smooth the biochemical reactions, and regulate and improve the metabolism.

The final stage of Embryonic Breathing is to bring Shén down to the Real Lower Dāntián, to unite with Qì. Qì stays at its residence and is stored to a very high level. This is called harmonization of Shén and Qì (Shénqì Xiànghé, 神氣相合). The two poles unite and become one, embodying the Wújí state, the beginning of life. I call this stage Wújí Breathing (WújíXí, 無極息). Lead the Shén down to the Real Lower Dāntián through the concentrated mind in coordination with breathing.

Two Ways of Leading Qì and Shén to the Real Lower Dāntián

There are two types of breathing that enable you to lead Qì and Shén to the Real Lower Dāntián for effective unification. When Qì is raised up to the brain, the Shén is

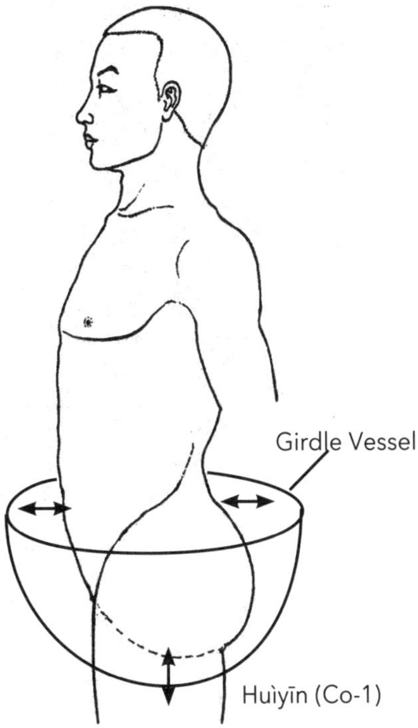

Figure 6-13. Embryonic Breathing

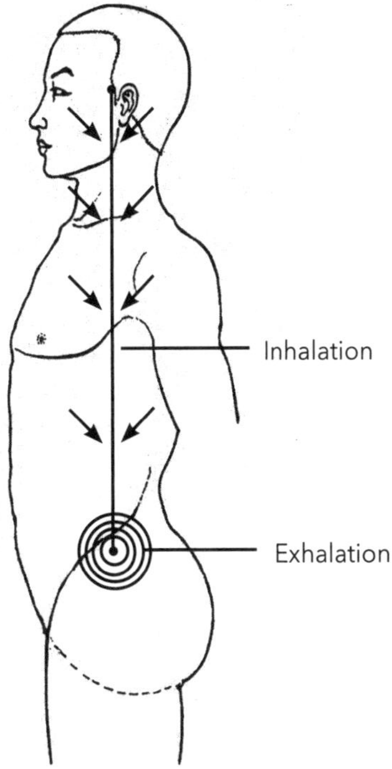

Figure 6-14. The Buddhist Way of Leading the Qì Down to the Real Lower Dāntián

excited, and the mind becomes scattered. Blood pressure and heartbeat rise as the manifestation of Qì is enhanced. But when Qì is led down to the Real Lower Dāntián, it is stored and stays there, and the mind is calmed and relaxed. The body cools down and blood pressure goes down. Shén is also led down by the calm mind.

Buddhist Way: Inhale deeply using the mind to lead Qì down through the Thrusting Vessel to the Real Lower Dāntián. Then exhale, keeping the mind there. When you inhale, the abdomen expands, while the Huìyīn gently pushes down. When you exhale, relax the abdomen and Huìyīn, and allow them to return naturally (Figure 6-14). Then a lot of Qì is led down to stay at its residence. The more you practice, the faster you can make it happen. This Buddhist technique is used to lower blood pressure, ease the excited mind, and slow down the heartbeat. It effectively relaxes both body and mind.

Daoist Way: Inhale to condense Qì into the center as you pull in your abdomen and Huìyīn. Guardian Qì (Wèiqì, 衛氣) shrinks and enhances Marrow Qì (Suǐqì, 髓氣). Once Qì is led to the Thrusting Vessel, exhale deeply while leading Qì down (Figure 6-15). While exhaling, push your abdomen and Huìyīn out gently, as you store Qì at the Real Lower Dāntián. This Daoist technique effectively cools the excitement of the body.

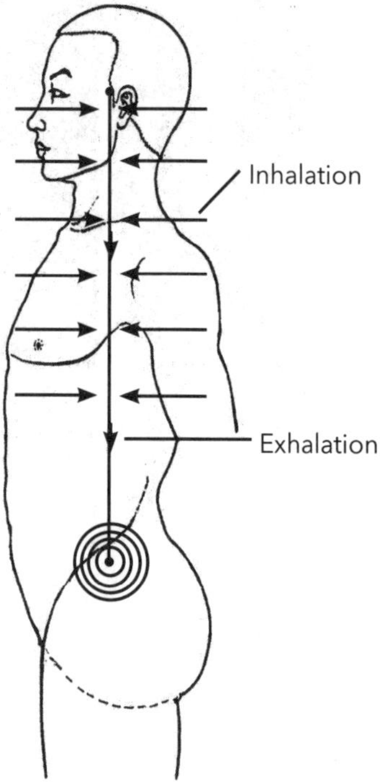

Figure 6-15. The Daoist Way of Leading the Qì Down to the Real Lower Dāntián

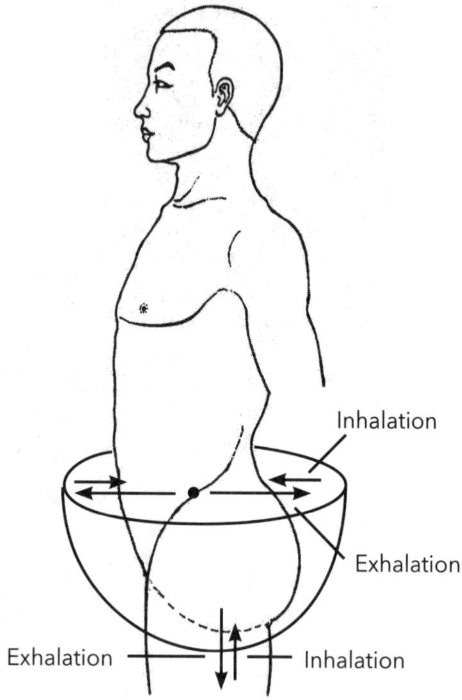

Figure 6-16. Girdle Vessel Breathing

Two Suggested Approaches:

1. Buddhist way first and then Daoist: This calms the mind and Shén first, then the calmed mind leads Qì inward.
2. Daoist way first and then Buddhist: This leads Qì inward to calm down the body and then the mind.

Each has advantages and disadvantages, depending on individual preference.

Having led the Qì down and stored it inside the Real Lower Dāntián, you must then keep your mind there, using two Embryonic Breathing practices. One is classified as Yáng and called Girdle Vessel Breathing (Dàimàixí, 帶脈息), while the other is classified as Yīn and called Marrow Breathing (Suǐxí, 髓息). Since Qì is led laterally when practicing these techniques, it is most effective to use Reverse Abdominal Breathing (Daoist breathing) instead of Normal Abdominal Breathing (Buddhist breathing).

Girdle Vessel Breathing (Dàimàixí, 帶脈息)

In this form you focus strongly on exhalation. When you exhale, the breath is long and slender, and firmly leads Qì outward from the Girdle Vessel. You gently push your abdomen out and Huìyīn down (Figure 6-16). The mind leads Qì out horizontally, a few feet or even yards. The body grows more Yáng and its Guardian Qì expands. To enhance the expansion of Qì, once you have exhaled completely, hold your breath for a few seconds and allow Qì to reach wherever the mind wishes. For even greater effect, also make the sound "Hā" while exhaling. When you inhale, relax, and allow the abdomen and Huìyīn to return to normal.

Qì manifestation in the Girdle Vessel is Yáng and makes your body and mind Yáng. Qì manifestation in the Thrusting Vessel is Yīn and calms down your body and mind. Using Girdle Vessel Breathing you can change the body's Qì from Yīn to Yáng. This strengthens your Guardian Qì and rids you of the feeling of cold. It is suitable for wintertime or when you are depressed. Naturally, it consumes your Qì.

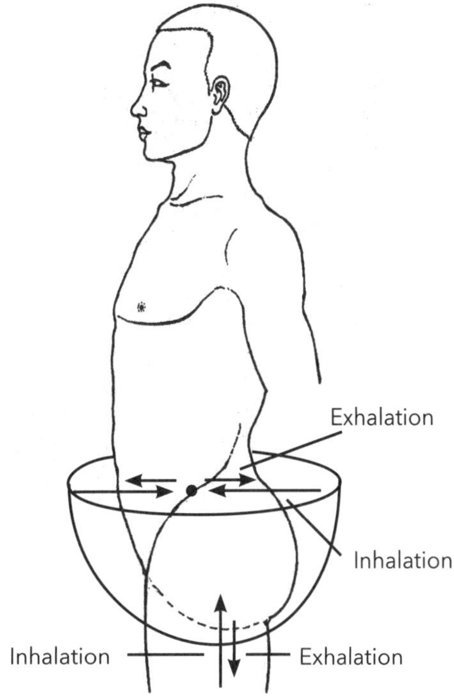

Figure 6-17. Marrow Breathing

Marrow Breathing (Suǐxí, 髓息)

Here, you focus strongly on inhalation. When you inhale, the breath is long and slender, and firmly leads Qì inward from the Girdle Vessel, as you draw your abdomen in and Huìyīn up (Figure 6-17). The mind continues to lead Qì in until it reaches the Yīn center of the Real Lower Dāntián. The body turns more Yīn, and the Guardian Qì shrinks. To lead the Qì in more effectively and keep it at the Real Lower Dāntián, once you have inhaled completely, hold your breath for a few seconds and allow the Qì to reach the Yáng center within the Yīn. When you exhale, relax, and allow the abdomen and Huìyīn areas to return to normal.

You are storing the Qì at the Real Lower Dāntián and also leading it into the bone marrow for Marrow Washing. Your Guardian Qì shrinks, weakening your resistance to cold, so you should not practice this in the winter. Instead, start in the spring and enhance the practice in the summer. When fall comes, change to Girdle Vessel Breathing to strengthen your Guardian Qì for the winter.

Conceiving the Spiritual Embryo, the Initiation of Enlightenment (Shéntāi Zhī Yùnyù, 神胎之孕育)

Here is a brief description of the method of conceiving the Spiritual Embryo (Shéntāi, 神胎) and leading it up to the Upper Dāntián to be born (Enlightenment). Please also refer to the next book, *Qìgōng Grand Circulation for Spiritual Enlightenment*.

Lead Fire Qì (Huǒqì, 火氣, Post-Heaven Qì) down from the Middle Dāntián (Zhōng Dāntián, 中丹田) and Water Qì (Shuǐqì, 水氣, Pre-Heaven Qì) up from the Real Lower Dāntián to meet at the Huángtíng (黃庭), the inner space between the diaphragm and the Real Lower Dāntián. This is called Kǎn and Lí. Yīn and Yáng Qì interact with each other, and the Spiritual Embryo (life) is conceived in the presence of the Shén, which is also led down to meet the Qì at the Huángtíng.

Summary of Embryonic Breathing:

1. Reverse Abdominal Breathing is more effective.
2. If inhalation and exhalation are of equal length, the body remains neutral.
3. If exhalation is longer than inhalation, it is Girdle Vessel breathing. Qì expands horizontally to build up Guardian Qì. It is also called Skin Breathing (Fūxí, 膚息) or Body Breathing (Tǐxí, 體息). The spirit is raised and the body energized. You should not practice this too much in the summer or when your body is already energized, as it can make your body too Yáng and can become harmful. You should practice it in the winter, so the Guardian Qì can expand against the cold.
4. If inhalation is longer than exhalation, it is Wújí Breathing. Qì is led to the Real Lower Dāntián and stored there, charging the biobattery. You should not practice this in the fall or winter, when you need stronger Guardian Qì to defend against the cold. Practice it in the summer and store the excess Qì.

Breathing's Yin and Yang 呼吸陰陽圖

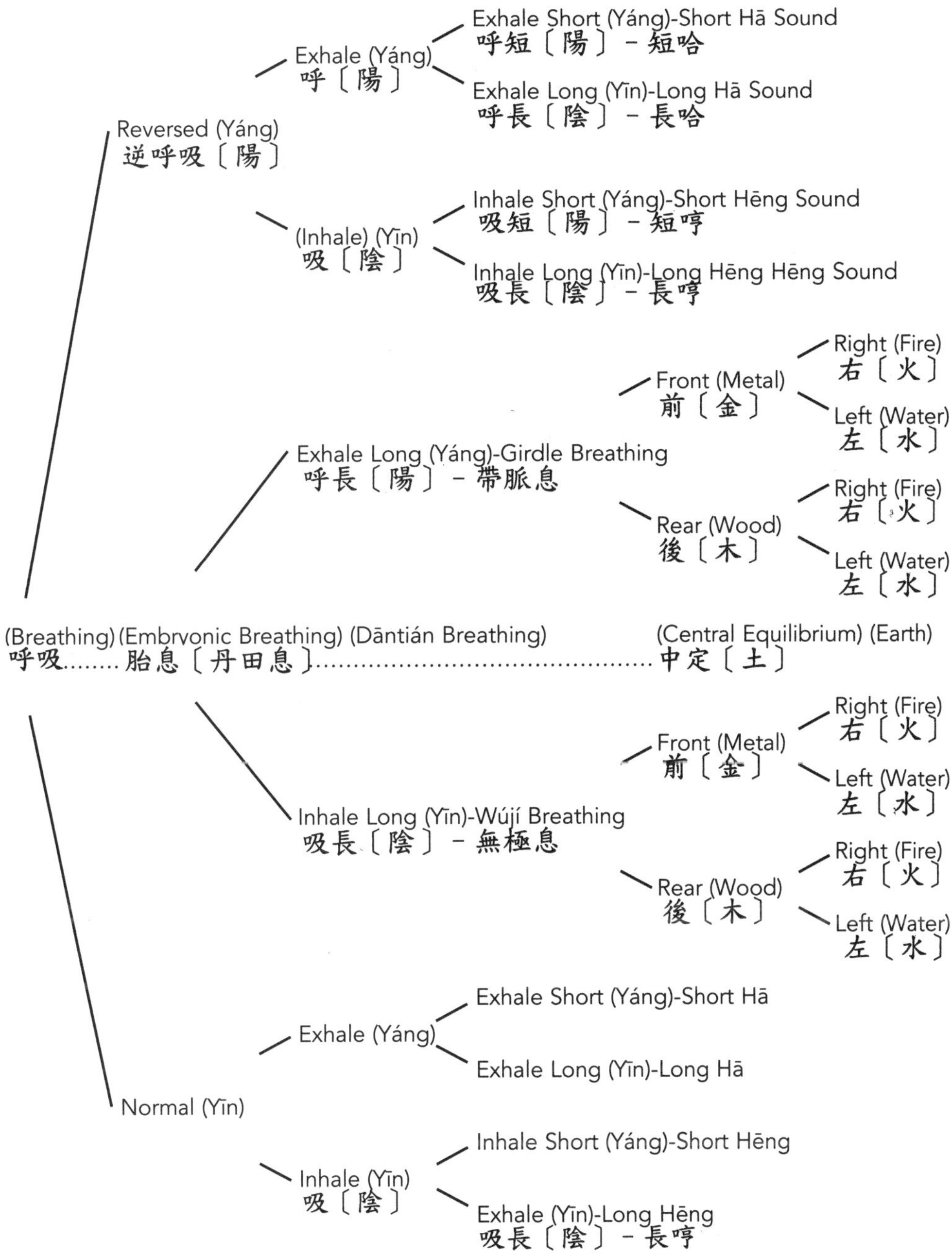

Figure 6-2. Breathing's Yīn and Yáng

References

1. 《道德經・十六章》：〝致虛極，守靜篤。〞

2. 《道德經・十六章》：〝致虛極，守靜篤；萬物并作，吾以觀其復。夫物芸芸，各復歸其根。歸根曰靜，靜曰復命。〞

3. 《道德經・六章》：〝谷神不死，是謂玄牝。玄牝之門，是謂天地根，綿綿若存，用之不勤。〞

4. 《道德經・十章》：〝載營魄抱一，能無離乎？專氣致柔，能如嬰兒乎？滌除玄鑒，能無疵乎？愛民治國，能無為乎？天門開闔，能為雌乎？明白四達，能無知乎？生之畜之，生而不有，為而不恃，長而不宰，是謂玄德。〞

5. 《靈劍子導引子午記注》：〝胎息者，抱一守中之法也。〞

6. "Animal Magnetism, The Strange Senses of Other Species," P. 32, *IEEE Spectrum*, March, 1996.

7. 《性命圭旨全書 》（大小鼎爐說）：〝黃庭為鼎，氣穴為爐。黃庭正在氣穴上，縷絡相連，乃人身百脈交會之處。〞元氣氤氳二穴之間，謂之〝小鼎爐。〞〝乾位為鼎，坤位為爐。〞即泥丸宮為鼎，下丹田為爐，謂之〝大鼎爐。〞

8. 《抱一函三秘訣》注云：〝兩腎之間，為我之根本，名曰藥祖丹基。〞

Chapter 7

Important Points in Meditation

7-1. Introduction (Jièshào, 介紹)

From the previous chapters, you have a sound map of how to practice Small Circulation without doubt and confusion. This can save you years of searching for the correct way. By preparing your journey both physically and psychologically, you lay a smooth path for your expedition. Before a long journey, first check your oil, map, flashlight, spare tire, weather report, and first aid kit to eliminate possible obstacles which may prevent you from completing your journey.

The first step is psychological preparation. Do you trust the theory? Do you have confidence you can complete the practice to its conclusion? Can you cope with the obstacles you will encounter? Most important of all, do you recognize why you want to practice? Are you aiming just for a peaceful mind, or for ultimate enlightenment? You should test yourself first. Sit quietly, keeping your mind calm and clear for thirty minutes a day, for a month, and see how you cope. This is not easy, and your greatest challenge is dealing with your mind, which is at the same time the most important factor in success. Without a clear, calm, and concentrated mind, you cannot lead the Qì, or accomplish the training. There are also important physical preparations for establishing a peaceful mind and making the practice flow smoothly.

Here we discuss some important preparations, such as choice of location, timing of meditation and orientation, common experiences one may encounter, and possible deviations and how to correct them. The traditional twenty-four rules of meditation are reviewed in the last section.

7-2. Preparations (Zhǔnbèi, 準備)

Preparation has mental and physical aspects. Are you forcing yourself to meditate? If so, it could take a long time to calm down. Be prepared for it. Do you have ego or expectations? You will probably be disappointed. When you meditate, you cannot set up a schedule of progress. If you do, you will be under pressure, and the mind will hinder the whole process. Is your mind peaceful before meditation? Do you get upset or excited before meditation? The point is to calm the mind before you meditate. You should meditate just to regulate your mind, if anything will stimulate it and lead it away from calmness and peace. Do not try to circulate Qì with a troubled mind.

Take a shower. Dirt and sweat seal the pores of your skin, making you uneasy and uncomfortable. It is best to shower or bathe half an hour before you meditate, to assist physical relaxation. Afterwards let your body return to normal from the stimulation of the water temperature.

Bowels. Go to the toilet before meditating. Tightness in the abdomen and bowels affects Qì flow at the Real Lower Dāntián, and your mind will be scattered and bothered. You should not go to the toilet directly after meditation, but should wait at least ten minutes. This gives your body time to digest Qì you have built and stored in your Real Lower Dāntián, which would otherwise be lost.

Clothing. When practicing Qìgōng meditation, don't wear artificial fibers such as polyester or rayon. These products were developed only in recent decades and our bodies have not adapted to them, having used natural materials for millions of years. Artificial fibers generate static, and this interferes with normal Qì circulation. This traps your energy, clouds your judgment, and makes you feel uneasy, impatient, depressed, or excited without reason. You may have a similar feeling before it rains, with low clouds and humidity, and a strong electric field between the clouds and the earth. Our emotions are also affected by the full moon, when the electromagnetic field between the moon and the earth is at its strongest.

So wear natural materials such as cotton or silk. Wear loose clothes, especially pants, for a comfortable, natural feeling, and to help Qì flow through the Real Lower Dāntián. This assists accurate sensing of your body's Qì.

Keep warm. In profound meditation, you are in the semi-sleeping state. Your body relaxes while your mind is awake, regulating the Qì circulation. Your heartbeat slows down and breathing becomes slower and deeper. As in sleep, inhalation is longer than exhalation, which shrinks Guardian Qì (Wèiqì, 衛氣) and lowers skin temperature. You can catch cold easily, so you should keep warm and comfortable. Cover your knees and ankles with a blanket of natural materials. In relaxation, the joints are open, which allows cold Qì, such as wind or moisture, to enter them. This weakens the immune system and can generate arthritis.

Meditation cushion. When you meditate, you should prepare a meditation cushion. To prevent excess Qì from entering the legs, it is very important that you cross them when sitting, which narrows the Qì path. Start with a cushion about six inches high, made from natural material like cotton, sitting for thirty minutes. Adjust the height for comfort, so you can sit for thirty minutes, using it for a week or so until you are satisfied with the height. Pay attention to your sitting posture, as incorrect posture can also generate discomfort.

Floor. The floor where you meditate is very important, and should not be too hard. Sit on a mat to ease pressure on the legs.

Light. If possible, sit in the dark. Uneven light can affect your judgment. For example, if the light to your right is stronger than to your left, you will feel stronger energy there. This can mislead your feeling and judgment. If you cannot sit in the dark, sit where the light is evenly diffused. Sitting under fluorescent light is not a good idea, as its strong electromagnetic radiation can affect your body's energy.

Electric field. You should sit away from any strong electric field, such as an electrical outlet, especially one in use. Use a sensitive compass to find a good spot in the house where the needle aligns with the earth's magnetic field. Do not use an electric blanket at all, as the electromagnetic field it generates is strong and harms Qì circulation, especially in your heart.

Humidity. Humidity can also affect your Emotional Mind. Too much can make you feel sticky and uncomfortable. Too little can cause static to build up around you. The most comfortable humidity for meditation is around 50–60 percent.

Temperature. Temperature is one of the main concerns. Extremes of heat or cold can affect your feelings during meditation. Avoid sitting close to a heater or air conditioner, as they affect your temperature significantly.

Noise. Most important of all during meditation is to prevent noise. Sudden loud noise can disturb your meditating mind and lead the Qì into the wrong path, which is dangerous and harmful. In meditation, your mind and body are extremely relaxed, and any slight noise can disturb you, tensing both mind and body. If you are leading Qì circulation, it can be led into the wrong path, damaging your nervous system or internal organs. Turn off your phone, silence the alarm clock, and place a sign at the entrance for people to see, to keep noise out of your meditation place.

7-3. Meditation Place (Jìngzuò Dìdiǎn Zhī Xuǎnzé, 靜坐地點之選擇)

For profound Qìgōng practice, one needs four things: money, partner, techniques, and place. So an appropriate location is important, not only for a peaceful mind for your cultivation, but also to obtain Qì from the natural surroundings. Choosing a good location for living, for burying the dead, and for Qìgōng practice is an important profession known as Fēngshuǐ (風水, wind-water).

Mountains are classified as fire (Lí, 離) and provide Qì, while water (Kǎn, 坎) soothes and cools your Qì, bringing you to a calm and harmonious state. To have harmonious Qì, live next to water, such as the ocean, rivers, or lakes. However, to obtain more Qì to nourish your body for Qì circulation and enlightenment meditation, find a suitable mountain.

The earth cooled down from a liquid state, spinning towards the east, so heavier materials such as metals tended to accumulate in the west of each landmass. Large mountain ranges in North and South America, and in Asia are located to the west (Figure 7-1). Qì is generally stronger in the mountains and more harmonious near the sea.

Finding the best place for spiritual cultivation has been a major challenge in establishing Buddhist and Daoist monasteries. An appropriate location shortens the time needed to reach the final goal of cultivation.

7-4. Best Time for Meditation (Jìngzuò Zhī Zuìjiā Shíkè, 靜坐之最佳時刻)

In general, you may meditate at any time. But at specific times, you benefit from it more, and Qì circulation will be more efficient. If you meditate when natural Qì is changing from Yīn to Yáng or vice versa, it enhances the achievement significantly, because the Qì in your body is also changing at this time. We age quickly and get sick due to irregular Qì being exchanged during these periods. The Complete Book of Principal Contents of Lífe and Human Nature (Xìngmìng Guīzhǐ Quánshū, 性命圭旨全書) says, “Zǐ (子, 11 pm to 1 am), Wǔ (午, 11 am to 1 pm), Mǎo (卯, 5 to 7 am), and Qiú (酉, 5 to 7 pm), these four periods are the time gates for entrance and exit of Yīn and Yáng.”[1] These are the best times for meditation. When your practice is well established, however, you can adjust the body’s Yīn and Yáng at any time and gain the same benefit, with a smooth and vital Qì flow. Huózǐshí (活子時) means time of vital Zǐ. Zǐ (11 pm to 1 am) is the best time of all for Marrow/Brain Washing.

The Qìgōng Dictionary illustrates Huózǐshí this way: “When practicing Qìgōng, shape and spirit are peaceful and calm, condense the spirit to the Qì cavity (Real Lower Dāntián). When you feel Qì moving there, then it is time to generate Yīn and Yáng.”2 The Daoist book Observing Vessels (Màiwàng, 脈望) says, “When you begin to build the foundation of generating Dān (Elixir or Qì), do not be restricted in the timing of Zǐ (11 pm to 1 am) and Wǔ (11 am to 1 pm). As long as there is movement in the calmness, then it is the time of Guǐ (end of calmness), which is the time of vital Zǐ.”[3] Guǐ (癸) is the last of the Ten Celestial Stems (Tiāngān, 天干), meaning that Yīn is ending, and Yáng is just starting.

Although the times for meditation are not very strict, it is advisable as a beginner to meditate according to natural Yīn and Yáng. Other than Zǐ, the best time is early morning until sunrise, the second best is sunset, and the third is at noon. Noontime meditation is only used to calm the body’s Yáng and to lead the Qì downward and inward for storage, since our body is extremely Yáng at this time. This is the best period for Embryonic Breathing, from noon until 2 pm, when natural Qì and the body’s Qì have passed extreme Yáng and are just beginning to cool down. Instead of sunset, you may also practice about one hour before sleeping.

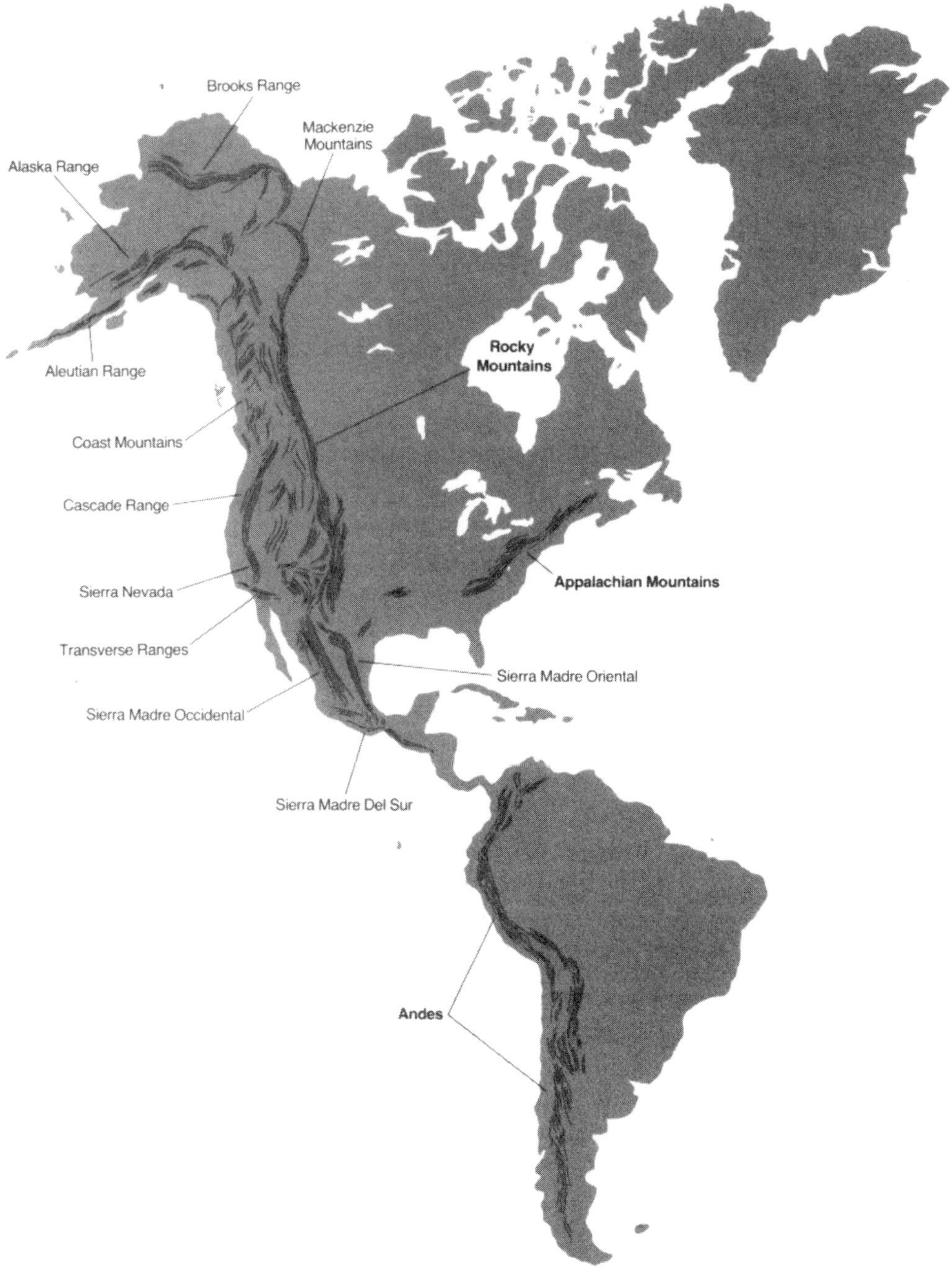

Figure 7-1. Map of South and North America

7-5. Meditation Orientation (Jìngzuò Zhī Miànduì Fāngxiàng, 靜坐之面對方向)

Our body's energy is always influenced by nature, especially by cosmic energy, solar energy, lunar energy, and earth energy. Earth energy includes the earth's magnetic field, the heat concealed below, electric charge in clouds, air energy, and all objects both living and inanimate. In choosing your location, consider the landscape, trees, water, and climate. This earth Qì directly affects the body's energy. Here we also discuss how to absorb Qì from the sun and moon, and from the earth's magnetic field. Since we do not understand cosmic Qì, it is not discussed here.

Chinese medicine classifies the front of the body as Yīn, and the back as Yáng. Qì is stored in front while it manifests at the back. External Qì is more easily absorbed by the front, while the back repels and rejects it. When exchanging Qì with your surroundings, the Yīn side absorbs while the Yáng side rejects. This is important when working with energy from the sun, the earth, and the moon.

Sun (Daytime). The early morning sun is gentle, soft, and nourishing, and easily absorbed by the body. Later in the day, its energy is stronger, and the body instinctively rejects it so as not to absorb too much. The sun's rays at sunset are also gentle and soft, but take energy with them, so it is a good time for cooling down instead of nourishing.

Earth (Nighttime). The Qì from the Earth's magnetic field starts at the geographic south pole (magnetic north pole) and returns to earth at the geographic north pole (magnetic south pole). If you face the south, you will be nourished by earth Qì, while if you face north, the earth Qì will reduce your Qì and therefore help you to calm down. This is discussed at length in the YMAA book, *The Root of Chinese Qìgōng*.

Moon (Nighttime). The three nights before the moon is full, and the night of the full moon itself, are a good time to face the moon and absorb Moon Qì for nourishing. The three days after the full moon are good for reducing or releasing Qì while facing the moon. To absorb more Qì from nature for your cultivation, you need to nourish (Bǔ, 補), or add fire. However, if you are already excited and energized and need to calm down, then simply maintain your Qì level or even allow nature to take some away. This is called releasing (Xiè, 洩), or adding water.

To summarize:

For Qì nourishment (Bǔ, 補) (Lí, 離)

1. Sunrise—face east to absorb Sun Qì
2. Noon—face south to absorb Earth Qì
3. Sunset—face east to stop the Qì from being drained by the sun
4. Night—face south to absorb Earth Qì
5. Night (3 days up to full moon)—face the moon to absorb its Qì

Preventing Qì nourishment or for releasing it (Xiè, 洩) (Kǎn, 坎)

1. Sunrise—face west to stop Qì being nourished by the sun
2. Noon—face north to release Qì to the earth
3. Sunset—face west to release Qì to the sun
4. Night—face north to release Qì to the earth
5. Night (2–3 days after full moon)—face the moon to release Qì to it

7-6. Common Experiences for Qìgōng Beginners (Chūxué Qìgōng Zhī Yībān Jīngyàn, 初學氣功之一般經驗)

There are common phenomena experienced in practice. Some are caused by improper posture, timing, or training methods. Since most beginners cannot generate significant Qì, they are usually harmless. But if you ignore them and continue to train incorrectly, you build bad habits which may eventually bring you harm. It is important to attend to them and understand their causes.

The mind is scattered and sleepy (Sànluàn Yǔ Hūnchén, 散亂與昏沉). The Daoist Níwánzǔ (泥丸祖) said: "For one hundred days, banish sleepiness. Sleepiness and confusion make the mind scattered and disordered, and you lose the real practice."[4] Having a scattered and disordered mind is one of the most common experiences of beginners, with their Yì (意) unable to control Xīn (心). Though Yì is strong, Xīn is even stronger, so first strengthen Yì and regulate Xīn, and analyze the causes and possible results of the disturbance.

If sleepiness is the result of fatigue, it is best to stop practicing, and relax or take a nap. Líe down comfortably, and pay attention to deep breathing as you bring your mind to the deep places of your body. Smoothly and slowly release the carbon dioxide, and every time you exhale, relax deeper. Breathing and heart rate slow down, and you feel rested, with your mind clear and your spirit fresh. Now raise your spirit, and keep it at its residence, centered and balanced.

Sleepiness can also result from relaxation and a scattered mind. Keep your mind inside and observe your inner self. Bring your mind back to the third eye, and raise your spirit. After a few minutes, bring your mind back to the Real Lower Dāntián for Embryonic Breathing. If you are sleepy, do not use your mind to lead the Qì, which can be as dangerous as driving a car in that condition.

Feeling cold (Fālěng, 發冷). Feeling cold during still meditation is very common. In moving Qìgōng you energize your body, so it is warm and more Yáng. But in still meditation you calm your mind and slow your breathing, reducing your heart rate and making your body more Yīn. In the winter, your body releases energy into the surrounding air more quickly than in the summer, and feeling cold can be more of a problem. So when you meditate in the early morning or in the winter, wear warm clothes and cover your legs, especially your knees, with a blanket.

Sometimes you feel cold even when warmly dressed and with the room at a comfortable temperature. This is most likely caused by your mind, which significantly influences Qì circulation in your body. Sometimes you may feel cold when nervous tension, emotional upset, or fear send a sudden chill through your body. Since your mind has such an effect on you, it is important to regulate it through meditation. You may also feel some part of the body suddenly colder or warmer. This is a common experience as Qì redistributes during deep relaxation, so do not be too concerned about it.

Numbness (Mámù, 麻木). Numbness is very common in Qìgōng still meditation. When you sit for a long time, your circulation slows down, reducing the blood supply to your legs. This is very common with beginners. You should not continue your meditation once concentration is affected. Stretch your legs and massage the bottom of your feet, especially the Yǒngquán (K-1, 湧泉), to speed the recovery of circulation. If you meditate regularly, you will find you can sit longer and longer without your legs becoming numb. Your body adjusts the blood supply to fit the new situation. After six months of regular practice, you should be able to sit at least thirty minutes without any problem. If your lower back feels stiff, adjust your posture by sitting on a higher cushion or a chair with back support.

Discomfort (Soreness and Pain) (Suāntòng, 酸痛). Discomfort is frequently caused by incorrect posture. Common places are the lower back, hips, and shoulders, caused by the wrong sitting height or posture. Correct the problems before they affect your concentration or cause injury, and regulate your body to a comfortable and natural state.

Part of the body feels hot (Bànbiān Shēnrè, 半邊身熱). Sometimes part of your body may feel hot, or just one portion feels cold while the rest feels hot. This usually happens when you are emotionally upset, sick, or recovering from illness. When you circulate unbalanced Qì, you may interfere with the body's efforts to achieve Qì balance. Simply relax and meditate on your Real Lower Dāntián, and be aware of your body and emotions.

Headache and eye ache (Tóutòng Yǎntòng, 頭痛眼痛). A common cause of headache during Qìgōng practice is failure to breathe smoothly. You may hold your breath without noticing it, causing Qì and blood flow to stagnate, which reduces oxygen supply to the head.

Eye ache is also common, for two main reasons. "The eyes watch the nose, and the nose watches the heart."[5] To keep your mind inside without being distracted by what is going on around you, restrain your vision. Focus your mind in your heart and regulate Xīn, your Emotional Mind. You do this with your mind, not your body. Don't actually stare at your nose, a major cause of eye ache.

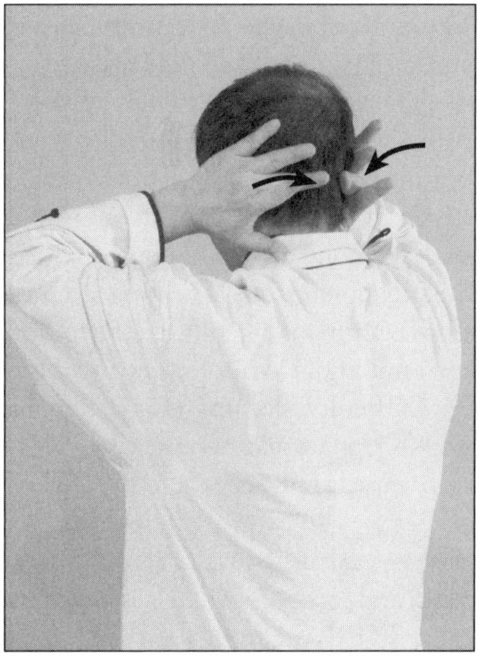

Figure 7-2

Your eyes may also ache when you focus the spirit (Shén) at its residence. Do this without using force. Lead the spirit back to its center firmly but gently. Mental force will cause not only eye ache but also headache.

Trembling body (Shēntǐ Dǒudòng, 身體抖動). Body trembling occurs spontaneously, mostly in the limbs, though sometimes also in the torso. During deep relaxation, extra Qì flows easily to activate muscles and causes them to tremble. Your upper body may sway by itself, following your breathing. These are good signs, indicating success in regulating your body, breathing, and mind, but you should not make it happen intentionally.

Warmth and sweating (Wēnrè Chūhàn, 溫熱出汗). In still meditation, even though you are not moving externally, you are exercising internally. When Qì increases significantly, it will manifest at the surface of your skin as warmth, even making you sweat. Be sure not to expose your sweaty body to a cold draft.

Fright (Shòujīng, 受驚). This is one of the worst things that can happen during Qìgōng meditation. It generally occurs for two reasons. Sometimes your mind is very clear but you cannot center it, and it may start to generate fantasy or illusion. This is called Entering the Demon (Rùmó, 入魔), or being bewitched. You may feel a cold draft and think it is an evil spirit, as your imagination generates thoughts to disturb you.

Unless you regulate your mind right away, you may start to believe the illusion and become very scared. The danger is that Yì no longer leads your Qì, disturbing your Qì circulation. If this happens during very deep meditation, it may cause you serious injury, so it is very important that your mind should be clear and calm, with emotions completely controlled.

If you experience this kind of fright, your Yì is too confused to lead your Qì correctly, so you should discontinue practice. There are several ways to help you collect yourself. The first is to cover your ears with your palms and tap the back of your head by snapping your index fingers off the middle fingers (Figure 7-2). This is called Beating the Heavenly Drum (Míngtiāngǔ, 鳴天鼓) and is one of the most common ways for your mind to find its center. You may drink some hot tea or coffee, wash your face with warm water, or take a shower. Alternatively, generate an Ăn (唵) sound in your brain, vibrating in the Spiritual Valley. This can often lead your mind into the spiritual center and stop the illusion.

This is called Righteous Sound (Zhèngyīn, 正音), commonly used to stabilize the spirit and keep it at the Mud Pill Palace.

The second type of fright happens when you realize your Qì has gone into the wrong path, called Entering the Fire (Zǒuhuǒ, 走火). For example, suddenly your heart starts beating fast or your head starts to ache. Your mind is disturbed, and you are confused and scared. If this happens, calm your mind and move it away from the trouble. The more you focus on the area of concern, the more Qì will flow there and stagnate, worsening the situation instead of helping it. Once your mind is calm, lead the Qì back to your Real Lower Dāntián. Sit still for a few minutes and gradually bring your mind back to your surroundings. Do not resume practice, but instead wait until the next session.

Difficulty sleeping (Fǎnyì Shīmián, 反易失眠). It is common to have difficulty sleeping for a while, because when you practice Qìgōng, your mind is energized and your spirit raised. This keeps you from falling asleep. Pay attention to your breathing, thinking every time you exhale that your body is becoming more and more relaxed. Inhale longer than you exhale to make the body more Yīn. Don't use Yì to lead Qì, but just breathe and relax, and soon you will fall asleep. You may also practice Embryonic Breathing, leading excited Qì down from your head to the Real Lower Dāntián. Then the mind becomes calm and the body relaxes.

Coughing (Késòu, 咳嗽). Beginners sometimes cough during practice. The most common reason is that breathing is not being regulated smoothly. You may be breathing too fast or holding your breath. Use Yì to regulate the breathing until it is no longer necessary.

The second possibility is that your body is not regulated correctly. For example, if you push your head too far back, the front of the throat will tense and cause you to cough.

The third possibility is that when you are in deep meditation, your heart beat slows, and body temperature drops. You feel cold, which may also cause coughing, so keep your body warm during meditation.

Sexual arousal (Xìngchōngdòng, 性衝動). It is normal to have sexual feelings and even to become aroused during meditation. Abdominal breathing increases Qì circulation in your lower body, stimulating the sexual organs. While this increases sexual desire, remember you are practicing Qìgōng to increase production of hormones to raise your spirit. You need to regulate your mind and not waste this extra supply through sexual activity.

Sexual arousal is a great problem in Marrow/Brain Washing Qìgōng, which trains methods of stimulating hormone production, so that hormonal essence can be converted into Qì to nourish the spirit and brain. People who do not understand the training, or whose willpower is weak, waste the achievement of their practice.

7-7. Common Sensations in Still Meditation (Jìngzuò Zhī Dòngchù Yǔ Jǐngxiàng, 靜坐之動觸與景象)

When you practice still meditation, regulating your body, breathing, and mind, you enter into deep meditation. Qì readjusts and balances itself, reaching even the smallest place in your body. You have feelings and visions, which cannot be experienced when you are not in meditation. The Chinese call them Qì scenery or Qì view (Jǐngqì, 景氣), and when you reach this point, it is called Enter the Scenery (Rùjǐng, 入景). Don't expect to experience all of these sensations, as they depend on the individual, the time of day, how deep you are in meditation, and even the environment in which you are sitting.

The Eight Touches (Physical and Sensory Phenomena, 八觸). The Eight Touches (Bāchù, 八觸) felt during Qìgōng practice, such as sensations of heat, someone touching you, or heaviness, are also called Touch Feel (Chùgǎn, 觸感) or Moving Touch (Dòngchù, 動觸). Some practitioners list them as moving (Dòng, 動), itching (Yǎng, 癢), cool (Liáng, 涼), warm (Nuǎn, 暖), light (Qīng, 輕), heavy (Zhòng, 重), harsh (Sè, 澀), and slippery (Huá, 滑). Others list them differently as shake (Diào, 掉), ripple (Yī, 猗), cold (Lěng, 冷), hot (Rè, 熱), float (Fú, 浮), sink (Chén, 沈), hard (Jiān, 堅), and soft (Ruǎn, 軟).

These are normal sensations in Qìgōng practice, even in the beginning. If you experience something, determine its cause. If it is the result of Qì redistribution, let it happen and don't worry about it. Otherwise, correct the circumstances causing them. For example, if you feel cold because the room temperature is too low, either put on more clothing or turn up the thermostat.

Don't expect these phenomena or look for them, and don't worry about them. Simply follow nature and let it happen, and continue your practice. Keep your mind clear and calm, and don't be distracted.

Sensations of movement or vibration (Dòngdàngjǐng, 動盪景). This is different from the above where one part of the body spontaneously starts to move or tremble. This sensation occurs in the False Lower Dāntián, and you might feel warmth there. After a couple of weeks, the area may start to vibrate by itself. This means Qì is becoming abundant there and it is time for your Yì to lead it through Small Circulation. This is often the first sensation, and it gives you confidence you are practicing correctly and making progress.

Sensations inside the abdomen (Xiǎofù Nèijǐng, 小腹內景). Once you feel warmth and vibration in your Real Lower Dāntián, the abundant Qì spreads out through your abdomen. The movement as you breathe increases circulation in your intestines and sometimes causes sounds and the release of gas. After a while, you feel warmth and other sensations throughout your abdomen, and the Qì flows smoothly and strongly.

Sometimes you sweat. Afterwards, these sensations disappear as all the channels in the abdomen open up, and Qì moves without stagnation.

The feeling of lightness (Piāorán Zhījǐng, 飄然之景). During deep meditation, with Qì circulating smoothly, your body may feel light and airy, and seems to disappear. This is very comfortable, but don't be distracted by it. Be aware of what is happening, but don't pay attention to it. To reach this stage, your body must be in deep relaxation, where breathing and heartbeat slow down to the minimum, and your mind is extremely calm and peaceful.

White clouds in the empty room (Xūshì Shēngbái, 虛室生白). You may suddenly feel your physical body disappear and blend with the surrounding Qì. It seems the room is empty, filled with a white cloud or fog. If you pay attention to this scenery, it disappears immediately, because your mind is not familiar with emptiness and generates an image of familiar, physical scenery to fill the void.

If you experience this white emptiness, be aware of it, but don't pay attention to it. It happens only when your mind is completely regulated in a highly concentrated and relaxed state. The Daoist Wùyīzi (悟一子) said, "If you wish to fill the abdomen with Qì, first empty the Xīn. If you wish to generate the White, first empty the room."[6] To accumulate Qì in your abdomen, first empty the Emotional Mind (Xīn). Only then can Yì (Wisdom Mind) start the fire (Qǐhuǒ, 起火) to build up the Qì. "White" here means simple, pure, light, and clean, like fog or cloud, and represents the disappearance of the physical body. To unite with the surrounding Qì, first let go of all objects, including your physical body.

Six other sensations (Líùjǐng, 六景). At a higher level of Qìgōng meditation, there are six other sensations you may experience. These are a). the False Lower Dāntián is hot as though it were on fire; b). the kidneys feel as though boiling in water, c). the eyes emit a beam of light, d). winds are generated behind the ears, e). an eagle is shouting behind your head, and f). your body is energized and your nose trembles. These are called Six Verifications (Líùzhǒng Yìngyàn, 六種應驗), because they verify correct meditation.

Six Transportations (Líùtōng, 六通). When you regulate and raise your spirit (Shén), it will be high and its supernatural Líng (靈) power will reach farther than any ordinary person's. Your mind will be able to communicate with the six natural powers:

- **Seeing the present.** Your mind is so clear it can analyze and understand events clearly and thoroughly. You see things from a neutral point of view, without being confused by Xīn, something most people cannot do.
- **Understanding the past and seeing the future.** You understand the past and predict the future. Since your mind is clear, you can analyze what happened, understand its causes and see the results. As your experience accumulates, you can predict the future, since people remain the same and history repeats itself.

- **Viewing the whole universe.** At the highest stage, your spirit senses the whole universe, including mountains, rivers, oceans, and the heavens. Your Qì unites with that of the universe, and you can exchange information freely.
- **Hearing the sounds of the universe.** Your spirit listens to and understands the sounds generated by variations of natural Qì, including wind, rain, waves, and many other things. You can also hear spirits and communicate with them.
- **Seeing a person's destiny.** After all this, you will be able to look inside a person's mind, personality, and true nature, and see his destiny. You will even be able to see his spiritual future, whether it involves enjoyment (heaven) or suffering (hell).
- **Knowing a person's thoughts.** Since you have energized your spirit and brain significantly, they are open to a much wider range of wavelengths. You will be able to match wavelengths with other people's minds and know their thoughts.

Daoist Wǔzhēnrén (伍真人) said, "Return to emptiness to combine with the Dào. After you reach steadiness and can leave your body, you can communicate with the powers of nature and transform into thousands of changes and ten thousand variations; nothing cannot be done."[7] This stage is Buddhahood or Enlightenment, where you can separate your spirit from your body and unite with nature, and have already reopened your third eye (Tiānyǎn, 天眼). Your spirit and the natural spirit have been unified as one (Tiānrén Héyī, 天人合一).

7-8. Deviations and Corrections (Piānchā Yǔ Jiǎozhèng, 偏差與矯正)

Once you accumulate Qì, especially at the False Lower Dāntián, be careful lest Qì deviate from the correct path and bring you into danger. This is caused by lack of knowledge, misunderstanding, or wrong training. Deviations are called Zǒuhuǒ Rùmó (走火入魔), which means Mislead the Fire and Enter the Devil. Mislead the Fire means to lead the Qì into the wrong path, and Enter the Devil means the mind enters the domain of evil. Serious problems or injury usually result. Here we discuss the causes of common Qìgōng deviations and how to correct them.

Causes of Deviations:

The Qìgōng style trained does not fit the individual or the circumstances. Every style of Qìgōng has its own special training methods and objectives. Each Qìgōng set was created by a knowledgeable Qìgōng master to train a specific group of people. When you choose a Qìgōng style for your training, first know your body's condition, the purpose of your training, and whether the Qìgōng style chosen is appropriate. For example, Iron Shirt (Tiěbùshān, 鐵布衫) Qìgōng is used to train people whose bodies are already stronger than average. If you are weak and force yourself to train Iron Shirt, you encounter difficulties and deviations. With Qìgōng styles for improving general health, such as The Eight Pieces of Brocade (Bāduànjǐn, 八段錦) and Five Animal Sports (Wǔqínxì, 五禽戲), you do not have to worry too much about deviations caused by choosing the wrong style. Such styles were created for average people, so you are safe so long as you follow the instructions.

Lack of a firm mind or a knowledgeable teacher. Find a knowledgeable teacher and stay with him, or there is a good chance you may be taught incorrect practices. Don't lose patience or confidence and change to another teacher, which may only increase your confusion. If you train Qìgōng without patience, perseverance, confidence, and a strong will, sooner or later confusion and deviations occur.

Anticipating phenomena. One common cause of deviation is expecting phenomena that you have heard about. Just because someone else has experienced something doesn't mean that you will experience it too. If you try to make it happen, you are likely to fall into wrong practices, and be misled by the wrong sensation or by illusion.

Body and mind are not regulated. Many practitioners encounter serious deviations caused by body tension. If your body is tired and your muscles are tense, first calm down and regulate your breathing to help your body relax and recover from fatigue. Any attempt to circulate Qì when you are tired is dangerous.

Deviations are also common when people circulate Qì before their minds are regulated. If you are excited or angry, your Yì is unsteady and it is dangerous to lead your Qì. If you cannot regulate your mind, you should not practice.

If you practice under these circumstances, your Qì can stagnate or enter the wrong channels. It is very common to experience headache or various pains. Regulating your body, breathing, and mind are basic requirements before you regulate Qì.

Losing patience. Don't lose patience during practice and use Yì aggressively to lead the Qì. This is very dangerous, especially for beginners. Take your time. Be patient and confident. Your understanding and experience grow with practice, until the time is right. Some beginners circulate Qì in Small Circulation before they really know what Qì is, or can move their abdomens easily. This only causes problems, like a child playing with fire.

Mixing imagination with Qìgōng exercises. Qìgōng is a science, not a religion or superstitious belief. Imagination will lead you to the wrong path. It is a major cause of fear and of Entering the Devil. Most people who have imagination lack scientific knowledge and understanding. They are confused and wonder what they are doing.

External interference. Some of the worst deviations are caused by external disturbances during Qìgōng meditation. For example, you are meditating when suddenly you are shocked by the telephone ringing, a loud noise, or a friend talking to you. Such things can cause serious injury, especially when you are circulating Qì in Small Circulation or practicing other higher levels of practice where great concentration is necessary. Before you practice, you should prevent all possible disturbances.

Believing non-professional opinions. A common failing is to believe and trust other people's judgment more than our own. We are especially open to advice from our friends. When you encounter a problem during practice, do not discuss it with anyone who is not experienced with Qìgōng. You can discuss it with your teacher or fellow students, but it is best not to talk about it with friends not practicing Qìgōng. You are likely to be much better qualified to evaluate things than they are.

Not following advice and rules of the Masters. At the end of this section, we discuss twenty-four rules you should observe while practicing Qìgōng, to avoid the most common and serious problems.

Though we have pointed out many possible sources of deviation and danger, you should not let this scare you away from practicing Qìgōng. Every practice always has some level of risk. For example, you would not ban swimming simply because some people drown, and you shouldn't refuse to drive a car even though many people are killed or injured by them. The proper approach to any of these things is to understand what you are doing, know the source of potential problems, define the training rules, and proceed cautiously.

Most deviations happen to those who generate a strong Qì flow, yet still do not understand and master the regulation of the body, breathing, and mind. Once you generate strong Qì in your body, you must know how to lead it, otherwise it may move into the wrong path and affect normal Qì circulation. This is harmful and even dangerous. That is why they are called deviations rather than phenomena, the term used earlier to refer to common experiences.

Deviations and corrections:

Headache. Earlier we discussed the headaches beginners have. Here we discuss the potentially serious headaches caused by excess Qì and blood, or lack of oxygen in the brain. Excess Qì and blood is usually caused by forced concentration, which means the mind is not regulated properly. Even when concentrating, Yì and body should be relaxed. If you force yourself to concentrate, your mind leads Qì and blood to the head, and you will become more tense and get a headache. If you can't sleep, it's no good trying to force yourself to sleep, just relax and let it happen.

The headache caused by lack of oxygen usually occurs when your breathing is not regulated properly. Beginners frequently concentrate Yì so hard that they unconsciously hold their breath. This reduces oxygen supply to the brain and causes headaches or dizziness. Regulate the breath until it is smooth and natural, which is regulating without regulating. Only then concentrate on leading Qì.

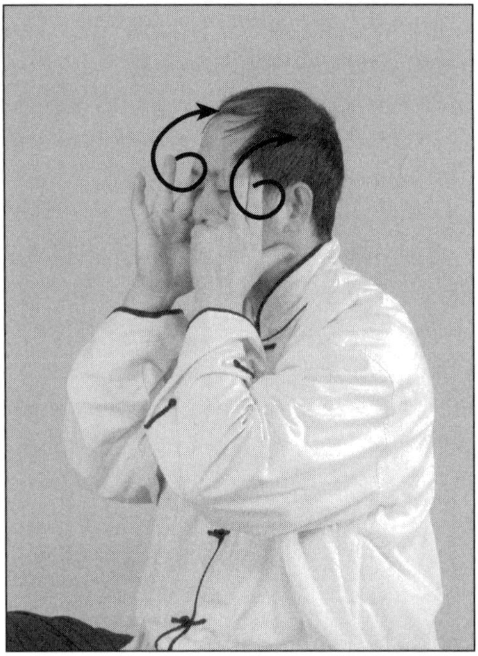

Figure 7-3

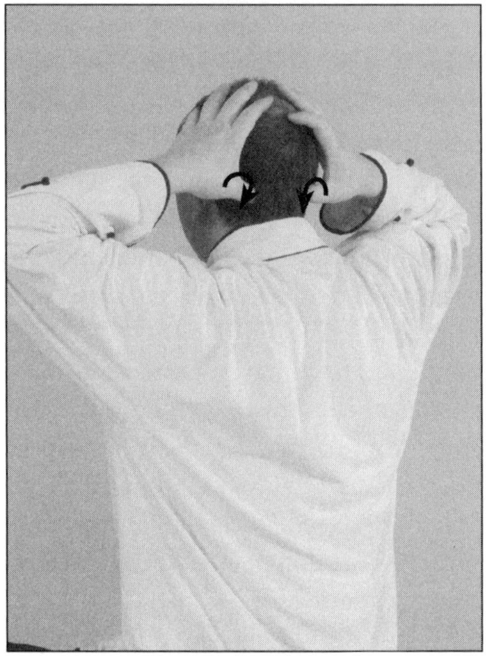

Figure 7-4

If you get a headache while practicing Qìgōng, immediately lead the Qì to the Real Lower Dāntián and, after a few breaths, stop training. With your breathing smooth, relax your body deeply. This opens the Qì channels in the neck, and excess Qì and blood in your head can disperse. Massage your temples (Figure 7-3), the Fēngchí cavity (GB-20, 風池, Wind Pond) (Figure 7-4), and the muscles at the back of your neck, pushing downward to lead the blood and Qì out of your head. Finally, place the center of your palm on the Bǎihuì cavity, lightly circle a few times and then follow the muscles down the back of the neck (Figure 7-5). Tap the head gently from the center to the sides, working from the front to the back. This leads stagnant Qì out to the surface of the skin (Figure 7-6). Then use the palms to smooth the hair back from the forehead to the back of the neck (Figure 7-7). Naturally, you may also brush it forward and down the Fire Path with your palms (Figure 7-8).

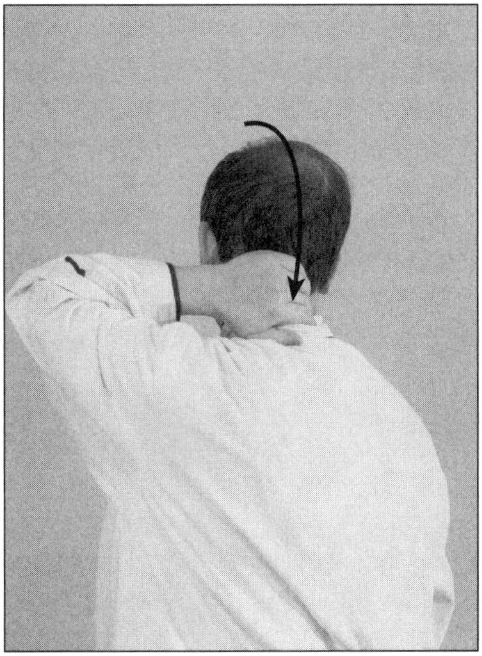

Figure 7-5

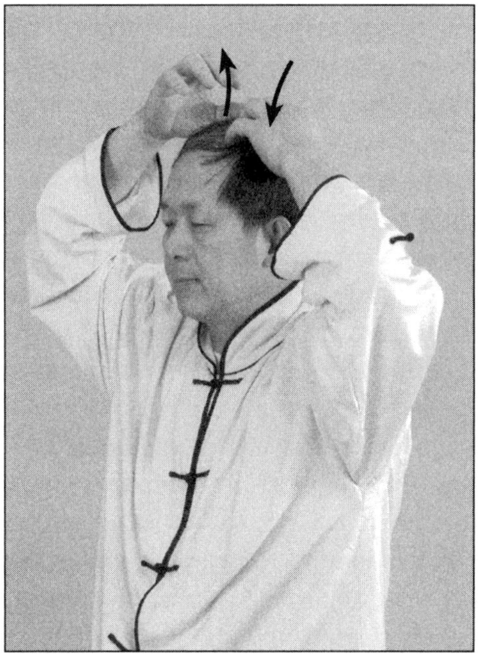

Figure 7-6

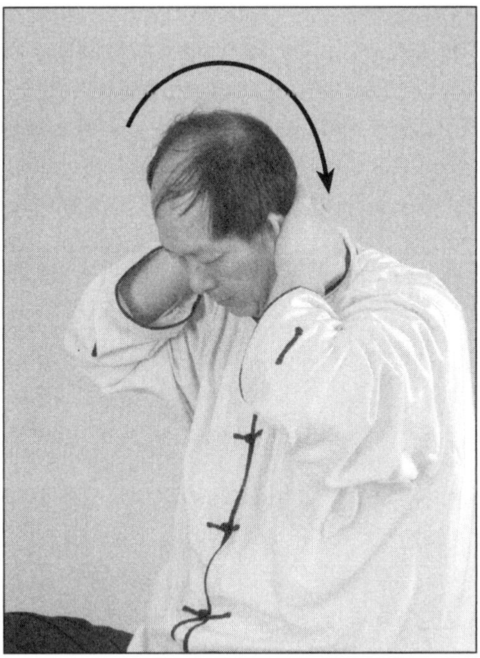

Figure 7-7

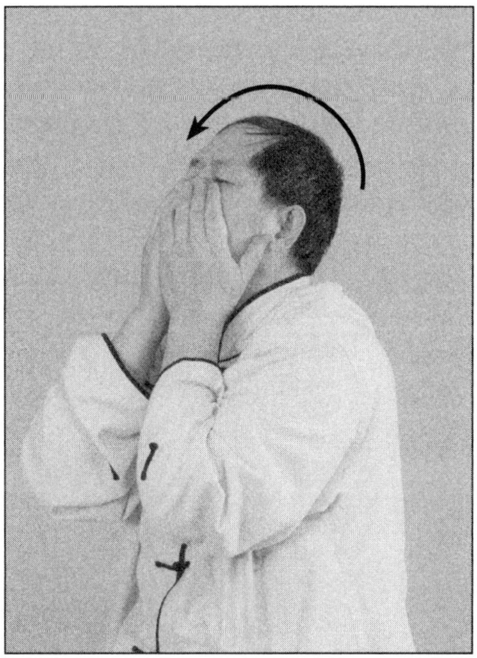

Figure 7-8

Stagnant Qì in the Upper Dāntián. When Qì stagnates in your Upper Dāntián, it feels like fly paper stuck to your third eye. This usually happens when you concentrate there very intensely. When you concentrate your spirit, your Upper Dāntián usually feels comfortably warm. If you feel uncomfortable, it means the Qì is stagnant. When this happens, massage your third eye and lead the Qì past the temples and down the sides of the neck (Figure 7-9).

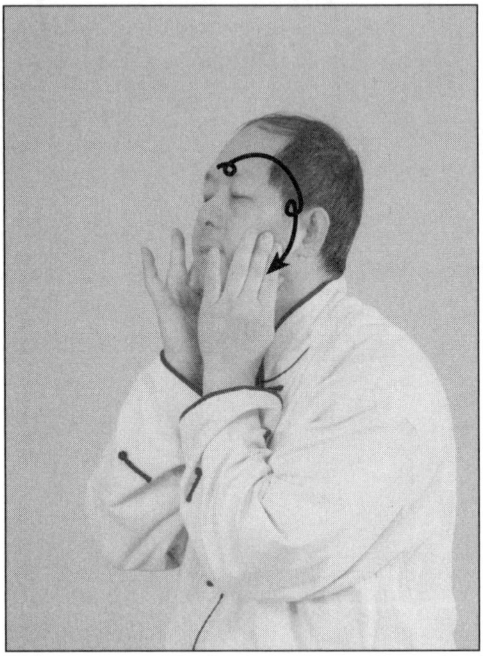

Figure 7-9

False Lower Dāntián feels distended and uncomfortable. This is more common with beginners and usually happens when you force your abdominal muscles in and out. When the muscles are tired, you can't control them. When training abdominal movement, remain soft and relaxed so Qì does not stagnate there. If your abdomen feels uncomfortable and Qì stagnates, massage it in a circular manner (following the bowel system) (Figure 7-10), then open your hands and brush the Qì down to the thighs (Figure 7-11).

Pressure and discomfort at the diaphragm. This usually happens if you don't regulate your breathing correctly. Reverse Abdominal Breathing can cause a feeling of pressure and discomfort, so start the session on a smaller scale, with smaller movements of the abdomen. There is a limit to how far you can move your abdomen without feeling pressure on your diaphragm. Discomfort means Qì is stagnant from pressure around the diaphragm. Stop training, fold your hands, and gently press in on the solar plexus a few times (Figure 7-12), then brush down and to the sides (Figure 7-13).

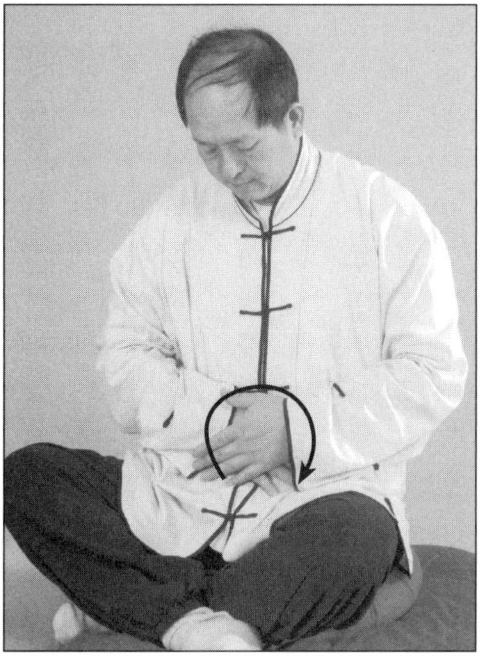

Figure 7-10

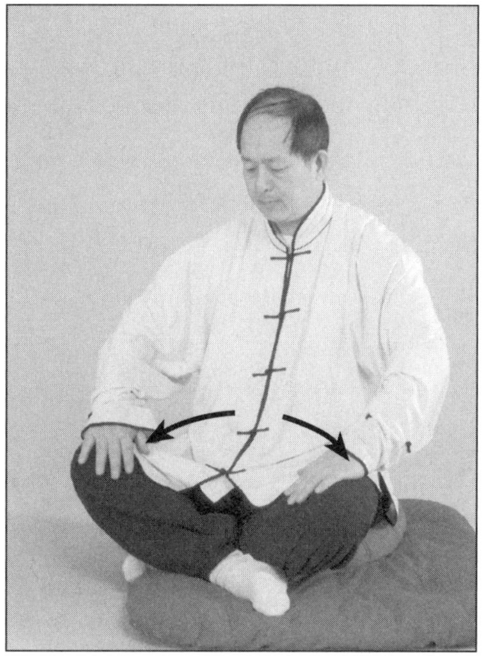

Figure 7-11

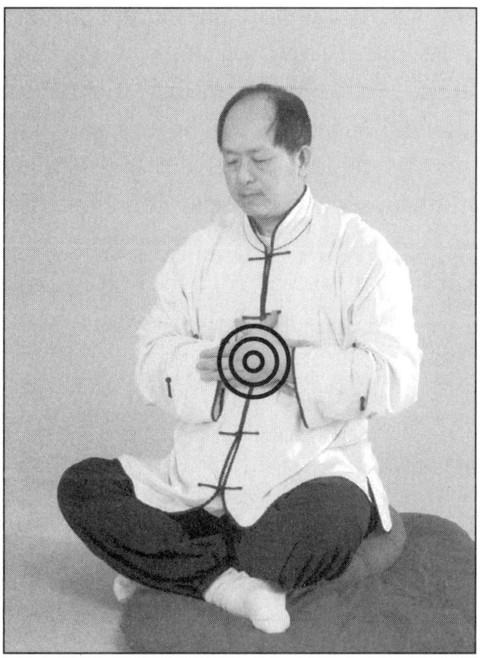

Figure 7-12

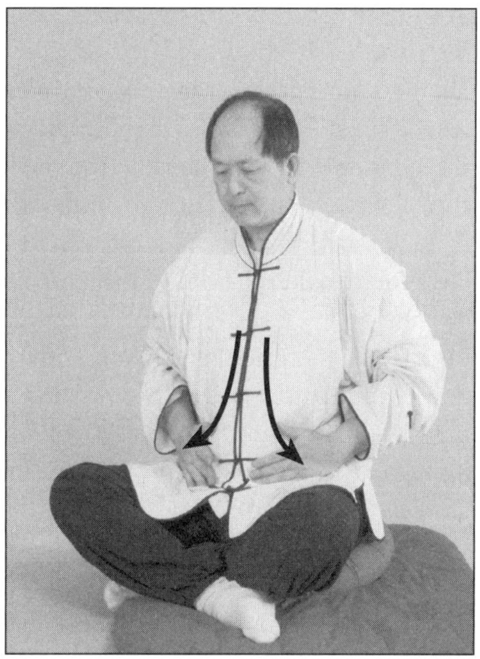

Figure 7-13

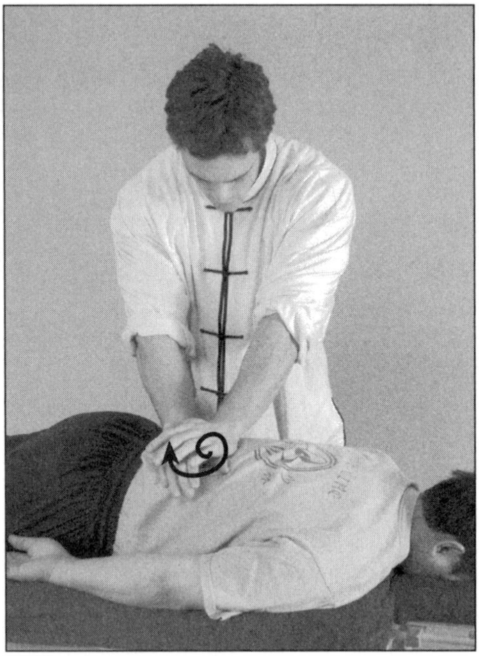

Figure 7-14

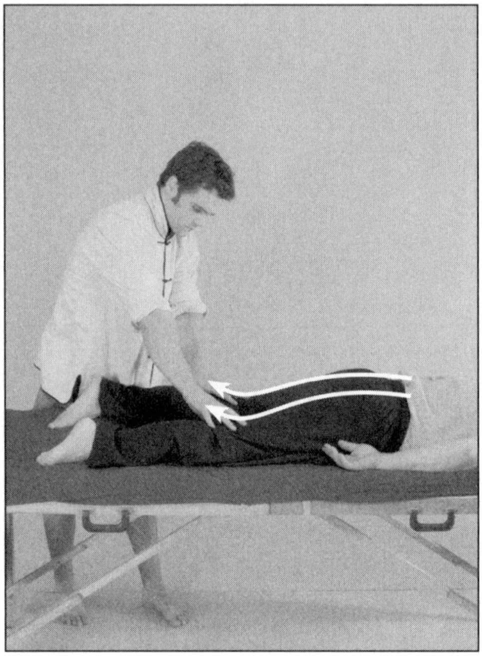

Figure 7-15

Back pain. Back pain in Qìgōng is usually caused by incorrect posture, especially during sitting meditation, causing Qì circulation to stagnate and increasing pressure on the muscles. If you have back pain, stop practicing immediately, or else you will only disturb your mind and make things worse. If possible, have someone massage the painful area (Figure 7-14), following the spine down to the hips (Figure 7-15). Spread the Qì to the sides of the body and down to the legs. You may gently lean your back against some support during meditation, but not against a wall or something that can drain your Qì. A comfortable couch can serve the purpose.

Nocturnal emissions. This happens when you accumulate Qì without keeping and circulating it. If you do a lot of Lower Dāntián exercises, Qì is abundant, your sexual organs are energized, and your body produces more hormones. This increases sexual desire and causes frequent erections, often without apparent cause. Without sexual activity, internal sexual pressure builds, and your body automatically releases it through nocturnal emissions. If you practice Qìgōng and semen is released automatically more than twice a month, it means you are not converting essence into Qì and circulating it properly. You need to coordinate the movement of your Huìyīn with your breathing.

This can also occur when Qì is depleted due to illness, excessive walking, or incorrect Qìgōng training. There is not enough Qì to keep the muscles functioning normally, and you occasionally experience nocturnal emissions. Massage your abdomen after practice until warm.

Qì circulates strongly by itself. Some people build Qì faster than their Yì can control it, which can be very dangerous and cause serious injury. Many Qìgōng students are impatient and try to regulate Qì before regulating body, breathing, and mind. When you feel Qì move by itself in Small Circulation, you are elated at the sign of progress. But if the Qì builds so much you cannot control it, you should stop practicing completely for a while. Practice regulating body, breathing, and mind until you are confident and understand what you are doing before you start regulating Qì. It is wisest to consult an experienced master. Qì may circulate by itself on a small scale, but usually not for too long before it stops by itself. This is nothing to worry about, and you should simply continue your practice with a calm and peaceful mind.

Qì entering the wrong path. This happens when your Qì is strong but your mind is scattered, and the Qì may go anywhere. It might make your internal organs too Yáng or too Yīn, and you could become ill. Qìgōng without a regulated mind is as dangerous as a car with a drunken driver. Always remember to regulate body, breathing, and mind before regulating Qì. If you are already ill because of Qìgōng practice, stop practicing immediately. Relax and get enough rest, and wait until the Qì regains its balance. You usually do not need to see a doctor, and if you keep calm and relaxed, it will balance itself. When you start again, begin with the most basic regulating exercises first, so that you do not repeat the problem.

If the Qì stagnates or enters the wrong path at the Three Gates (Sānguān, 三關) during Small Circulation, the situation can be very dangerous. You should treat it seriously and pay attention to avoiding injury. I urge you to read section 5-5 again about these three gates and the dangers involved, and understand the remedies for the problems.

Stiff tongue. When the tongue is stiff in Qìgōng practice, Qì can stagnate in the Small Circulation. Practice relaxing your tongue as the tip lightly touches the roof of your mouth. Do this naturally and comfortably before practicing Small Circulation.

7-9. Twenty-Four Rules for Qìgōng Practice (Qìgōng Liànxí Èrshísìzé, 氣功練習二十四則)

The twenty-four rules which have been passed down are based on study and experience by generations of Qìgōng masters, and you should observe them carefully. Where they do not fit today's lifestyle, judge wisely. They are summarized here for your reference and consideration.

Don't be stubborn about plans and ideas (Yùzhí Wàngniàn, 預執忘念). This is one of the easiest mistakes for beginners to make. When we take up Qìgōng we are enthusiastic and eager. However, sometimes we don't learn as fast as we would like to and become impatient, and try to force things. Sometimes we set up a schedule for ourselves, such as: today I want to make my Lower Dāntián warm, tomorrow I want to get through the tailbone cavity, by such-and-such day I want to complete the Small Circulation. This is the wrong way to go about it. Qìgōng is not an ordinary task you set for yourself. You cannot make a progress schedule for it. This only makes your thinking rigid and stalls your progress. Everything happens when the time is ready. If you force it, it will not happen naturally.

Don't focus on discrimination (Zhuóyì Fēnbié, 著意分別). When you practice, don't focus on the various phenomena or sensations which occur. Be aware of what is happening, but center your mind where it is supposed to be for the exercise you are doing. If you let your mind go where you feel something interesting happening, the Qì will follow and interfere with your body's natural tendency to rebalance itself. Don't expect anything to happen, and don't let your mind wander around looking for various phenomena. Nor should you judge the phenomena, such as asking "Is my Lower Dāntián warmer today than it was yesterday," or "Where is my Qì now?" When your mind is on your Qì, your Yì is there also, and this stagnant Yì will not lead the Qì. Be aware of what is happening, but don't pay attention to it. When you drive a car, you don't watch yourself steer and work the pedals and shift gears. Simply think of where you want to go and let your body automatically drive the car. This is called Regulating Without Regulating.

Avoid miscellaneous thoughts remaining on origins (Zániàn Pānyuán, 雜念攀緣). This is a problem of regulating the mind. The Emotional Mind is strong, and every idea is connected to its origin. If you cannot cut the ideas off at their source, your mind is not regulated, and you should not try to regulate Qì. You will also find that, even though you stop the flow of random thoughts, new ideas are generated during practice. For example, when you notice your Lower Dāntián is warm, your mind immediately recalls where this is mentioned in a book, or how the master described it, and you start to compare your experience with that. Or you may start wondering what the next step is. These thoughts lead you away from peace and calm, and your mind ends up Entering the Devil (Rùmó, 入魔). It becomes confused, scattered, and often scared, and you will get tired quickly.

Xīn should not follow the external scenery (Xīnsuí Wàijǐng, 心隨外景). This is also a problem of regulating the Xīn. When your Emotional Mind is uncontrolled, any external distraction leads it away from your center and toward the distraction. Train yourself so that noises, smells, conversations and such will not disturb your concentration. Be aware of what is happening, but your mind remains calm, peaceful, and firmly on your cultivation.

Regulate sexual activity (Rùfáng Shījīng, 入房施精). A man should not have sexual relations at least twenty-four hours before or after practicing Qìgōng, especially in Small Circulation. The conversion training is a very critical part of these practices, and if you practice Qìgōng soon after sex, you harm your body significantly. Sex depletes your sperm and the Qì level in the lower portion of your body. Practicing Qìgōng under these conditions is like doing heavy exercise right after sex. When your Qì level is abnormal, your feeling and sensing are not accurate either, and your Yì can be misled. You should wait until the Qì level returns to normal before you resume Qìgōng practice. Only then will the Essence-Qì conversion proceed efficiently.

One major purpose of Qìgōng is to increase the conversion and use this Qì to nourish your body. Once a man has built up a supply of Qì, having sex will only pass this Qì on to his partner. Many Qìgōng masters insist that you should not have sex three days before and four days after practice.

During sexual relations, the woman usually gains Qì while the man loses Qì during ejaculation. The woman should not practice Qìgōng after sex until her body has digested the Qì she has obtained from the man. There are certain Daoist Qìgōng techniques which teach men how to avoid losing Qì during sexual activity and how women can receive Qì from the man and digest it. We leave the discussion of this subject to Qìgōng masters who are qualified and experienced in it.

Don't be too warm or too cold (Dàwēn Dàhán, 大溫大寒). The temperature of the room in which you are training should be neither too hot nor too cold. You should practice in a comfortable environment which will not disturb your mind and cultivation.

Beware of the five weaknesses and internal injuries (Wǔláo Ànshāng, 五癆暗傷). Five weaknesses are those of the Yīn organs, namely heart, liver, lungs, kidneys, and spleen. When any of them is weak, you should proceed very gently. Qìgōng practice is an internal exercise directly affecting these five organs. Excessive exertion does not build up strength and may cause serious injury.

Internal injuries disturb your internal Qì circulation. Practicing Qìgōng may exacerbate your problem and interfere with the natural healing process. Certain Qìgōng exercises are designed to heal internal injuries, but to use them properly you need a deep understanding of the Qì situation of your body.

Avoid facing the wind when sweating (Zuòhàn Dāngfēng, 坐汗當風). Don't practice facing the wind, especially cold wind. When you practice Qìgōng you are exercising both internally and externally. With your pores wide open, you are vulnerable and liable to catch cold.

Don't wear tight clothes and belt (Jǐnyī Shùdài, 緊衣束帶). Always wear loose, comfortable clothes during practice, and keep your belt loose. The abdomen is the key area in Qìgōng practice, and anything which limits movement of this area interferes with your practice.

Don't eat too much greasy and sweet food (Tāotiè Féigān, 饕餮肥甘). Regulate your eating while practicing Qìgōng. Greasy or sweet food increase Fire Qì, scattering your mind and letting your spirit stray from its residence. Eat more fruit and vegetables, and abstain from alcohol and tobacco.

Don't hang your feet off the bed (Báchuáng Xuánjiǎo, 跋床懸腳). In ancient times the most common place for Qìgōng practice was sitting on the bed. Since most beds were high, if you sat on the edge of the bed your feet would hang above the floor. When you practice Qìgōng, your feet should touch the floor, or else all your body weight presses down on the lower part of your thighs and reduces Qì and blood circulation.

Don't practice with a full bladder (Jiǔrěn Xiǎobiàn, 久忍小便). You should go to the toilet before starting your practice. If you need to go during practice, stop your practice to do so. Holding it in will disturb your concentration.

Don't scratch an itch (Sāozhuā Yǎngchù, 搔抓癢處). If you itch for some external reason, such as an insect biting you, do not be alarmed, and keep your mind calm. Let your Yì lead the Qì back to the Lower Dāntián. Breathe a couple of times, and gradually bring your consciousness back to your surroundings. Then you may scratch or think of how to stop the itching. However, if the itching is caused by Qì redistribution, don't move your mind there. Simply ignore it and let it happen. Once it reaches a new balance, the itching stops. Scratching this kind of itch disturbs your mind, while your hands interfere with the natural rebalancing of your body's Qì.

Avoid being disturbed or startled (Cùhū Jīngjì, 猝呼驚悸). If this does happen, calm down your mind, and refrain from losing your temper. Now prevent it from happening again. Most important is learning to regulate your mind when you are disturbed.

Don't take delight in the scenery (Duìjǐng Huānxǐ, 對景歡喜). It is very common during practice to notice something happening inside of you. Perhaps you feel Qì moving more strongly than ever before, or you sense your bone marrow, and feel elated and excited. This is a very common trap, as your concentration is broken and your mind divided, which is dangerous and harmful. You need to be aware of what is going on inside you without getting excited.

Don't wear sweaty clothes (Jiǔzhe Hànyī, 久著汗衣). Sweaty clothes make you feel uncomfortable, affecting your concentration. It is better to change into dry clothes before resuming practice.

Don't sit when hungry or full (Jībǎo Shàngzuò, 飢飽上坐). You should not practice Qìgōng when hungry or when your stomach is full. When you are hungry, it is hard to concentrate, and when you are full, your practice affects your digestion.

Heaven and Earth strange disaster (Tiāndì Zāiguài, 天地災怪). Your body's Qì is directly affected by changes in the weather. It is not advisable to practice when there is a sudden change of weather, because it interferes with your body's natural readjustment to the new environment. Nor can you sense and control your Qì flow as you do normally. You should remain emotionally neutral when you do Qìgōng, and even during a natural disaster like an earthquake, remain calm so that your Qì stays under control.

Listen sometimes to true words (Zhēnyán Ǒutīng, 真言偶聽). You need confidence when you practice Qìgōng. You should not listen to advice from inexperienced people who are not familiar with the condition of your body. Some people listen to classmates explaining how they reached a certain level, or how they solved a certain problem and then blindly try to use the same method themselves. Everyone has a different body, with a different state of health, and everyone learns differently. When the time comes to learn something new, you will understand what you need. Play it cool, and always have confidence in your training.

Don't lean and fall asleep (Hūnchén Qīngyī, 昏沉傾欹). Discontinue Qìgōng training when you are sleepy. Leading Qì with an unclear mind is dangerous. Your body will not be regulated, tending to lean or droop, which interferes with Qì circulation. It is better to rest until you regain your spirit.

Don't meditate when too angry, happy, or excited (Dànù, Dàlè Rùzuò, 大怒、大樂入坐). When your mind is scattered, Qìgōng will bring more harm than peace.

Don't keep spitting (Tǔtán Wúdù, 吐痰無度). It is normal to generate a lot of saliva while practicing Qìgōng, which should be swallowed to moisten your throat. Spitting wastes it and disturbs concentration.

Don't doubt and become lazy (Shēngyí Xièdài, 生疑懈怠). You need confidence in the methods of practice. Doubt leads to laziness and discontinuing the practice. Then you will not be successful.

Do not ask for speedy success (Bùqiú Sùxiào, 不求速效). Qìgōng practice is time-consuming and progress is slow. To reach your goal, you need patience, a strong will, and confidence. Let your practice proceed naturally.

References

1. 《性命圭旨全書・王子喬胎息訣》：〝子、午、卯、酉四時，乃是陰陽出入之門戶。〞

2. 習煉氣功中，形神安靜，凝神入氣穴，覺丹田氣動，陰陽生發之時。

3. 《脈望》：〝下手立丹基，休向子午推，靜中才一動，便是癸生時，謂之活子時。〞

4. 泥丸祖曰：“百日之中忌昏，昏迷散亂失卻真。

5. 眼觀鼻，鼻觀心。

6. 悟一子曰：〝欲實其腹，先虛其心，欲生其白，先虛其室。〞

7. 伍真人云：〝還虛合道，出定以後，倏出倏定也可，六通十通皆能，千變萬化，無所不能。〞

Chapter 8

Small Circulation Meditation Practice

8-1. Introduction (Jièshào, 介紹)

After studying the theory of Small Circulation, practice it with caution. Always go back and ponder it. During practice, you may have new questions or doubts, and the best way to find a solution is pondering the theory which has been derived from past experience. After finding a possible answer, go back and put it into practice. From repeating this process, you become wiser and more proficient. Theory is like a map. The more you understand it, the easier and more safely you can approach your goal.

Often, theory alone is not enough, and you need guidance from an experienced teacher. There are different approaches to a problem, and many paths can lead to the same goal. The more you open your mind, the more you learn and experience on the way to becoming a real expert of Small Circulation. You should not be concerned with dignity and pride, but remain humble and learn from experience. Filter ideas and adopt those which are appropriate for you.

Since Small Circulation is so important for spiritual cultivation, different practice methods have been developed by different cultures. It is called Microcosmic Orbit in Indian Yoga, where its methods are different from those used by Chinese Qìgōng. The methods used in Buddhist and Daoist monasteries also differ from each other. Although the methods differ, the theory and the goal remain the same.

The most important factor for successful practice is training your feeling. Deep feeling leads to profound communication between your spirit and body. It connects with the subconscious mind and raises the spirit.

There was a wise king in Korea who had a fifteen-year-old son. This son had grown up comfortably in the palace, with all of the servants' attention. This worried the king, who believed his son would not be a good king to care for his people. So he summoned a wise old man, living deep in the woods.

In response to this call, the old man came to the palace. He promised to teach the prince to be a wise, good king, and took him to the deep woods. After they arrived there, the old man taught him how to find food, cook, and survive in the forest. Then he left him there alone, but promised to return a year later.

A year later, when the old man came back, he asked the prince what he thought about the forest. The prince replied, "I am sick of it. I need a servant. I hate it here. Take me home." The old man said, "Very good. That is good progress, but not enough. Please wait here for another year, and I will be back to see you again." Then, he left again.

Another year passed, and the old man came back to the woods, asking the same question. This time the prince said, "I see birds and trees, flowers, and animals." His mind had started to accept his environment, and he recognized his role in the forest. The old man was satisfied and said, "This is very good progress, but not enough, so you must stay here for another year." This time, the prince did not even seem to mind.

Another year passed, and the old man returned. This time, when the old man asked the prince what he thought, the prince said, "I feel birds, woods, fish, animals, and many things around me here." This time, the old man was very happy and said, "Now I can take you home. If you can feel the things happening around you, then you will be able to concern yourself with the people's feelings, and you will be a good king." Then he took him home.

When you do anything, you must put your mind into it, feel it, taste it, and experience it. Only then may you say that you understand it. Without this deep feeling and comprehension, the arts you practice or create will be shallow and lose their essence.

In this chapter, we finally reach the keys of practice. In Sections 8-2 to 8-6, we discuss the methods of regulating the body, breathing, mind, Qì, and spirit in Small Circulation. Because the Original Essence (Yuánjīng, 元精) is one of the keys to success, we review the concept of regulating it in Section 8-7. Then we summarize how to recover from deep meditation in Section 8-8. Finally, we discuss how to use meditation to heal yourself in Section 8-9.

8-2. Regulating the Body (Tiáoshēn, 調身)

The first step is to sit correctly, comfortably, and naturally for at least thirty minutes. If you cannot sit still that long, you may have difficulty leading the Qì safely. When you lead the Qì in Small Circulation meditation, your mind must be comfortable and focused. If it is disturbed by an uneasy posture, it can scatter, so you should not advance further. First learn to sit correctly and patiently. Most important is to cultivate the mood and joy of meditation. You regulate the body to establish a very relaxed, comfortable, natural feeling, so your mind can concentrate on regulating. Start with only five minutes, and gradually increase it.

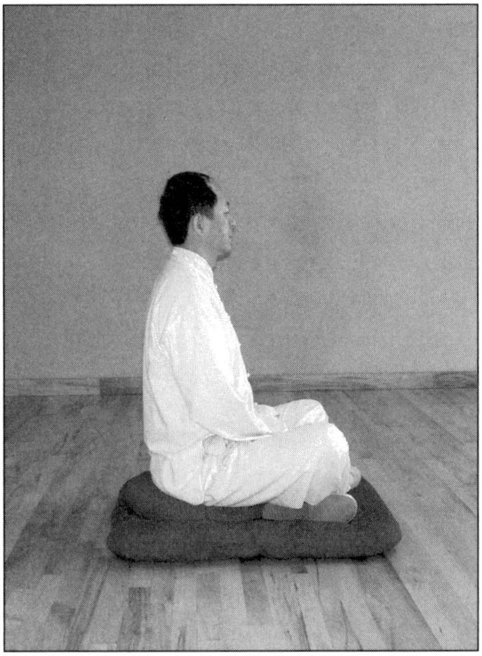

Figure 8-1. Sitting Meditation Posture

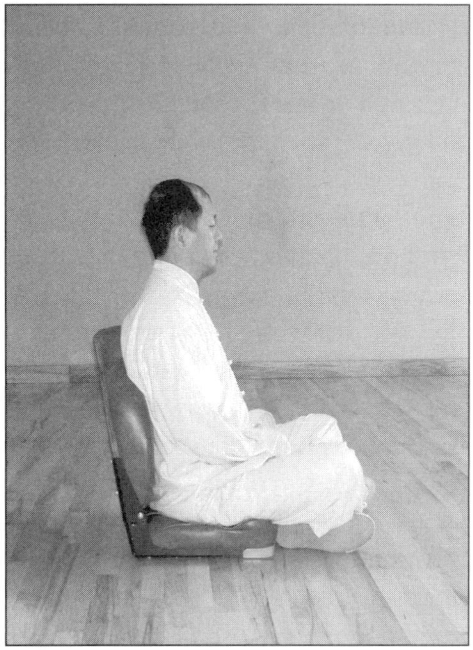

Figure 8-2. Sitting Meditation on a Fishing Chair

Torso. The correct posture of the torso is very important to make the body balanced, centered, and relaxed. Only then can the Qì circulate smoothly without stagnation, and the mind can easily lead the Qì to circulate naturally.

This also applies to the neck and the head. The neck must relax to allow Qì and blood to flow easily to the brain. It is the junction where Qì and blood are exchanged between the head and torso, and when it relaxes, the brain obtains ample nourishment. The head must also be comfortable. First relax the mind, then the head can relax too.

In meditation, keep the torso upright and the head as though suspended from above. You should not lean forward, backward, or sideways. Improper posture makes the torso tense and scatters your mind. This is especially true for beginners, who may easily lean forward and fall asleep, which can lead to lower back pain, or block Qì circulation. You should not stiffen the torso when you keep it upright. It should be relaxed so the Qì can circulate smoothly.

Practice for some time on a meditation cushion (Figure 8-1). If you continue to experience tightness in the torso, especially your lower back, sit on a chair which supports your back (Figure 8-2). Alternatively, sit on a couch or sofa which provides good support while not restricting your Qì flow, and is not so comfortable that you fall asleep (Figure 8-3). If you are too tired to practice, simply lead the Qì to the Real Lower Dāntián, and take a short nap. Don't keep struggling, which may bring more harm than good.

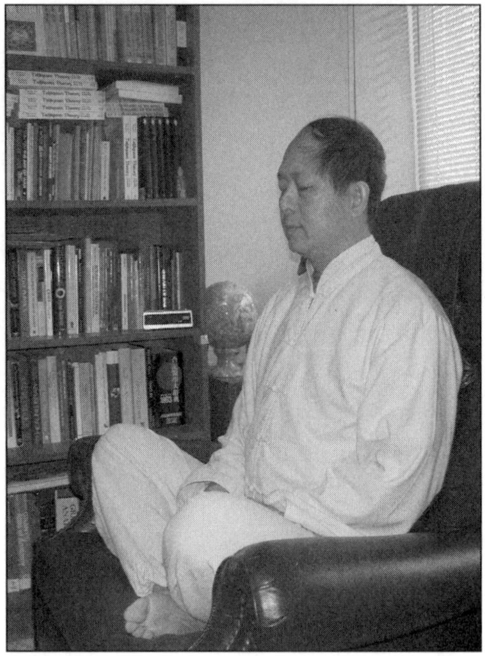

Figure 8-3. Sitting Meditation on a Couch

Hands. The hands should be placed comfortably on your legs in front of your abdomen. It does not matter which hand is on top, as long as they feel comfortable and natural. Some teachers claim a man should place the right hand on top while women place the left hand on top. The most important thing is to feel balanced. The Qì circulating on either side of the body is not perfectly balanced, nor is the body itself. Heart and spleen are on the left, while the liver is on the right. Hands, legs, and feet are not the same length. Due to this imbalance, Qì circulation is not balanced either. The mind adjusts the feeling of unbalanced Qì in the body, so body and mind can coordinate with each other. If you force left-handed people to change to using the right hand, they experience emotional and mental imbalance, and children often develop a stutter.

Placing the hands in front of the lower abdomen is called Wògù (握固) which means to Hold and to Firm. In *Dào Dé Jīng*, Chapter 55 (道德經・五十五章), it says, "When the bones are weak and the tendons soft, then Wògù."[1] When your body is weak, the first thing you should do is to store abundant Qì at the Real Lower Dāntián. Wògù helps keep your mind there. Then Qì is not led outward, and can be preserved and stored.

To enhance the feeling of firming the Qì, various ways of holding the fingers were taught. *The Thesis on the Origins and Symptoms of Various Diseases* (*Zhūbìng Yuánhòu Lùn*, 諸病源候論) said, "What is Wògù? It is to use the four fingers of both hands to hold the thumb."[2] That means holding the thumb in the four fingers in front of the Lower Dāntián (Figure 8-4). *The Necessary Book of Entering the Daoist Religion* (*Dàomén Tōngjiào Bìyòng Jí*, 道門通教必用集) said, "Wògù is using the thumb to nip the middle of the middle finger and the four fingers are gathered at the center."[3] The finger nail of the thumb presses the middle of the middle finger while the other four fingers are holding it (Figure 8-5). In fact, this is only a trick to help beginners concentrate the mind at the Lower Dāntián.

Various hand forms are used in Buddhist meditation. These are called hand stamps (Shǒuyìn, 手印). In Daoist society, it says, "There are two different purposes for hand posture. First, concentrate the mind and spirit on the Shǒuyìn, persevere and finally obtain the steadiness of Chán. Second, after forming the Shǒuyìn, the mind and spirit are

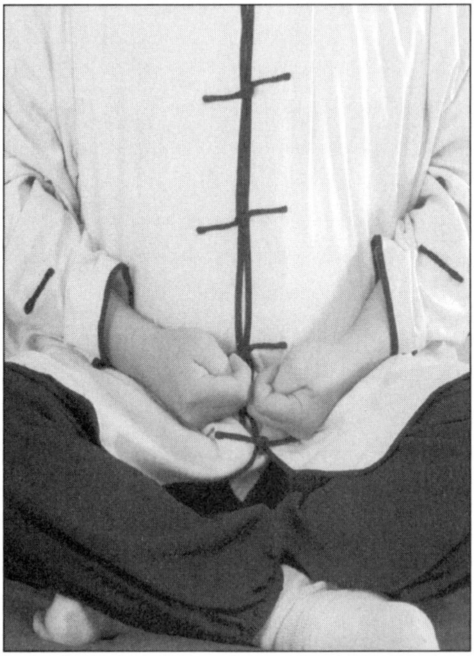

Figure 8-4

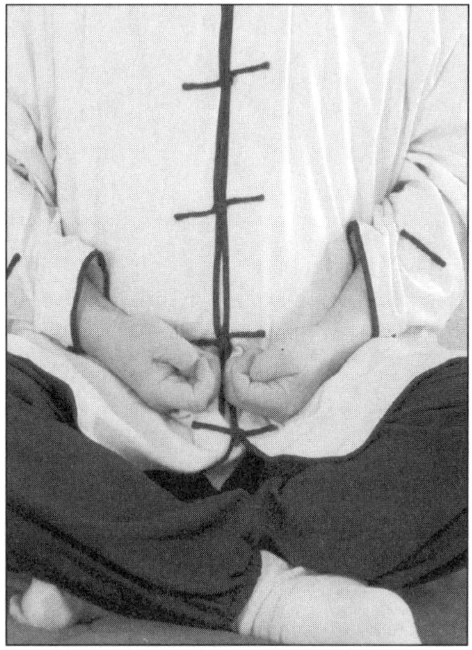

Figure 8-5

on the breathing, to reach the highest level and become the Buddha."[4] Hand posture or Shǒuyìn helps one calm the mind and concentrate on the Lower Dāntián and the breathing. Again, this is a trick to regulate the mind and breathing. The Buddhist classic *The Classic of Tuóluóní* (*Tuóluóní Jíjīng*, 陀羅尼集經) said, "There are various body stamping techniques in chanting, if using hands to make Shǒuyìn and chanting, it can easily be effective."[5] Chanting is very common in different religions, to achieve the state of hypnosis and harmony. Meditation is considered self-hypnosis in Chinese Qìgōng practice. Through chanting and different hand stamps, Buddhists reach a high level of meditation.

Legs. When you sit for Small Circulation, the legs should be crossed comfortably (Figure 8-6). This prevents stronger Qì flow to the legs. Since man has walked for millions of years, the Qì naturally flows there strongly, instead of in the Small Circulation path. To prevent the stronger Qì flow from injuring the legs, they should be crossed, blocking it at the hip area. In this way, Qì flow is stronger and more efficient in the Governing and Conception Vessels. Another way of restraining the strong Qì flow to the legs is to stand with the knees bent (Figure 8-7). This is how the ancient Shàolín martial monks (Sēngbīng, 僧兵) practiced Small Circulation.

Crossed legs are called Jiéjiā Fūzuò (結跏趺坐) in Buddhism.[6] You must keep searching for the most comfortable and stable posture, so your mind can concentrate fully. In the beginning, when you cross your legs, don't place one on top of the other. This pressure causes numbness of the bottom leg. Place them slightly apart. A comfortable

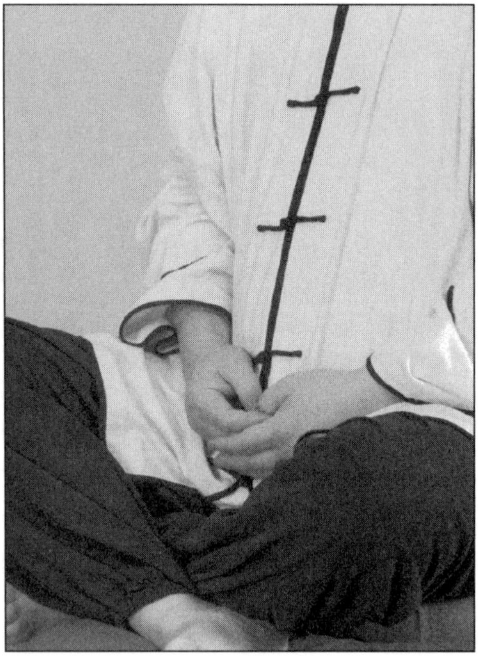

Figure 8-6

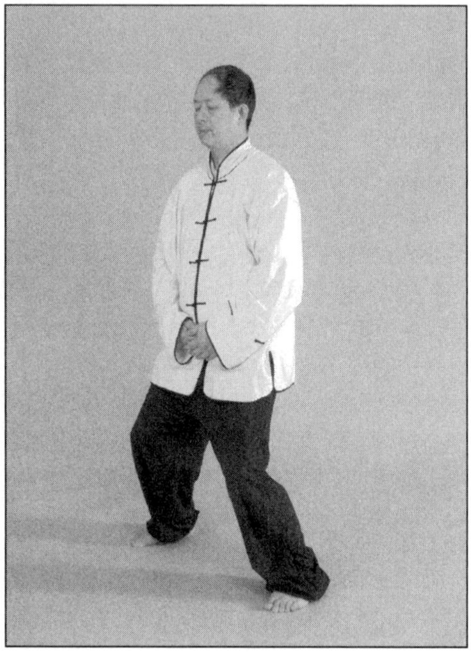

Figure 8-7

cushion of the proper height reduces the problem, and also eases tension in the lower back. You should sit on a thick, comfortable mat to prevent the pressure from the floor generating numbness of the legs. The material used for sitting and wearing should be natural fabrics.

Eyes and Tongue. The eyes should be comfortably closed. To keep the thoughts from imagination and fantasy, teachers often have a beginner keep his eyes slightly open. After you have meditated for a long time, it will be easier to lead the Qì if you close your eyes. Then you can feel deeper and more clearly into the deep places of your body.

The tongue should gently touch the palate (Figure 8-8). This connects the Yīn Conception Vessel and Yáng Governing Vessel and allows Qì to pass. *The Red Wind Marrow* (*Chìfēngsuǐ*, 赤風髓) said, "The secret trick is closing the two eyes, half dropping the curtain (eye lid), and the head (tip) of the red dragon (tongue) touches the palate of the mouth upward."[7] The Mirror of Cui's (Method) of Entering the Herb (Cuīgōng Rùyào Jìng, 崔公入藥鏡) said, "The silver river (Milky Way) separates the meeting of Yīn and Yáng. It must rely on the magpie bridge to cross. Man's tongue is regarded as a magpie bridge". When training Gōng, the tongue touches the palate of the mouth to connect Yīn and Yáng."[8]

You need to provide comfortable and natural conditions for relaxation, Qì circulation, and spiritual cultivation. When you are relaxed, Qì can circulate smoothly. Then you can achieve balance and be centered. When you are centered, you can be rooted.

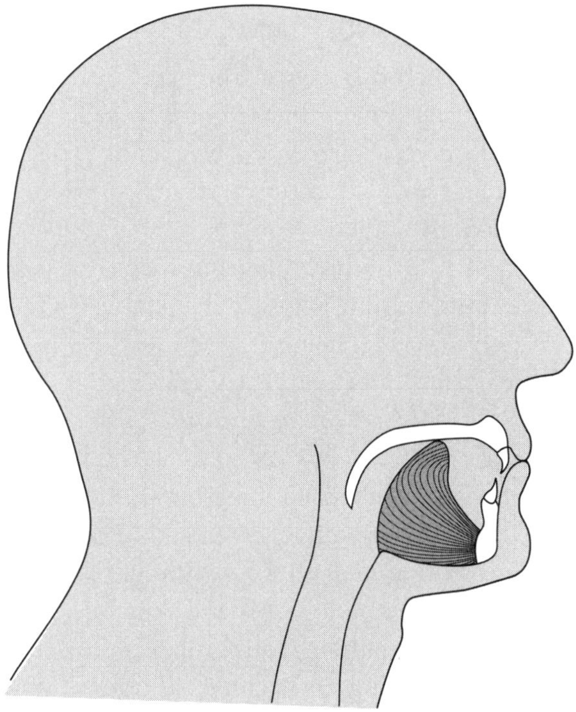

Figure 8-8. Tongue Position

Only then can you raise up the spirit of vitality for spiritual cultivation. Relaxing, balancing, centering, rooting, and finally raising up the spirit form a chain of sequential connections.

Once you regulate your mind to a deeper level, regulation of the body can also be more profound. The goal is to feel the bone marrow and internal organs, and relax them. At this level, you feel any Qì imbalance. For example, if you have an injury to your right shoulder or back, you feel the body tends to turn right when you reach a highly relaxed state. This is because the muscles of the right side of the body are tighter. Let the turning happen by itself. Once it reaches its maximum, relax it and allow it to return to its original state. From this practice, you can easily heal your injuries. This kind of mind and body communication is called 'Gōngfū of internal vision' (Nèishì Gōngfū, 內視功夫).

Once you reach a good level of regulating the body, you should increase regulation of the breathing. Even then, you continue to regulate your body, because the two are closely related.

8-3. Regulating the Breathing (Tiáoxí, 調息)

Remember, the goal is to absorb oxygen and expel carbon dioxide efficiently. Then the body has plenty of oxygen for production of new cells, and can remove dead cells from the deep places in the body. When you have plenty of oxygen, your energy is high, because it is the vital element for combustion and energy production. To generate strong Qì, you must breathe correctly and efficiently.

To produce abundant Qì, the breathing must be soft and slender, and the body relaxed. Then, oxygen consumption is low and metabolism is efficient. *Dào Dé Jīng*, Chapter 10 (道德經・十章) said, "Focusing the breathing to reach softness, can it be soft like a baby?"[9] When breathing is soft, the Qì circulation becomes soft and smooth. *The Complete Book of Principal Contents of Life and Human Nature* (*Xìngmìng Guīzhǐ Quánshū*, 性命圭旨全書) said, "Focus on making the breathing soft and the spirit stays long. The real breathing (Embryonic Breathing) is long, gentle, and slow. Breathe softly to return the Original Qì. Unlimited spiritual fountain will flow naturally."[10] This implies that one produces unlimited Qì flow through correct Embryonic Breathing, where "Exhaling is slender and inhaling is soft and slow."[11]

When you practice correct breathing, you regulate it until regulating is no longer necessary. That means correct breathing has become natural and smooth. *Easy Understanding of Daoist Talking* (*Dàoyán Qiǎnjìn*, 道言淺近) said, "Regulating the breathing must regulate until the real regulating is stopped… To condense the spirit and regulate the breathing, you need a peaceful mind and harmonious Qì."[12] *The Complete Book of Principal Contents of Life and Human Nature* (*Xìngmìng Guīzhǐ Quánshū*, 性命圭旨全書) said, "Regulating the breathing, must regulate until the real regulating ceases. Training the Shén, must train until the spirit is no longer necessary for the training."[13] When you regulate your breathing or train your spirit, first use your mind and spirit to make it happen. However, after long practice, everything becomes natural and happens automatically. Then, no more regulating is necessary.

You should follow the following procedures to achieve Embryonic Breathing:

1. **Normal Abdominal Breathing** (Zhèng Fùhūxī, 正腹呼吸)
   When you inhale, expand your abdomen while pushing your Huìyīn (Co-1, 會陰, perineum) out gently and softly (Figure 8-9). When you exhale, withdraw your abdomen and hold up your Huìyīn (Figure 8-10). Huìyīn is the gate which controls the Qì at the Real Lower Dāntián, letting it be stored or released. Your tongue touches the palate of your mouth to connect the Conception and Governing Vessels. In Normal Abdominal Breathing, you lead the Qì through the twelve primary channels to the four limbs. This makes you feel natural and relaxed.

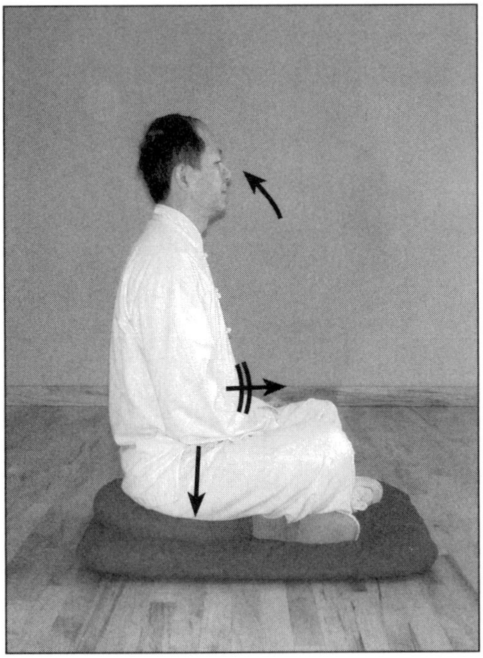

Figure 8-9

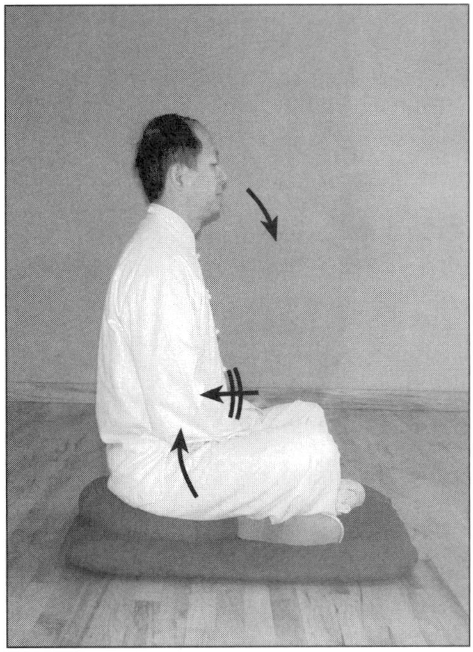

Figure 8-10

Start with small abdominal movement until you feel comfortable, gradually increasing the scale. Do not tense, which causes Qì circulation to stagnate. After long practice, your mind can control the abdominal muscles, so they stay relaxed even though the abdominal movements are big. This accomplishes the first step of Embryonic Breathing.

2. **Reverse Abdominal Breathing** (Fǎn Fùhūxī, 反腹呼吸)(Nì Fùhūxī, 逆腹呼吸) When you can control the abdominal muscles easily and naturally from Normal Abdominal Breathing practice, you begin Reverse Abdominal Breathing. When you inhale, withdraw your abdomen and hold up your Huìyīn (Figure 8-11). When you exhale, push your abdomen and Huìyīn out, gently and softly (Figure 8-12). Reverse Abdominal Breathing leads Qì from the twelve primary channels laterally through the muscles to the skin to strengthen Guardian Qì, and also to the bone marrow to enhance marrow Qì and to nourish and clean the marrow.

   As with Normal Abdominal Breathing, start with small abdominal movements to keep the area relaxed, proceeding gradually and carefully. When you can control the movement, you increase its scale while remaining relaxed. Then you can lead the Qì in from the body to the Dāntián and out from the Dāntián to the whole body.

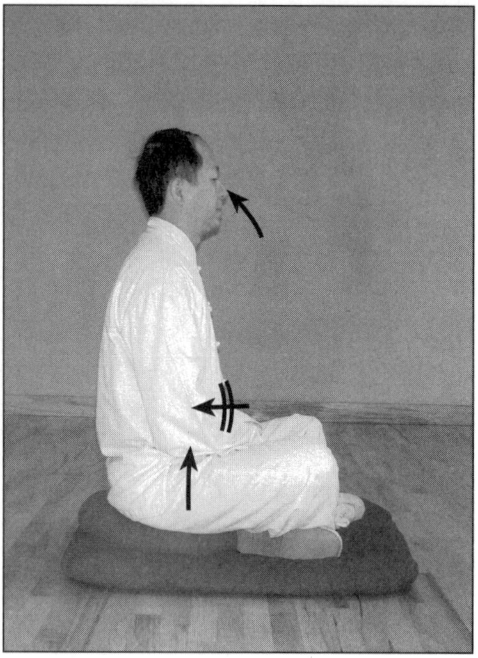

Figure 8-11

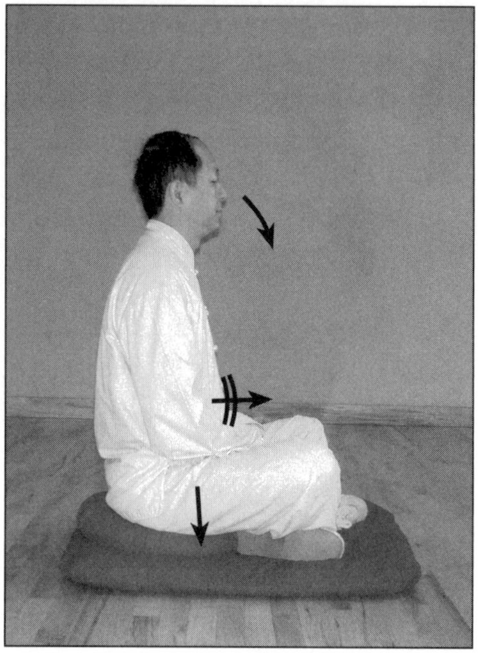

Figure 8-12

3. **Embryonic Breathing** (Tāixí, 胎息)
   Embryonic Breathing is used to store Qì in the Real Lower Dāntián and to strengthen the Guardian Qì through Girdle Vessel Breathing (Dàimài Hūxī, 帶脈呼吸). This is achieved by keeping the mind there. It is commonly called Yìshǒu Dāntián (意守丹田) which means to keep the mind at the Dāntián. When the mind is there, the Qì is led there and stays in its residence (Qìshè, 氣舍). When the mind's focus is elsewhere, Qì is led away and consumed. To store the Qì through Wújí Breathing, you should inhale longer than you exhale, practicing in the spring and summer. If you strengthen Guardian Qì through Girdle Vessel Breathing, your exhalation should be longer than inhalation. The Girdle Vessel Breathing should be done in the fall and winter, when strong Guardian Qì is important to protect against the cold.

Since you are leading Qì laterally to the skin and bone marrow, you must use Reverse Abdominal Breathing. The only difference is that when you inhale, the abdomen and lower back withdraw at the same time, while holding up Huìyīn. When you exhale, the abdomen and lower back expand, at the same time pushing your Huìyīn down, softly and gently.

Again, you start from a small scale of movement, until you control the muscles efficiently, then increase it. After long practice, every movement becomes natural, easy, and automatic without too much mental effort, as you achieve real regulating. Slowly and gradually your mind shifts to the Real Lower Dāntián and remains there at the center of your body.

Before Small Circulation, practice Embryonic Breathing for a few minutes. If you inhale longer than exhaling, you lead Qì to the Real Lower Dāntián and calm yourself down. This calms down your mind and stores Qì for the circulation practice.

In Nèidān Qìgōng practice, the Real Lower Dāntián is called Qì Cavity (Qìxuè, 氣穴). Above it is the Yellow Yard (Huángtíng, 黃庭), the tripod (cooking utensil) in which the herb is cooked. When Kǎn Water Qì from the Real Lower Dāntián is mixed with Lí Fire Qì at the Huángtíng, the Spiritual Baby Embryo (Shéntāi, Shèngtāi, or Língtāi, 神胎、聖胎、靈胎) is conceived. This interaction of Water and Fire is called Kǎn and Lí (坎離). Once this Spiritual Baby Embryo is ready, it is led to the spiritual residence (Shénshì, 神室, Upper Dāntián) for further cultivation, and later leaves through the third eye to unite with the natural spirit.

The *Complete Book of Principal Contents of Life and Human Nature* (*Xìngmìng Guīzhǐ Quánshū*, 性命圭旨全書) said, "Huángtíng is the tripod and the Qì cavity is the furnace. Huángtíng is right above the Qì cavity and they are connected with each other by Luò. This is the meeting place of hundreds of channels in the body." The Original Qì condenses between the two cavities in the Small Tripod Furnace (Xiǎo Dǐnglú, 小鼎爐). "The position of Qián (乾) is tripod while the position of Kūn (坤) is furnace." If this concept is applied to the Circulation Meditation, the brain (Níwángōng, 泥丸宮 or Upper Dāntián, 上丹田) is Qian (tripod) while the Lower Dāntián (Xià Dāntián, 下丹田) is Kūn (furnace).[14] *The Verification Thesis of Golden Immortal* (Jīnxiān Zhènglùn, 金仙証論) said, "Those who pick up the herb (Qì) to transport the cyclic heaven (Small Circulation) should start the fire at the Kūn furnace (Real Lower Dāntián). Ascend to the Qian head (tripod) and descend to the Kūn abdomen (furnace). This is what the ancients meant by using Qiánkūn as the cooking tools. Whenever Shén and Qì rise and fall, the tripod's Qì exists." When there is Shén and Qì, you have furnace and tripod. Without Shén and Qì, there is neither furnace nor tripod.[15]

Therefore, when you start the fire in the False Lower Dāntián and accumulate it in the Real Lower Dāntián, breathing significantly influences how the Qì builds up. If you build it up slowly with long, gentle technique, it is called Scholar Fire (Wénhuǒ, 文火). If you build it up quickly with short, fast, heavy breathing, it is called Martial Fire (Wǔhuǒ, 武火). *Anthology of Daoist Village* (*Dàoxiāngjí*, 道鄉集) asked, "What is scholar fire? It is to keep and to exist. Do not extinguish and do not assist."[16] In Scholar Fire cultivation, it seems the breathing is there but not there. It is like cooking with a very small fire to simmer the food.

The Daoist book *The Record of Reaching the Mystic with Heavenly Nature of Wind and Moon* (*Xìngtiān Fēngyuè Tōngxuán Jì*, 性天風月通玄記) said, "Among the calmness, there is movement of the fire. This is the right time to refine the large returning (Dàhuán, 大還) (i.e., nourish the Shén with Qì). When Qì is picked up, it is the herb, and within the herb, there is fire. If asked for Martial Fire, raise up the wind strongly, if asked for Scholar Fire, Embryonic Breathing slow and soft."[17] When you meditate, your body is in an extremely calm state. You build up the fire at the Real Lower Dāntián, then lead it up to the brain to nourish the spirit. Martial fire is generated from quick, heavy breathing, while scholar fire is produced from slow, gentle Embryonic Breathing.

Since Embryonic Breathing is vital in storing Qì for spiritual cultivation, you should study this subject first, as described in the previous YMAA book, *Qìgōng Meditation—Embryonic Breathing*.

8-4. Regulating the Emotional Mind (Tiáoxīn, 調心)

The way you regulate your mind depends on your purpose. But no matter what the purpose is, the general rule is simple: When the mind is calm and peaceful, it can be centered at the Qì residence, leading Qì to stay there; when the mind is elsewhere, it leads Qì out to be manifested and consumed.

You regulate your mind according to your purpose. The first purpose for regulating the mind in Small Circulation is to store abundant Qì at the Real Lower Dāntián. Qì in the eight vessels is raised and the twelve primary Qì channels are regulated, so the whole body's vital energy is strong, healthy, and in high spirits. The second main purpose of practicing Small Circulation is to lead the Qì to circulate smoothly in the Conception and Governing Vessels. This strengthens the body and is crucial to the Muscle/Tendon Changing practice.

In Small Circulation meditation, first lead your mind from the Third Eye to the Mud Pill Palace. This calms down random thoughts and leads it into the state of emptiness. You are regulating your Emotional Mind to set it free from the bondage of the seven emotions and six desires described earlier. If you have difficulty regulating this Emotional Mind by paying attention to your third eye and leading it to the Mud Pill Palace, you may simply focus on your breathing.

The normal procedure of taming the Emotional Mind has three steps. "The eyes observe the nose, and the nose observes the Xīn (Emotional Mind)."[18] Focus your vision inside by closing your eyes, then pay attention to the breathing. The breathing gradually regulates the Xīn.

Make the inhalation long, soft, and slender, and allow the exhalation to happen slowly by itself. This calms down your mind and body. With clear inner feeling, you bring your mind to the Jiūwěi (Co-15, 鳩尾, Middle Dāntián) and continue regulating your mind, assisted by the breathing. To cool down the body's emotional and physical fire, you must first cool down the Middle Dāntián, which is the center of the Post-Heaven Fire Qì. Once you cool down this fire center, you can lead your physical and mental bodies to a very calm and peaceful state.

After this, shift your mind to the Real Lower Dāntián. This is Embryonic Breathing, which slowly leads Qì to its residence. The physical body will not be energized further, and it starts to cool down. Continue Embryonic Breathing for a while until you feel Qì has accumulated to a comfortable level. Then it is said you have grown the herb (Chǎnyào, 產藥), meaning you have built up a fire.

Producing the herb at the Real Lower Dāntián depends on the movement of the tricky gate, Huìyīn. Huìyīn can lead the Qì to the Real Lower Dāntián and store it there (Yīn), and can also lead it to the physical and mental bodies to manifest it (Yáng). Reverse Abdominal Breathing leads the Qì to store it at the Real Lower Dāntián. Then your mind can circulate it. This is Picking up the Herb (Cǎiyào, 采藥).

Set yourself free from lingering emotional bondage, which confuses the present and sows doubt about the future. This is caused by lack of understanding of the meaning of life. Recognize yourself, be aware of yourself and your environment, and let your mind awaken to comprehend occurrences. Then you can set yourself free from bondage. Confucius (Kǒngzǐ, 孔子) said, "Once the knowing (self-recognition) has stopped, then there is steadiness. After steadiness, then it can be calm. When it is calm, then it can be peaceful. When it is peaceful, then you can think. Once you can think, then you will gain."[19] This is the process of building up self confidence in life or in any study. Without it, your mind will wander and be confused, and your Emotional Mind will not be governed by the Wisdom Mind.

The final goal is called the righteous mind (Zhèngniàn, 正念), the mind of no mind (Wúniàn, 無念), or the real mind (Zhēnniàn, 真念). The mind is completely separated from emotional thoughts. It is said in The Complete Book of Principal Contents of Lífe and Human Nature (Xìngmìng Guīzhǐ Quánshū, 性命圭旨全書), "If one desires to cease the initiation of the Xīn (Emotional Mind), one must start from the thought of no thought."[20] To reach this stage, body and mind must be extremely calm and empty. *Dào Dé Jīng*, Chapter 16 said, "Reach the extreme emptiness, and keep the profound calmness."[21] When this stage is reached, the Yīn and Yáng in the body interact in harmony with each other, generating the Yáng essence of life. *The Complete Book of Principal Contents of Lífe and Human Nature* (*Xìngmìng Guīzhǐ Quánshū,* 性命圭旨全書) said, "(When) there is nothing in your mind, it is emptiness. When no more thought arises, it is calmness. Reaching emptiness to its extremity, keeping calmness to its profundity, Yīn and Yáng interact naturally. Then the Yáng essence is generated."[22]

In *Anthology of Daoist Village* (*Dàoxiāngjí*, 道鄉集), it is said, "When Xīn (desire) is generated, then observe its crux. When no Xīn (Wúxīn, 無心) is generated, then observe the marvelousness. These words describe the applications of the Dào. The saying that 'if desire is generated, then observe the crux,' is actually the application of the saying that 'if no desire is generated, then observe the marvelousness.' The saying that, 'if desire is generated, then observe the marvelousness (of the Dào),' is, in fact, the core of the saying that, 'if desire is generated, then observe the crux.' 'If there is desire, then observe its crux,' means having an intention of doing. It is the time when the spirit and Qì return to the body. 'There is no desire, and observe the marvelousness (of the Dào),' means there is no intention of acting. This is the state of no others, no self, no mountain, no river, grass, or trees, mixed and indistinguishable, no sense and no feeling."[23]

This paragraph discusses the two states of meditation, the state of desire and the state of no desire. In the state of desire, or intention, your Emotional Mind leads Qì to fulfill your desire and to nourish and raise your spirit. Then, you are paying attention to the methods (crux) of leading and cultivating. The other state is the state of no desire. This is the state of Wújí, of no extremity and no thought. When you reach a profoundly calm state, it is "the thought of no thought." In this state, you are part of nature and forget yourself and nature, both becoming indistinguishable. Your spirit blends and unites with the natural spirit. This is the state of Unification of Heaven and Man (Tiānrén Héyī, 天人合一), the end and the origin of life.

When you practice Small Circulation in the state of Embryonic Breathing, your mind is at the center. If you have a desire to store Qì at the Real Lower Dāntián or expand it to the Girdle Vessel (Dàimài, 帶脈), you have an intention. However, once you have reached a very deep level, the stage of "regulating of no regulating," then you have the "thought of no thought." You are in the extremely calm Wújí state, which allows you to be in harmony with nature.

However, when you are in the state of using the mind to lead Qì in the Conception and Governing Vessels, you have an intention. Once you reach the state of "regulating of no regulating," everything becomes natural and you enter "the thought of no thought."

8-5. Regulating the Qì (Tiáoqì, 調氣)

Regulating the Qì in Small Circulation practice can be divided into two parts. The first part is, through Embryonic Breathing, to build up abundant Qì and to store it in the Real Lower Dāntián. The second part is using the mind to lead the Qì to circulate smoothly in the Conception and Governing Vessels. Here we focus on methods of circulating the Qì in the Conception and Governing Vessels.

There are many paths of Small Circulation, but here we focus only on the path of circulating the Qì in the Fire Path. This is the safest and most important path, most favored by beginners and experienced practitioners alike. It follows the natural path of Qì circulation and strengthens the Qì circulation in the body. Most Small Circulation practitioners follow the Fire Path exclusively.

There are also many ways of circulating the Qì in the Fire Path. Buddhists accumulate Qì at the Lower Dāntián and lead it to circulate using Normal Abdominal Breathing. However, Daoists prefer using Reverse Abdominal Breathing. The Daoist method is more aggressive, since the mind is more actively involved in leading the Qì, so it is classified as a Yáng method compared with the Buddhist method, which is classified as Yīn. I only practiced the Buddhist method for three years, starting when I was 16 years old. After more than thirty years of practicing the Daoist method, I have more experience in that technique. Here, I will share with you what I have experienced of Daoist Small Circulation techniques.

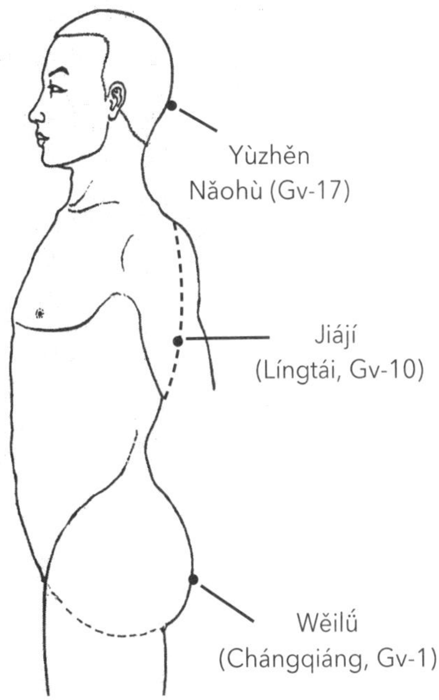

Figure 8-13. Three Gates (Sānguān): Yùzhěn, Jiájí, and Wěilǘ

The most important point in Small Circulation practice is that there are three dangerous gates (Sānguān, 三關) which, according to experience, could cause serious injury, especially for beginners. They are called 1). Chángqiáng (Gv-1, 長強) (medical society) or Wěilǘ (尾閭) (Tailbone, Daoist society), 2). Língtái (Gv-10, 靈台) (medical society) or Jiájí (夾脊) (Daoist society), and 3). Fēngfǔ (Gv-17, 風府) (medical society) or Yùzhěn (玉枕) (Jade Pillow, Daoist society) (Figure 8-13). How to lead the Qì past these three gates was kept secret in ancient practice. Next, I share what I believe are the safest and most natural ways to do so.

To start, you should keep the mind at the False Lower Dāntián and Start the Fire for at least five minutes. Not only is the fire built, but your mind also gradually moves from outside the body to internal feeling. If you inhale longer than exhale, you can easily calm down. However, if you know Embryonic Breathing, then you may use it instead, paying more attention to the inhalation.

After five to ten minutes of False Lower Dāntián Breathing or Embryonic Breathing, you should notice a distinct feeling of warmth in the area. You may also feel vibration if the False Lower Dāntián is used. Don't be alarmed, as all of these phenomena are very common.

Keep your tongue touching the center of your palate gently. This is called Dā Quèqiáo (Yínjiāo, Build the Magpie Bridge,) which allows you to connect the Conception (Yīn) and Governing (Yáng) Vessels in your mouth. Daoists call this place Shàng Quèqiáo (Yínjiāo, Upper Magpie Bridge), while the Huìyīn, which also connects the two vessels, is called Xià Quèqiáo (Lower Magpie Bridge, 下鵲橋).

To help beginners lead Qì past the first gate, Chángqiáng, I teach what I call Small Small Circulation (Xiǎo Xiǎozhōutiān, 小小周天). The key is to lead the Qì by keeping the mind ahead of it. When the mind is on the Qì, the Qì stagnates. The mind should not be on the Qì.[24] Place the mind one or two cavities ahead of the Qì, and then it can be led.

In Small Small Circulation, you inhale, keeping your mind at the Lower Dāntián, then exhale to lead the Qì to the Huìyīn. Inhale and lead the Qì upward from Huìyīn to Mìngmén (Gv-4, 命門), and then return to the Lower Dāntián or Real Lower Dāntián (Figure 8-14). Repeat the cycle.

When you practice, you should ignore the existence of the Chángqiáng cavity. The more you focus on this gate, the more the Qì stagnates there.

You may experience that your Qì moves faster than your mind. In this case, it is just like leading a cow with a rope, but instead the cow walks ahead of you. This means your mind is not leading the Qì, so practice until you can do it effectively. Slow down your breathing, and move your Huìyīn up and down slowly. Your mind needs to be calm, peaceful, and concentrated. You should practice for a few months until you are proficient in it.

Next, you circulate Qì in the regular path of Small Circulation. You lead it up the spine step by step, advancing a few cavities at a time. When you reach a certain point, you must turn and lead the Qì back to the Real Lower Dāntián. There are various turning points which you can use, which are normally kept secret in different styles. If you choose the correct point, the danger can be significantly reduced. Do not push to make it happen, but take your time, otherwise your ego and anxiety can obstruct and endanger you. Take it easy and enjoy the practice. The following turning points are considered the safest for practice:

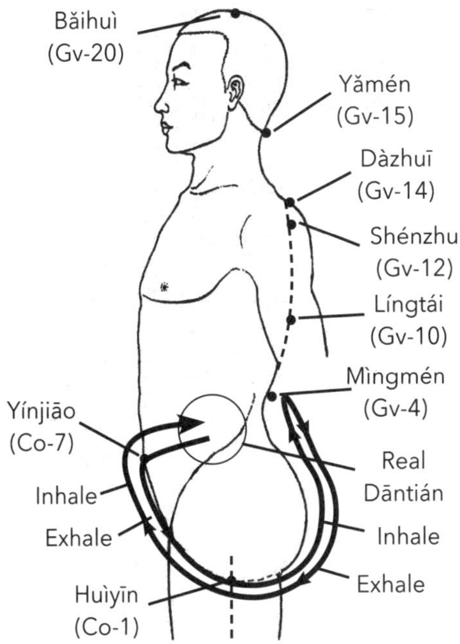

Figure 8-15. Real Dāntián-Yínjiāo-Huìyīn-Mìngmén-Huìyīn-Yínjiāo-Real Dāntián

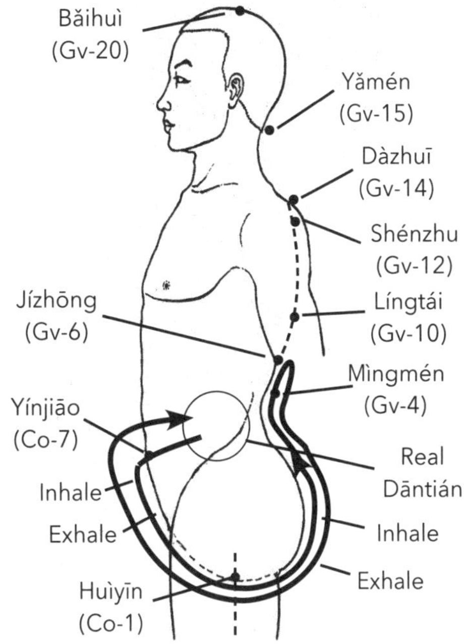

Figure 8-16. Real Dāntián-Yínjiāo-Huìyīn-Jízhōng-Huìyīn-Yínjiāo-Real Dāntián

1. **Mìngmén** (Gv-4, 命門). Use Mìngmén as the first turning point. Since Mìngmén connects to the Real Lower Dāntián, if there is any stagnation, Qì can easily return through this cavity.
   First exhale and lead the Qì to the Huìyīn, then inhale and lead it up to the Mìngmén. Exhale again to lead Qì back to the Huìyīn, and finally inhale and lead it back to the Real Lower Dāntián (Figure 8-15). There is a simple rule to coordinate your breathing with leading the Qì. Whenever you lead Qì out from the Dāntián, you exhale, and whenever you lead it back to the Dāntián, you inhale.
2. **Jízhōng** (Gv-6, 脊中). Once you can lead the Qì to the Mìngmén easily, you extend the path by leading it up to the Jízhōng, which means "spinal center." Use this cavity for a turning point because it is away from the vital cavity Língtái (Gv-10, 靈台), the second tricky gate. First exhale and lead Qì to the Huìyīn, then inhale and lead it up to the Jízhōng. Exhale and lead it down to the Huìyīn, and finally inhale and lead it back to the Dāntián (Figure 8-16).

3. **Shēnzhù** (Gv-12, 身柱) or Dàzhuī (Gv-14, 大椎). Again, after you have practiced for a while and feel comfortable leading the Qì to the Jízhōng, then can you proceed to lead it to the Shēnzhù or Dàzhuī cavity. These cavities are chosen because if the Qì is stagnant there after practice, it can easily be dispersed into the arms to prevent any problem. Between Jízhōng and these two cavities is the dangerous Língtái cavity. The method of dealing with this gate is to ignore it. The more you focus on it, the more Qì is led there and enters the heart. Ignore it and pay attention to the Shēnzhù or Dàzhuī cavities. First exhale and lead the Qì to the Huìyīn, then inhale and lead it up to Shēnzhù or Dàzhuī. Exhale and lead it back to Huìyīn, and finally inhale and lead it back to the Dāntián (Figure 8-17).
4. **Yǎmén** (Gv-15, 啞門). The next step is leading the Qì to the Yǎmén, or Mute Door, located at the rear center of the neck. One moves the neck all the time, so any Qì stagnation there can be removed easily before it causes harm. First exhale and lead the Qì to Huìyīn, then inhale and lead it up to the Yǎmén. Exhale and lead it down to Huìyīn, and finally inhale as you lead it back to the Dāntián (Figure 8-18).
5. **Bǎihuì** (Gv-20, 百會). Above Yǎmén is the Fēngfǔ (Gv-16, 風府) or Jade Pillow (Yùzhěn, 玉枕), the

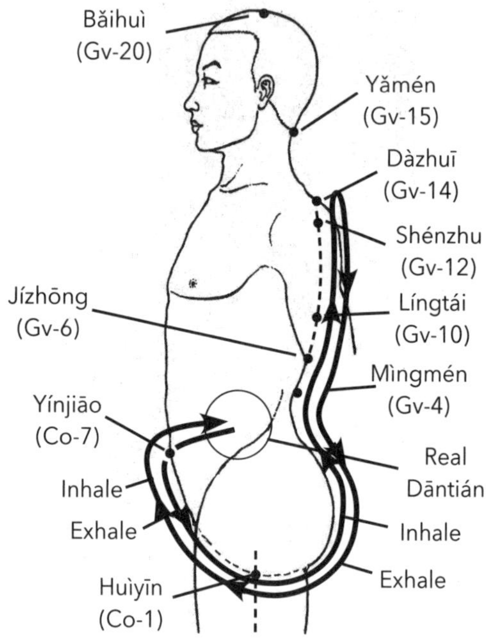

Figure 8-17. Real Dāntián-Yínjiāo-Huìyīn-Dàzhuī-Huìyīn-Yínjiāo-Real Dāntián

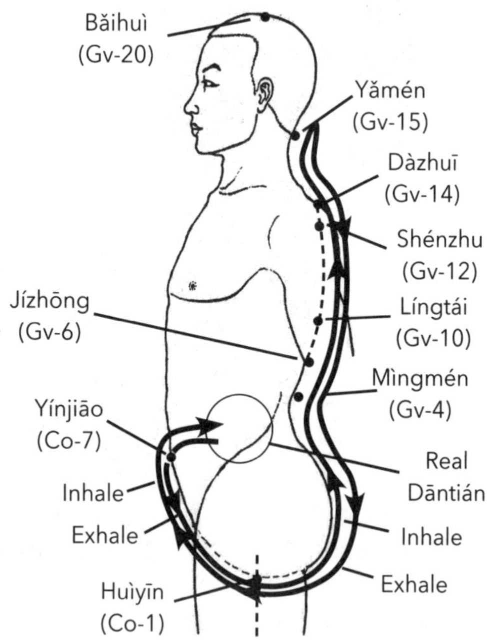

Figure 8-18. Real Dāntián-Yínjiāo-Huìyīn-Yǎmén-Huìyīn-Yínjiāo-Real Dāntián

third tricky gate, which you ignore. The more you pay attention to it, the more Qì stagnates there. Simply lead the Qì to Bǎihuì, the "hundred meetings" which is connected to the central energy line. When the spirit is raised up at this cavity, the whole body's Qì can be governed efficiently, and any stagnation easily led away. First exhale and lead the Qì to Huìyīn, then inhale as you lead it up to Bǎihuì. Exhale and lead it down to Huìyīn, and finally inhale and lead it back to the Dāntián (Figure 8-19).

6. **Palate** (Shàngè, 上顎). The palate of the mouth is the Qì junction of the Yīn (Conception) and Yáng (Governing) vessels. There you change your inhalation to exhalation and lead the Qì down the front of the body to Huìyīn to complete the cycle. You first exhale and lead Qì to Huìyīn, then inhale to lead it up past Bǎihuì and down to the palate of the mouth. Exhale and lead the Qì down the front of the body to Huìyīn (Figure 8-20). While leading it down past Yīnjiāo (Co-7, 陰交), you are also leading more Qì from the False or Real Dāntián to join the Qì flow to enhance its circulation.

Now you have completed the Small Circulation. You should continue circulating for twenty minutes or more, depending on your condition. How fast should the Qì be led by the mind? This depends on each individual's technique. Ancient documents described

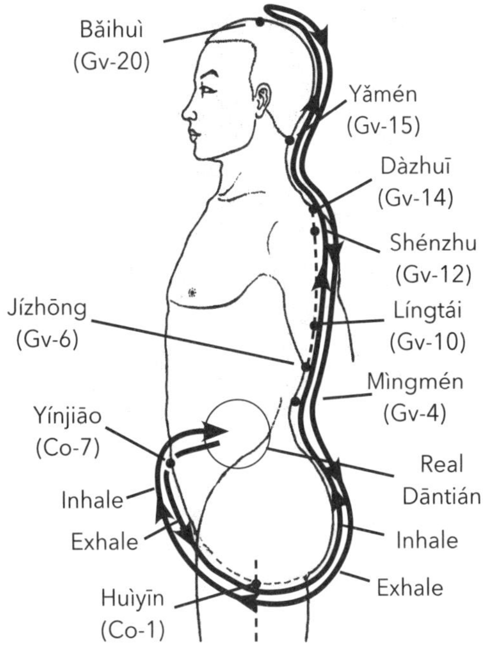

Figure 8-19. Real Dāntián-Yínjiāo-Huìyīn-Bǎihuì-Huìyīn-Yínjiāo-Real Dāntián

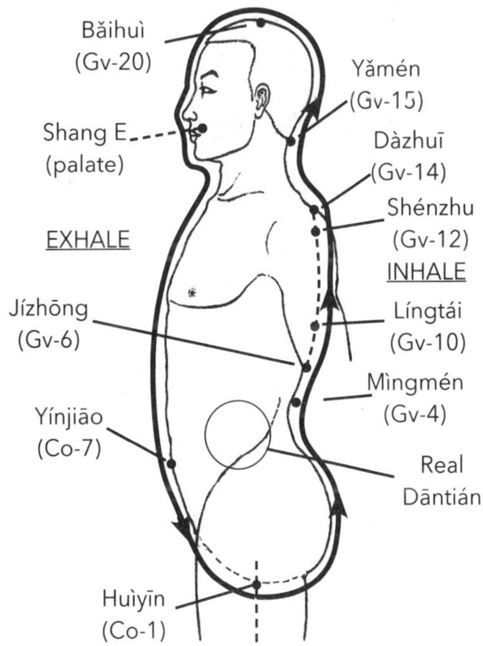

Figure 8-20. Small Circulation

three ways of leading the Qì in Small Circulation, called Héchē (River Vehicles, 河車). From Wěilǘ to Jiájí was classified as "Sheep Vehicle" (Yángchē, 羊車), and its Qì movement should be slow. From Jiájí to Yùzhěn was classified as "Deer Vehicle" (Lùchē, 鹿車), and the Qì movement should be fast. Finally, from Yùzhěn to Níwán is classified as "Bull Vehicle" (Niúchē, 牛車), and the Qì movement should be strong. These three ways of Qì's transportation are commonly called Sānchē (三車) which means "Three Vehicles."[25] This is only for your reference. The most important of all is your feeling.

If you enjoy it and feel comfortable, you may meditate for a couple of hours. However, if you feel uneasy even just for a short time, you should stop and try again later. You should not force yourself to sit long, if it causes you more tension and discomfort. I would like to remind you of a few important points:

1. When you lead Qì to a cavity, do not focus on its exact location. Simply pay attention to the area. This is different from acupuncture, in which the accuracy of the needling is very important. In meditation, if you pay too much attention to the exact location, your mind stagnates together with the Qì. Simply pay attention to the area, and the Qì will be led smoothly.
2. The Conception Vessel is Yīn, while the Governing Vessel is Yáng. They regulate the six Yīn and six Yáng primary channels independently. To prevent the Yīn vessel from becoming more Yīn, when you lead Qì in it, you exhale (Yáng) to balance the Yīn. Similarly, when you lead Qì in the Governing Vessel, you inhale (Yīn) to stop it becoming too Yáng. This balances the Qì status when you meditate. Huìyīn is used as the turning point when you change the breathing from exhalation to inhalation, and the palate is the turning point as you change it from inhalation to exhalation.
3. Often, to make the breathing more smooth and natural, a master teaches his student two-cycle breathing. If one-cycle breathing for Small Circulation is too urgent and uncomfortable, you may add another inhalation and exhalation. From my personal experience, the best place to add this extra breath is in front. That means when you exhale to lead the Qì down from the palate, instead of leading it to the Huìyīn directly, first exhale to Yīnjiāo (Co-7, 陰交), then inhale and lead the Qì into the Real Lower Dāntián. Finally, exhale again and lead the Qì to Huìyīn to complete the cycle (Figure 8-21).
4. Remember a simple rule. When you practice Small Circulation, do not hold your breath. Inhale and exhale smoothly and naturally. Whenever you hold your breath, you tense your body and mind, and this causes Qì stagnation.
5. If you cannot yet control the abdominal area, don't lead the Qì, as it means your mind is still regulating your abdominal breathing. If you lead the Qì regardless,

your stomach and abdominal area will be tense and uncomfortable. This hinders the meditation process. You should practice abdominal breathing for a while until it becomes very natural, smooth, and comfortable.

6. While meditating, pay attention to your back. It can become tense after meditating for a while. First regulate your body until it is regulated. Then regulate your breathing until it is regulated. Only then have you provided good conditions for your mind to lead the Qì. Take it easy and be natural. Whenever your body is tense, the Qì circulation becomes stagnant.

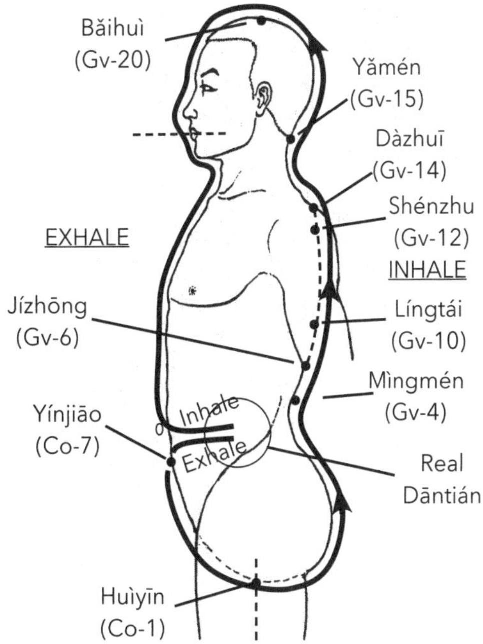

Figure 8-21. Small Circulation (Two Respirations)

8-6. Regulating the Spirit (Tiáoshén, 調神)

Regulating the Spirit is the final stage of Qìgōng regulating. In different schools, the purposes of spiritual regulating are also different. For example, within medical Qìgōng, Regulating the Spirit aims simply to raise the spirit of vitality for healing purposes. For martial arts Qìgōng, Regulating the Spirit raises one's awareness and fighting morale. In the scholar group, the spirit is regulated until it reaches extreme calmness and peace.

To reach this state of peace, scholar Qìgōng practitioners strive to be free from emotional bondage. *Dào Dé Jīng*, Chapter 1, said, "Always maintain the state of no desire, so can see its marvelousness."[26] Chapter 16 said, "Attain the insubstantial extremity, and maintain true calmness."[27] What is the "insubstantial extremity?" It is what is defined as spirit. *All Application Secrets of Real Holy Embryonic Spirit* (*Zhūzhēn Shèngtāi Shényòng Jué*, 諸真聖胎神用訣) said, "What is spirit? It is the application of insubstantiality and nothingness."[28] Spirit is invisible, empty and intangible. It is the master of being, residing in our physical form.

However, in religious society, regulating the spirit is intended to give birth to the Spiritual Embryo, to open the third eye for enlightenment or Buddhahood. Buddhists and Daoists also strive for emotional emptiness, or freedom from emotional bondage. The Buddhist classic *Sixth Ancestor's Lecturing Classic* (*Liùzǔ Tánjīng*, 六祖壇經) said, "Bodhi does not have a tree originally, nor is there a shining mirror in front. There are no objects there originally, so how can they be contaminated by dust or mud (objects or emotions)?"[29] "Bodhi" is a special Buddhist term which refers to the ultimate wisdom, developed from a high level of spiritual cultivation. "Tree" means all the physical objects around us and mirror reflects the emotional reactions to events. If there is neither object nor emotional disturbance in your mind, how can you be disturbed by the emotional dust or mud?

Spirit is called Yuánshén (Original Spirit, 元神). This spirit was born originally in physical form and resides in the brain. The book *A Detailed Outline of Basic Herbs (Běncǎo Gāngmù,* 本草綱目) clearly points out, "Brain is the residence of Original Spirit."[30] The brain is also called Upper Dāntián (Shàng Dāntián, 上丹田) by Daoists. The book *Observing Vessels* (*Màiwàng*, 脈望) said, "The brain is the Upper Dāntián, the palace where the Original Spirit resides. If one firms the Original Spirit and keeps it residing in its original residence, then the golden Qì is raised and the real breathing steady automatically. This is what is said, when one knack opens, a hundred knacks will open. When the big gate is passable, then hundred gates are passable."[31] The Original Spirit resides at the Mud Pill Palace, the center of the brain where the pineal and pituitary glands are situated. These two glands are shaped like small mud pills. The Daoist book *Further Study of Cān Tóng Qì* (*Cāntóngqì Fāhuī*, 參同契發揮) said, "Follow the real breathing's to and fro, allow the real Qì to ascend and descend freely. From morning till evening, the Original Spirit should always reside in Mud Pill."[32] Again, it is first very important to read and understand the book *Qìgōng Meditation—Embryonic Breathing*.

Original Spirit is also called Valley Spirit (Gǔshén, 谷神), because the space between the two hemispheres of the brain forms a valley which generates echo and resonance. This space is also called Spirit Valley (Shéngǔ, 神谷). *Dào Dé Jīng*, Chapter 6 said, "Valley spirit does not die, it is called Xuánpìn. The door of Xuánpìn is the root of heaven and earth. It is as though it were existing. When used, it will not be exhausted."[33] Daoists believe the spirit does not die with the physical body. The spirit finds a new body and enters it for reincarnation. Xuánpìn (玄牝) means the creation of life from the combination of the physical object and the invisible spiritual energy. From Xuánpìn, millions of lives are born. Therefore, Xuánpìn is the root of the physical world. If we know how to keep this spiritual force strong, it will last forever. Spirit is called Original Spirit or Valley Spirit, and its residence is the brain, Upper Dāntián, Spiritual Valley, or Mud Pill Palace.

To Buddhists and Daoists, the final goal of Regulating the Spirit is to open the third eye and allow the spirit to communicate with the external spiritual world. This is called the Unification of Heaven and Man (Tiānrén Héyī, 天人合一). The third eye is also called Heavenly Eye (Tiānmù, 天目), as explained in the Daoist book *The Illustration of Cultivating the Truth in Wǔdāng* (*Wǔdāng Xiūzhēn Tú,* 武當修真圖): "Under the Míngtáng, the upper mid-place of the line between the two eyebrows, there is a spiritual light emitted here; it is called heavenly eye."[34] Míngtáng (明堂) means the forehead.

The third eye is called Yìntáng (M-HN-3, 印堂) by medical society and Heavenly Yard (Tiāntíng, 天庭) by the general public.

The third eye is the door for the spirit to exit and enter the Spiritual Valley. The Daoist book *Seventh Bamboo Label of Bookcase* (*Yúnjí Qīqiān*, 云笈七籤) said, "The place between the two eyebrows is the (precious) jade door of Mud Pill."[35] The third eye is the door to the Mud Pill Palace, the residence of Original Spirit.

There is an ancient document which describes the cultivation of spirit in Small Circulation:

Anthology of Daoist Village
《道鄉集》 (Dàoxiāngjí)

Small Circulation should be practiced after the real seed enters the furnace, at the time the Yáng fire (Qì) just starts to produce. Follow the opportunity (timing) of this production and growing, use the spirit to lead, and use the breathing to blow (fan the flames). When the fire receives the leading of the spirit and the blowing of the breath, it ascends naturally. But you need not be confined by the diagrams for divination (in Bāguà) or restricted by the time. When there is an opportunity to ascend, then lead it up. When there is an opportunity for steadiness and calmness, then allow it to be steady and calm. It does not matter how, always lead when there is movement (of Qì), and stabilize when there is calmness. If there is no movement and you lead, it is useless. If there is no calmness and you stabilize, it is harmful. It does not matter whether it is movement or calmness, each must follow its opportunities. In this case, it is coordinating with the natural (Dào). Though using the spirit to lead, yet you should not observe (concentrate), and though using the breathing to blow, it should not be stagnant. When Qì starts to move and ascend, the Original Spirit condenses in Xuánguān (tricky gate, Real Lower Dāntián). Then use some spirit (mind) to lead the ascending Yáng fire, and use the breathing to enhance it. It is not because the breathing can (make Qì) ascend by following the Yáng fire. It is just using the function of inhalation (to lead Qì to ascend). When exhaling, then follow the natural way. Though the function of the exhaling breath is downward, however, when the Yáng fire receives the pressure of the real breathing, it will turn and ascend. It is only when using spirit and breathing. I follow its (Qì's) ascending and descending. Therefore, the Yáng fire begins from Xuánqiào (Huìyīn) and ends at Xuánqiào to complete a cycle. This is called the heavenly cycle.

小周天，行于真種入爐之後，陽火發生之時，順其生發之機，以神而引，以息而吹，火受神息引吹，自然上升。但不必論其爻象，限其時刻，有上行之機，則引上行，有定靜之機，則聽其定靜。總是動而后引，靜而后定。不動，引之無益；不靜，定之有損。無論動靜，均須順其機而為之，方合乎自然也。雖有神引，亦不可看，雖以息吹，亦不可滯，當升機發動之時，元神仍凝玄關，稍分其神，以引上升之陽火，息之吹逼，非息能隨陽火上升也。不過稍作用于吸機，呼則順其自然，息機雖向下，而陽火受真息壓迫，反轉而上升也，用神用息，不過如是，余則聽其自升自降而已。因此，陽火發于玄竅，止于玄竅，經過一周，故曰周天。

In Small Circulation practice, first you build up the Qì (Fire) through Abdominal Breathing. You focus your mind and spirit at the False Lower Dāntián to initiate the seed fire. Through Abdominal Breathing for some time, abundant Qì accumulates. The abdomen first feels warm and later starts to vibrate by itself. This state is called Chǎnyào (產藥). Next, you lead this Qì to circulate in the vessels. This stage is called Cǎiyào (采藥), or Picking up the Herb. "Herb" here means Qì or elixir. When you reach this stage, the Qì will have an intention to move. Use your mind and spirit to lead Qì to the Huìyīn, and then up the Governing Vessel to reach the Upper Dāntián. When your mind leads the Qì, you should coordinate it with the breathing. Breathing is regarded as the strategy of Qìgōng practice, which significantly enhances the leading of the Qì.

When you use your mind to lead the Qì, you should not concentrate but simply pay attention and lead it gently. When your breathing enhances Qì circulation, it should be smooth and natural, otherwise it becomes stagnant. Though you are using your mind to lead the Qì, do not forget that mind and spirit should always be kept in the Real Lower Dāntián. It is the same as travelling away from home; your mind should always be concerned for your family at home.

Xuánguān (玄關) means Lower Dāntián, and Xuánqiào (玄竅) means Upper Dāntián. Though you are inhaling, you are leading the Qì upward, and after passing the Upper Dāntián, you allow Qì to flow down the Conception Vessel in coordination with the natural exhaling. Finally, complete the Small Circulation circuit.

When you reach a profound meditative state, you are as though asleep and as though awake. It seems you are sleeping, but your conscious mind is still aware in a drowsy state, and the Qì in the brain is strong. The Daoist document *A Comparative Study of the Zhōu's Yì* (*Zhōuyì Cāntóng Qì*, 周易參同契) said, "When a truthful person reaches the stage of marvelousness, it seems to be there and seems not to be there. It is like a great deep gulf, suddenly sinks and suddenly floats. When it retreats, it spreads and maintains its position."[36]

When you reach this stage after long practice, you open your third eye and reach enlightenment. We will discuss this more in the next book, *Qìgōng Grand Circulation for Spiritual Enlightenment*.

8-7. Regulating the Essence (Tiáojīng, 調精)

In Qìgōng and medical society, Jīng (精, Essence), Qì (氣), and Shén (神, spirit) are three precious treasures of life. If you preserve Original Essence (Yuánjīng, 元精), inherited from your parents and absorb Post-Birth Essence (air and food) correctly, you have a firm foundation to generate abundant Qì. When this Qì nourishes the brain, the spirit is raised to a high level, and you will have a long, healthy life. This process is necessary to attain Buddhahood or enlightenment.

What is the Original Essence? It is the foundation of one's life (Shēngmìng Zhīběn, 生命之本). It is formed from the Original Qì of nature. Through the mother's body, a new life is born, and the Original Essence is carried with it. The document *Discussing Extraordinary Balance* (*Lùnhéng. Chāoqí*, 論衡·超奇) said, "Heaven has the natural endowment of Original Qì; when man absorbs it, it becomes Original Essence."[37] Comparative Study of Ancient Documents (Gǔwén Cāntóng Qì, 古文参同契) said, "The Original Qì that is abundant and refined is called Original Essence."[38]

Original Essence also means the hormones or sperm stored in a man's testicles. When a man abuses his sexuality, he loses too much Original Essence. This weakens the function of his kidneys because the Original Essence is stored there. The kidneys with adrenal glands are called Internal Kidneys, while testicles are called External Kidneys. These internal and external kidneys are connected and closely related. When the Qì level in one is weakened, the other is affected as well. For this reason, techniques to preserve and control the ejaculation of sperm are a major task in Qìgōng training. *The Complete Book of Principal Contents of Life and Human Nature* (*Xìngmìng Guīzhǐ Quánshū*, 性命圭旨全書) said, "Those who refine the essence, it is to refine the Original Essence. It is to draw the original Yáng from Kǎn. When the Original Essence is firmed, then sperm is not released during intercourse."[39] The groin area is considered Yīn, as water, and called Kǎn (Water). The penis is considered Yáng within Yīn in the groin area.

One method of firming this essence right after meditation, has been recorded and passed down to us:

Original Explanation of Not Using Herbs (Secrets of Golden Elixir) (Wāng, Áng, Qīng Dynasty)

《勿藥元詮・清・汪昂輯》(Wùyào Yuánquán)

金丹秘訣

One rubs and one holds, left and right change hands. The achievement of Nine-Nine (eight-one times), the real Yáng will not be released. Shù (7 to 9 pm) and Hài (9 to 11 pm) two periods, the Yīn strengthens, while the Yáng weakens, one hand holds up the External Kidneys, one hand rubs under the navel. Left and right change hands, eighty-one times each. Half month, the sperm is firmed. The longer the better.

一擦一兜，左右換手，九九之功，真陽不走。戌、亥二時，陰盛陽衰之候，一手兜外腎，一手擦臍下，左右換手，各八十一，半月精固，久而彌佳。

Use one hand to hold the testicles. Hold up your Huìyīn throughout the process. Inhale and exhale normally with deep relaxation. Then use the other hand to rub the area between navel and groin with a circular motion. Circle for eighty-one times and then change hands and repeat in the other direction. This firms the essence and increases hormone production.

Qìgōng emphasizes techniques of increasing hormone production in the adrenal glands, sex glands, and pituitary and pineal glands. When the production of Original Essence (hormone) is strong and healthy, the life force Qì is strong and the spirit is high. For ways to increase hormone production in the adrenal glands, please refer to the YMAA book, *The Root of Chinese Qìgōng*. We will describe methods of producing growth hormone and melatonin in the book *Qìgōng Grand Circulation for Spiritual Enlightenment*.

8-8. Recovery from the Meditative State (Jìngzuòhòu Zhī Huīfù, 靜坐後之恢復)

Correctly recovering from meditation is most important. If you don't do it correctly, you may experience headache (mental imbalance) or some physical tightness, especially in the spine. Correct recovery methods remove Qì stagnation caused by meditation.

The methods of recovering from meditation are both mental and physical. The trick is to reverse the normal regulating process of meditation. First regulate your mind, then your breathing, and finally your body. Here I introduce the general methods of recovery that have been passed down, or gained through my personal experience.

Regulate the Mind, Qì, and Breathing. The first step in recovery from meditation is keeping your mind calm. Slowly awaken from your semi-hypnotic state. It seems that you have just woken up from a deep sleep, yet your conscious mind is still in control.

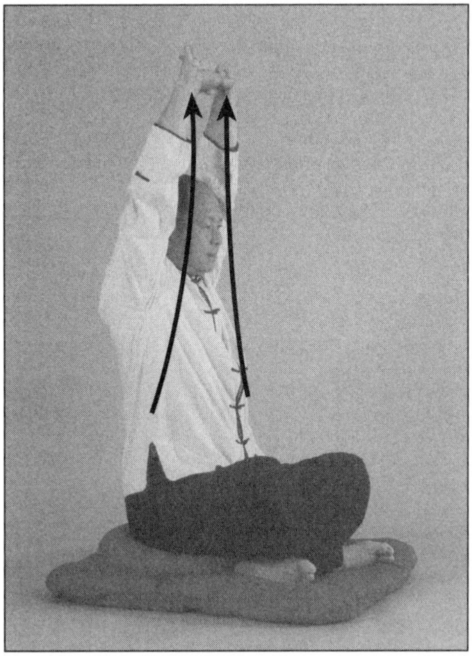
Figure 8-22

Bring your mind to the Real Lower Dāntián. This is very important. Your mind leads your Qì back there, removing it from the path of Small Circulation, where it could otherwise stagnate. Real Lower Dāntián is the residence of Qì, so the first step is to return the Qì there to prevent disturbance. This is the same as the treatment in case of shock, if suddenly awakened from deep meditation.

Keep your mind in the Real Dāntián, and resume Embryonic Breathing for a couple of minutes until you feel that the Qì has returned. After Embryonic Breathing, you may practice a few minutes of Skin Breathing, if you know it well. Try to exhale longer than you inhale. This leads the Qì to the skin surface and rouses the body from the sleeping state.

Then move your mind to the Upper Dāntián, and relocate your spiritual center. Sit there for a couple of minutes. When you do this mentally, you wake yourself up completely and comfortably.

Remember, when mentally recovering from your meditative state, you should not resist or speed up the process. You should take it easy. Be natural and comfortable. From this, you obtain great satisfaction, peace, and harmony.

Regulate the Body. After bringing your mind back to the concrete world, you should then regulate your body and arouse it from sleep. Through correct movement, you disperse stagnant Qì that may be caused by long sitting or improper posture. Next, some effective movements and stretches are recommended.

Upward Torso Stretching. First stretch your torso. Interlock your hands and push upwards (Figure 8-22). This stretch loosens any tightness of the torso or spine caused by long sitting. After your hands have reached the highest position, stay there, inhale deeply and then exhale. Inhale again and lower your arms. Repeat twice.

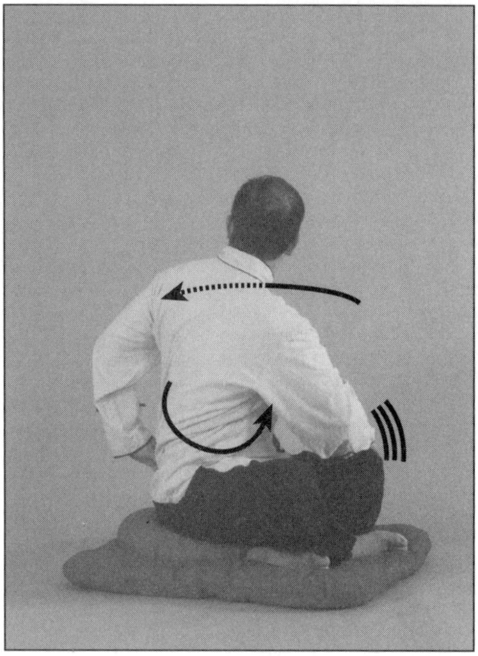

Figure 8-23

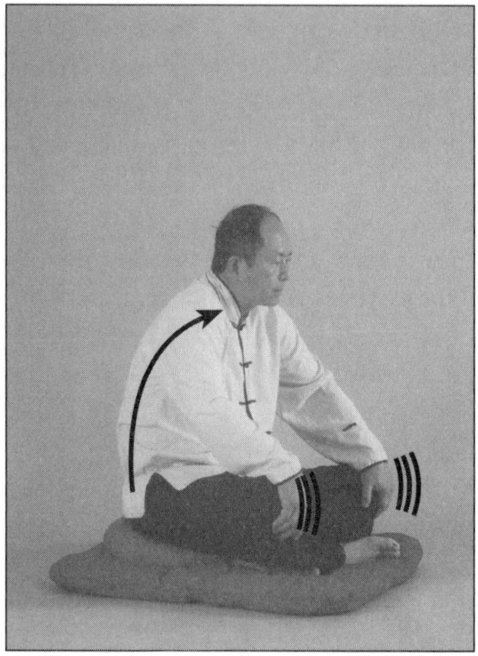

Figure 8-24

Sideways Torso Twist. After the upward stretch, twist your torso sideways. Turn your body to the left first, and use your right hand to pull your left thigh while pushing your left shoulder backwards (Figure 8-23). Stay in this position, inhale and then exhale. Next, repeat on the other side.

Spine Waving. Next, loosen your vertebrae, section by section, from the sacrum up to the neck. Place your hands on your knees, and pull them to generate a waving spine motion (Figure 8-24). When you begin to pull, the lower torso is thrust forward, and you inhale deeply. When the waving motion reaches the upper spine, you exhale. Move comfortably and naturally, with the spine movement of a sigh. When you are depressed or feel great emotion stuck in your body, you generally inhale deeply, with the "Hēng" sound, and generate a waving motion from the lower back. When the motion reaches the upper torso, you exhale. This is the most natural torso movement and it allows you to relax the torso and release any trapped emotional energy.

Loosening the Shoulders. Next, loosen the upper spine, and remove any stagnant Qì there. Slowly move your shoulders clockwise in a big circle at least six times (Figure 8-25). When they circle forward, inhale deeply, and when they circle backward, exhale deeply. After you complete the clockwise circling, reverse the direction and repeat for the same number of times. However, this time you should inhale deeply when you circle backward and exhale when you circle forward. To lead stagnant Qì down and loosen up the torso,

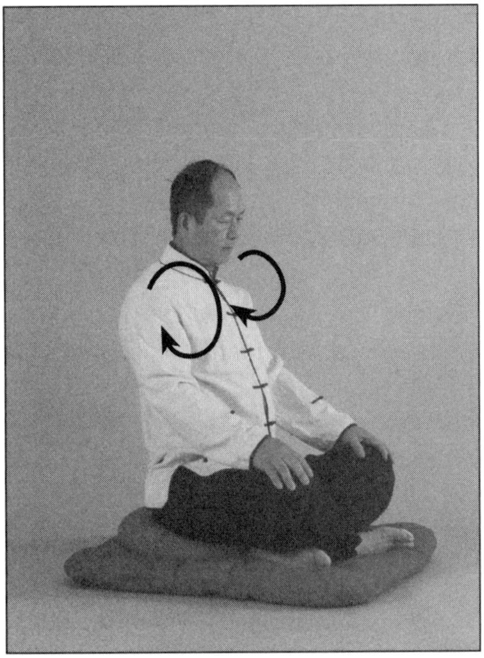

Figure 8-25

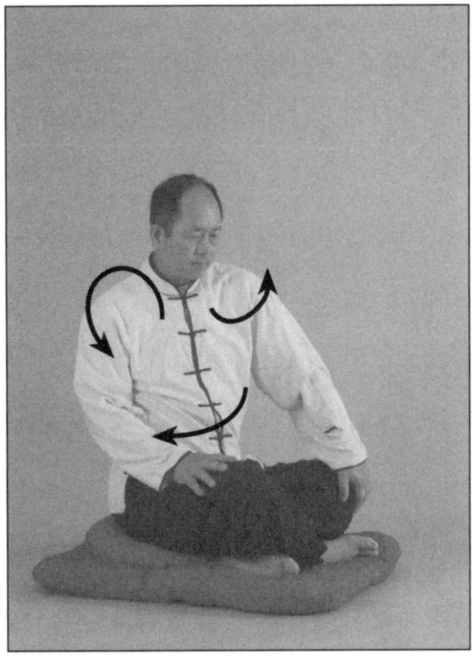

Figure 8-26

you may circle one shoulder forward and the other one backward (Figure 8-26). Repeat six times, then reverse direction. In this case, you may coordinate your breathing any way you choose.

Turning the Head. To loosen the neck, slowly turn your head to the sides (Figure 8-27). Exhale deeply, and inhale when it turns forward. Turn to each side at least six times.

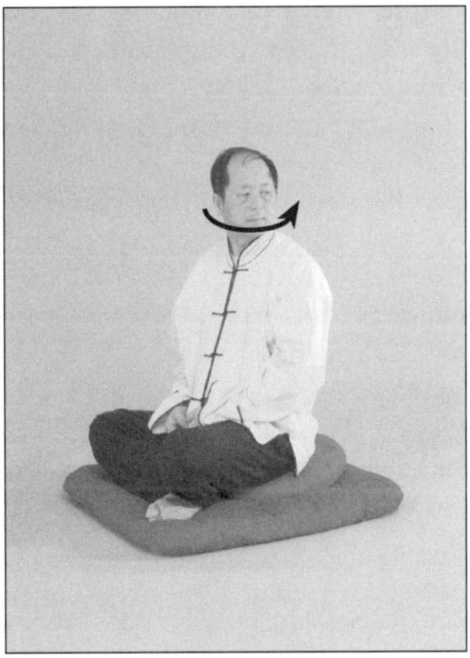

Figure 8-27

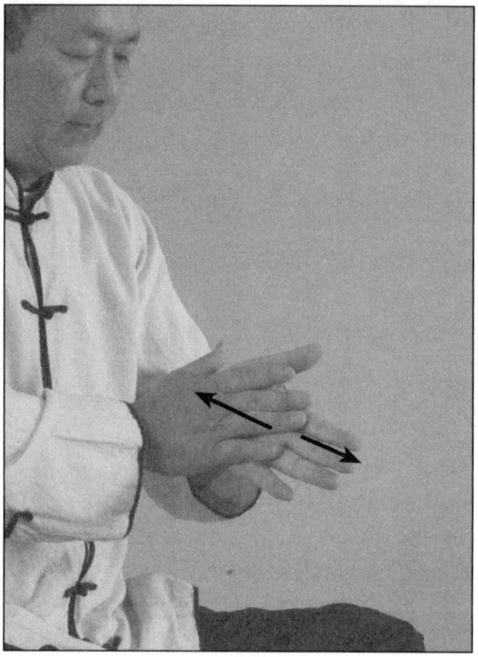

Figure 8-28

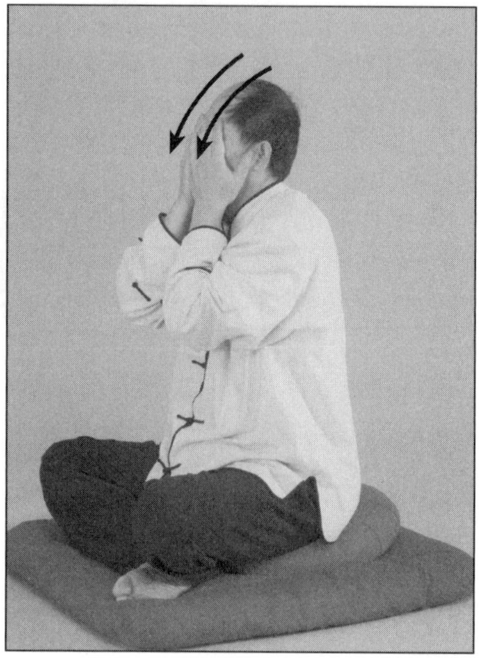

Figure 8-29

Massage the Head. After loosening the neck, rub your hands until they are warm (Figure 8-28). Then brush the face downwards twenty-four times, using the palms (Figure 8-29). This massage is called Washing the Face (Xǐliǎn, 洗臉). It rejuvenates the skin with enhanced Qì and blood circulation.

Immediately after Washing the Face, use the palms to brush the hair from the forehead backward to the neck twenty-four times (Figure 8-30). This is called Combing the Hair (Shūtóu, 梳頭). It keeps your hair healthy and looking young.

Next, rub your hands until they are warm again and use the base of your thumbs to cover your eyes (Figure 8-31). This is called Ironing the Eyes (Tàngyǎn, 燙眼), which nourishes degenerating eyes. Also massage your eyes with a circular motion to improve the Qì circulation.

Next, use your thumb and index fingers to massage the ears for a few minutes (Figure 8-32). Different parts of the ears are related to different organs (Figure 8-33). Massaging them keeps the internal organs healthy. Then cover your ears with the

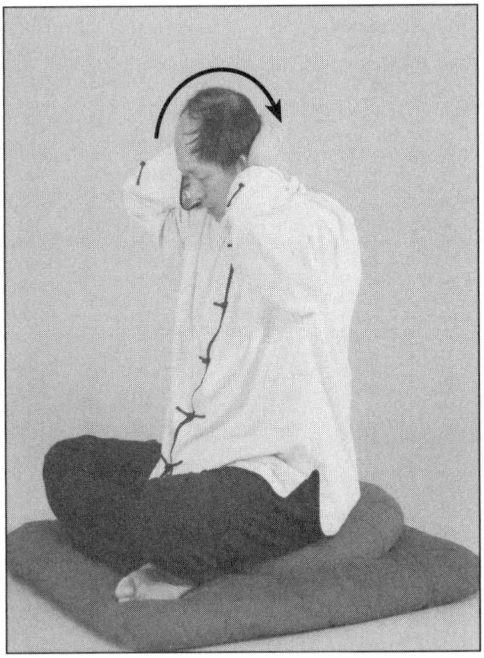

Figure 8-30

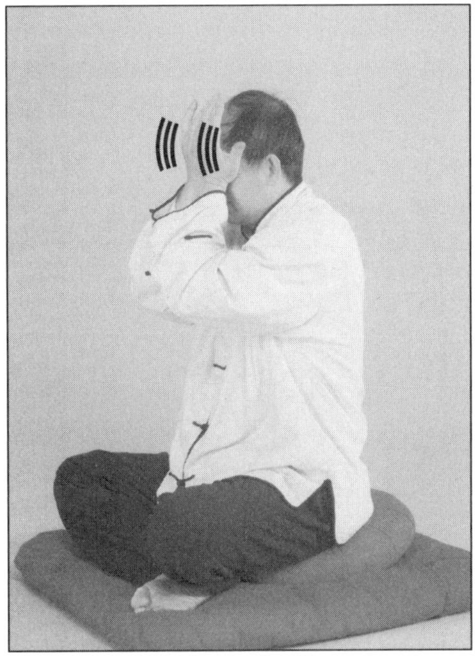

Figure 8-31

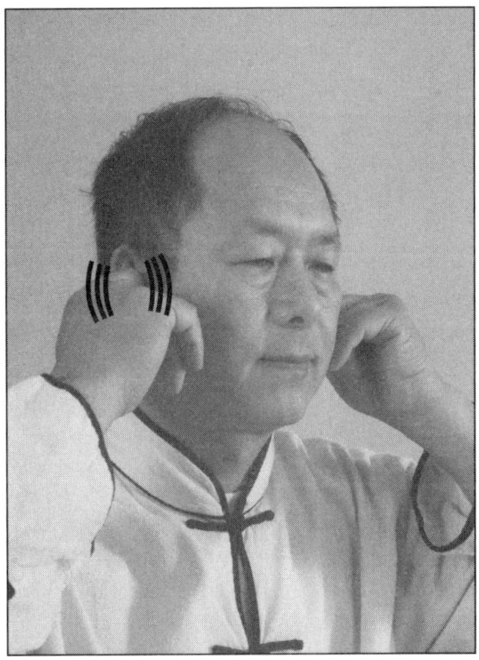

Figure 8-32

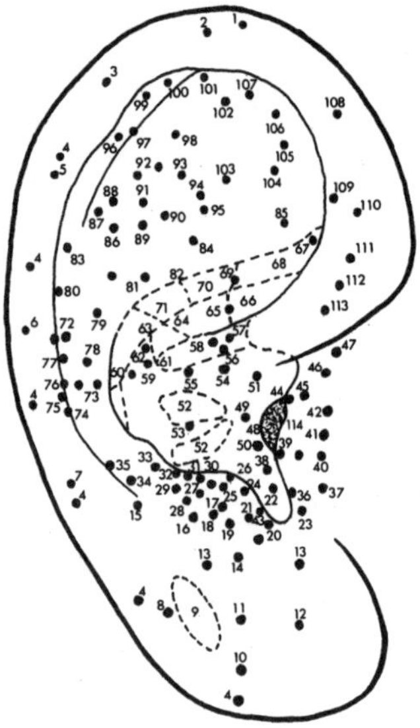

1. Pt. Ear Apex
2. Pt. Tonsilla
3. Pt. Ganyang
4. Helix
5. Pt. Ganyang
6. Pt. Tonsilla
7. Pt. Tonsilla
8. Pt. Auris Interna
9. Pt. Facies and Bucca
10. Pt. Tonsilla
11. Pt. Oculus
12. Anesthetic points for tooth extraction
13. Pt. upper and lower Mandible
14. Pt. Lingua
15. Pt. Nephritis
16. Pt. Vertex
17. Pt. Taiyang
18. Pt. Hypophysis
19. Pt. Emphysema
20. Pt. Oculus (Astigmatism)
21. Pt. Frons
22. Pt. Hormone
23. Pt. Oculus (Glaucoma)
24. Pt. Subcortex
25. Pt. Pingchuan
26. Pt. Testis
27. Pt. Excitation
28. Pt. Nervus
29. Pt. Occiput
30. Pt. Encephalon
31. Pt. Vertigo
32. Pt. Brain Stem
33. Pt. Collum
34. Pt. Glandula Thyroidea
35. Pt. Clavicula
36. Pt. Endocrine
37. Pt. Hypertension
38. Pt. Bronchiectasis
39. Pt. Glandula Suprarenalis
40. Pt. Hunger
42. Pt. Thirsty
43. Pt. Ovarium
44. Pt. Tragic Apex
45. Pt. Pharyngo Larynx
46. Pt. Cor (Xinzang)
47. Pt. Auris Externa
48. Pt. Sanjiao
49. Pt. Bronchus
50. Pt. Glandula Parotis
51. Pt. Cardia
52. Pt. Pulmo
53. Pt. Cor
54. Pt. Ventriculum
55. Pt. Ptosis
56. Pt. Fulcram
57. Pt. Diaphragm
58. Pt. Mid-crus Helicis
59. Pt. Jisong
60. Pt. Lien
61. Pt. Uterine Appendages
62. Pt. Lowering Blood Pressure
63. Pt. Duodenum
64. Pt. Intestinum tenue
65. Pt. Appendix Vermiformis
66. Pt. Intestinum Crassum
67. Prostata
68. Pt. Vesica Urinaria
69. Pt. Ureter
70. Pt. Ren
71. Pt. Pancreas and Gall Bladder
72. Pt Shoulder
73. Pt. Glandula Mammaria
74. Pt. Art. Humeri
75. Pt. Thorax Externa
76. Pt. Shoulder Ache
77. Pt. Subaxilla
78. Pt. Thorax
79. Pt. Abdomen
80. Pt. Appendix Vermiformis
81. Pt. Lumbago
82. Pt. Appendix Vermiformis
83. Pt. Cubitus
84. Pt. Nates
85. Pt. N. Ischiadicus
86. Abdomen
87. Pt. Lower Abdomen
88. Pt. Genu
89. Pt. Fever
90. Pt. Cavum Pelvis
91. Pt. Popliteal Fossa
92. Pt. Sura (Calf)
93. Pt. Shenmen
94. Pt. Hepatitus
95. Pt. Guguan
96. Pt. Carpus
97. Pt. Allergy
98. Pt. Art. Coxae
99. Pt. Digitas Manus
100. Pt. Appendix Vermiformis
101. Pt. Digitum Pedis
102. Pt. Malleolus
103. Pt. Asthma
104. Pt. Os
105. Pt. Uterus
106. Pt. Esophagus
107. Pt. Calx
108. Pt. Hemorrhoid
109. Pt. N. Sympathetica
110. Pt. Organa Genitalia Externa
111. Pt. Urethra
112. Pt. Anus
113. Pt. Lower Rectum
114. Pt. Nasus Internus

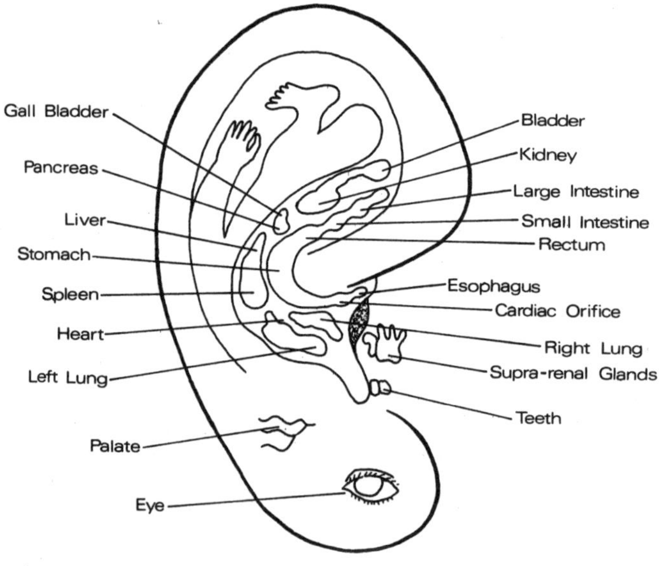

Figure 8-33. Acupuncture Points in the Ear

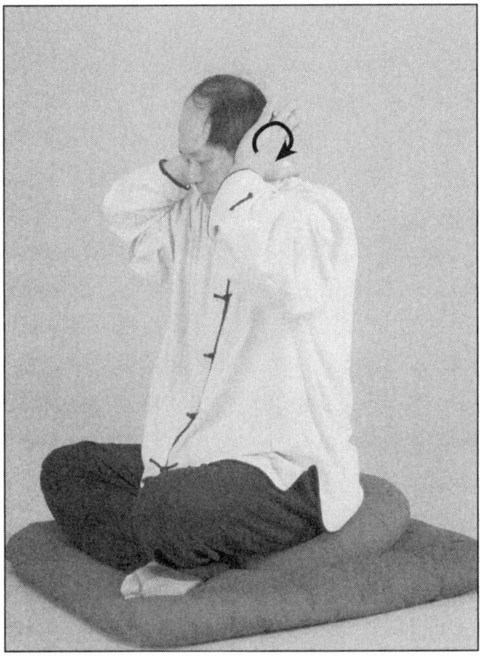

Figure 8-34

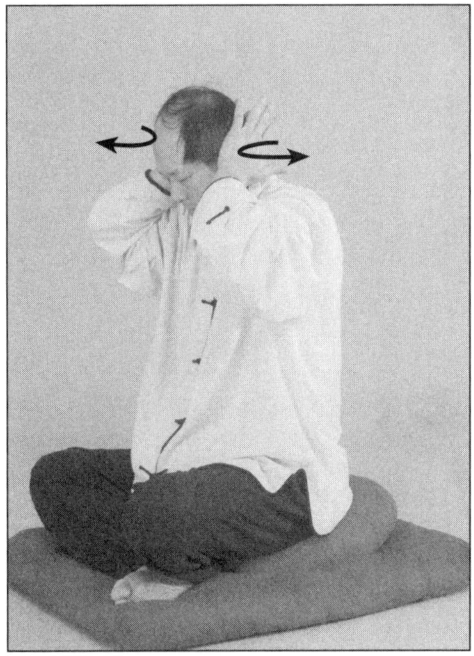

Figure 8-35

palms and circle ten times on each side (Figure 8-34). This improves the circulation of Qì and blood in the deeper parts of the ears. Finally, press the ears and pop them several times (Figure 8-35). This stimulates the eardrums and improves their circulation. All these are simple ways of maintaining the ears in a healthy condition.

Next, use your index finger and thumb to rub and press down along the sides of the nose and then sideways (Figure 8-36). This releases pressure built up in the frontal sinus.

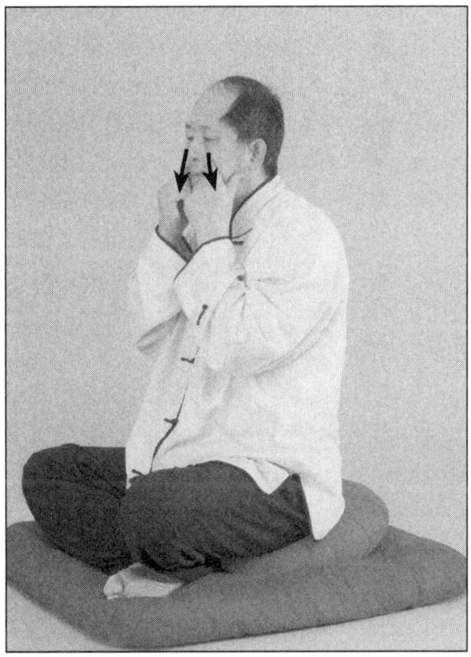

Figure 8-36

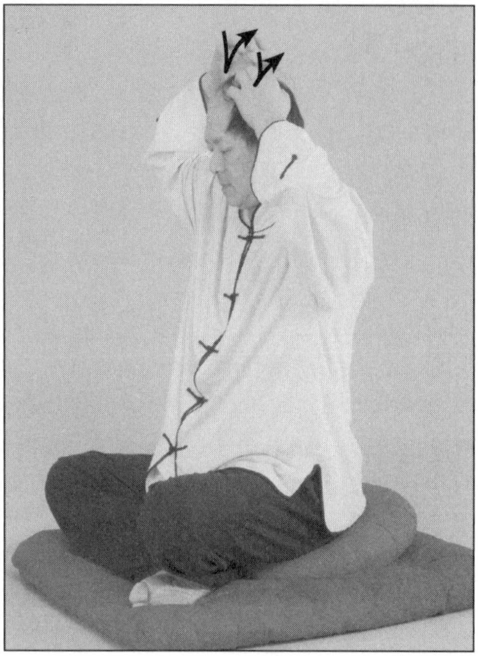

Figure 8-37

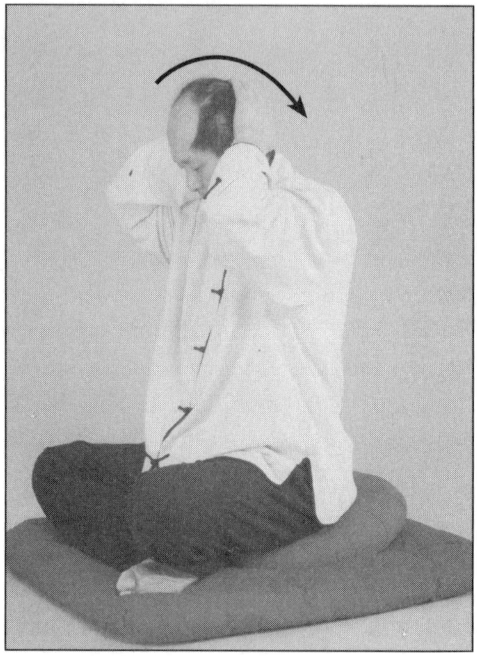

Figure 8-38

Finally, use the fingertips to tap your head from front to back and from the center to the sides for a few minutes (Figure 8-37) This tapping action leads the Qì accumulated inside the head to the skin surface. After tapping, use both hands to brush your head lightly from the front backward (Figure 8-38).

Massage the Three Yīn Channels on the Legs—Spleen, LívER, and Kidneys. After sitting for a long time, Qì and blood may be stagnant in the hip and knee areas. To remedy this, straighten your legs and bend forward to stretch them out (Figure 8-39). Massage them from the thighs to the bottom of the feet, especially the insides of the legs where the three Yīn channels are located. After massaging for a couple of minutes, use your thumb to press the Sānyīnjiāo cavity (Sp-6, 三陰交) (Figures 8-40 and 8-41). Sānyīnjiāo means Three Yīn Junction, and is the junction of the three Yīn channels: spleen, liver, and kidneys. Press in for five seconds, then release. Repeat three times. This leads Qì down from the hips.

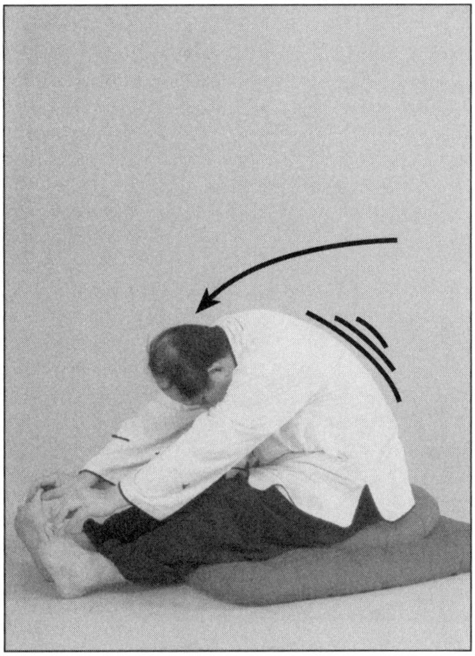

Figure 8-39

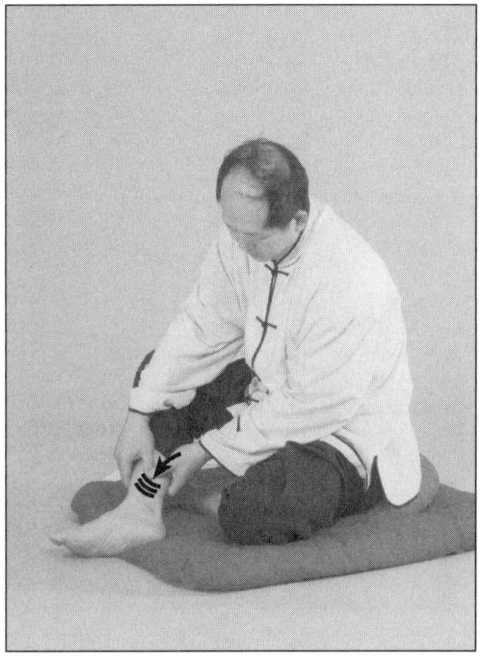

Figure 8-40

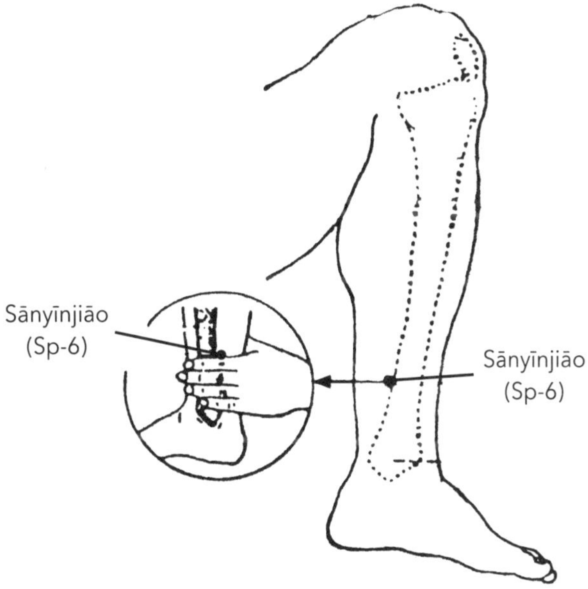

Figure 8-41. The Sānyīnjiāo (Sp-6) Cavity

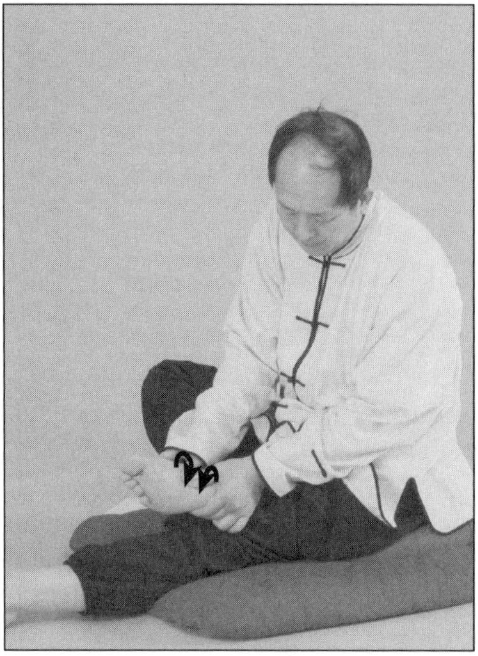

Figure 8-42

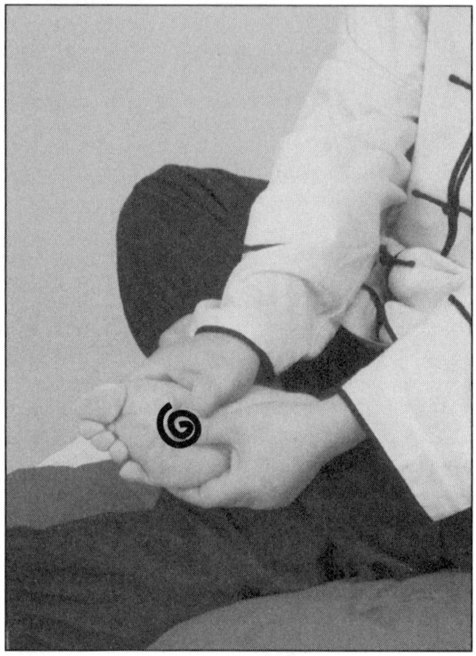

Figure 8-43

Next, massage the soles of the feet where the two Yīn vessels, Yīn Heel and Yīn Línking Vessels (Yīnwjuēmài, Yīnwéimài; 陰蹻脈・陰維脈), end (Figure 8-42). Finally, massage the Yǒngquán cavity (K-1, 湧泉) for a few minutes (Figure 8-43).

Chanting. Often right after meditation, a meditator makes specific chanting sounds. This leads the Qì down to the Lower Dāntián. These chanting sounds are commonly used for healing purposes as well. Three of the most common ones used are Ǎn (唵), Ā (阿), and Hōng (吽). The use of these three sounds has been recorded in a Buddhist classic, which I would like to translate for your reference.

Classic of Positioning the Image into the Extreme Calmness[40]

《安象三昧儀經》(Ānxiàng Sānmèiyí Jīng)

After chanting these real words (Buddhist classic), imagine the perfectness of the Buddha's image. Then use Ǎn, Ā, Hōng, three words, and place them on the image. Place the word Ǎn on the crown, place the word Ā on the mouth, and place the word Hōng in the heart.

誦此真言已，復想如來如真實身諸相圓滿，然以唵阿吽三字，安在像身三處，用唵字安頂上，用阿字安口上，用吽字安心上。

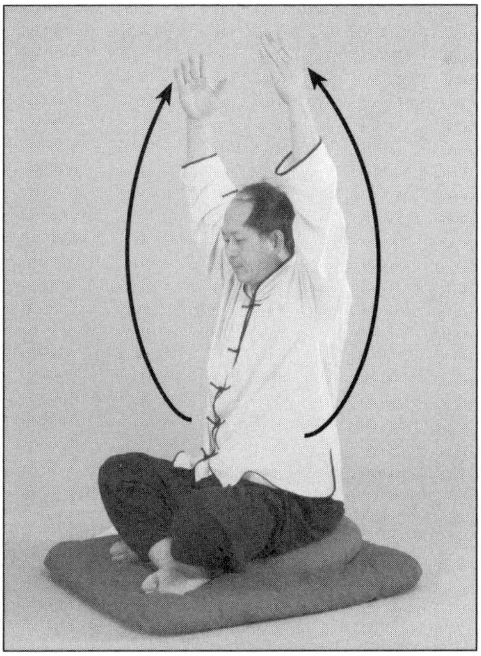

Figure 8-44

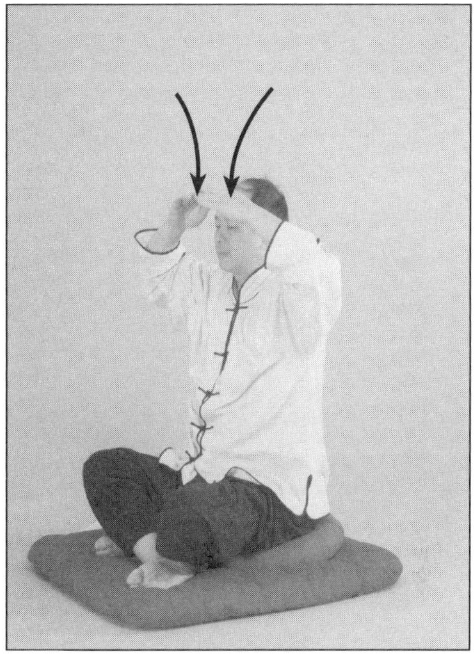

Figure 8-45

It is common for a Buddhist to imagine a likeness of Buddha in his mind and then perform some chanting or meditation. This brings him to a profound level of peace and calmness. The three words, Ăn, Ā, and Hōng, are also commonly used right after chanting of the Buddhist scriptures or deep meditation.

Many meditators use the "fourth word" to lead Qì down to the Lower Dāntián. The fourth word does not have sound, and the word itself does not exist. It only exists in the mind right after chanting the third word, as you lead the Qì downward to return to its residence at the Lower Dāntián. That means returning your being to the Wújí state.

First, inhale deeply while raising up your arms from the sides of your body, with the palms facing upward (Figure 8-44). When both hands reach their highest point, start to exhale, lowering the hands with the palms facing downward, while making the sound of Ăn (唵) (Figure 8-45). You feel a strong vibration at the back of your brain when the sound of Ăn is made. Continue to exhale, lowering your hands until they reach the level of the mouth, then change the sound into Ā (阿), and continue to lower them (Figure 8-46). When the Ā sound is made, the throat vibrates strongly. Continue exhaling as you lower your hands until they reach the sternum, then change the sound to Hōng (吽) (Figure

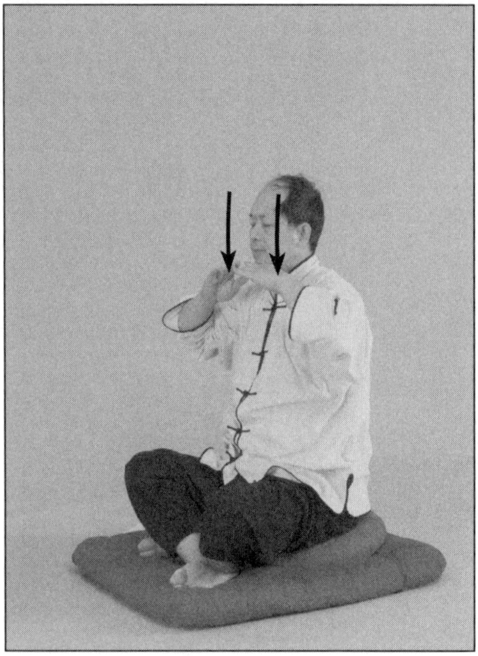

Figure 8-46

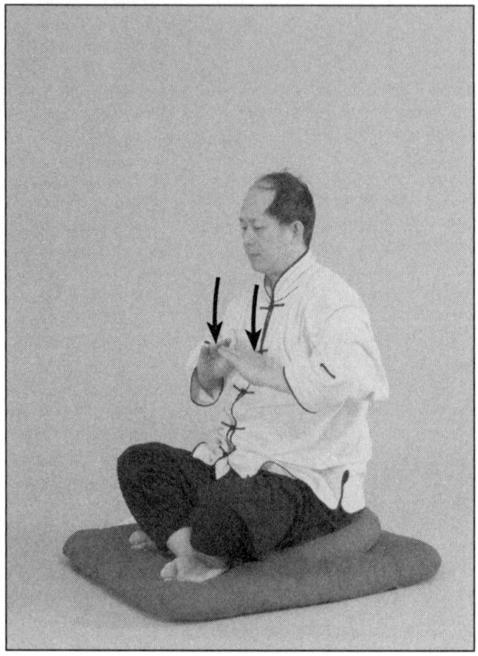

Figure 8-47

8-47). When this happens, you feel a strong vibration in your upper chest. Finally, keep quiet while still exhaling, and use the mind to lead the Qì down to the Lower Dāntián to complete the chanting process. You may repeat the whole process three times.

The positions where you change the words of your chanting are at the Yìntáng (M-HN-3, Upper Dāntián), Tiāntū (Co-22), Jiūwěi (Co-15), and Qìhǎi (Co-6) (Figure 8-48). These four cavities are four of the 7 major corresponding gates of the body.

If necessary, walk for a few minutes. If you wish, after you have finished the recovery massage and exercises, you may walk or simply lie down to rest for a few minutes.

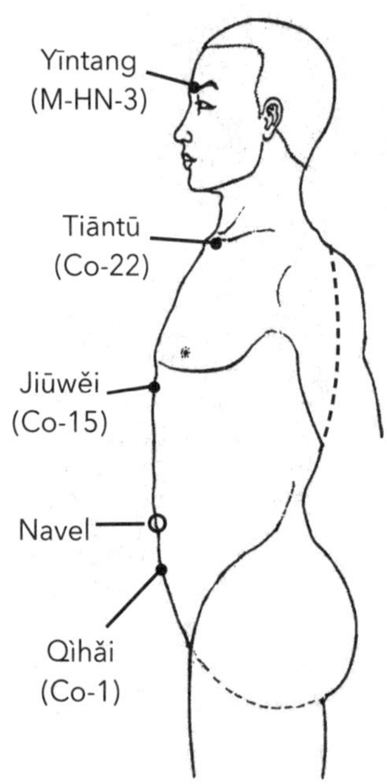

Figure 8-48. Yīntang (M-HN-3), Tiāntū (Co-22), Jiūwěi (Co-15), and Qìhǎi (Co-6)

8-9. Meditation and Healing (Jìngzuò Yǔ Zìliáo, 靜坐與自療)

There are a few ancient documents which record how you can use Small Circulation Meditation for effective self-healing. The theory is very simple. Since your mind can focus on and feel the affected area, it can lead the Qì there to improve circulation of Qì and blood. This is no different from physical massage, which also improves the circulation of Qì and blood. To improve them through meditation is much harder. You need to have reached a high level of meditation to effectively lead the Qì for healing. Next, I will translate some ancient documents about healing through meditation. First, one about Sealing the Breath (Bìqì, 閉氣).

Vessel Viewing
《脈望》(Màiwàng)

Sealing the Breath does not mean to hold and choke the breath. It means the spirit is steady and the Qì harmonious, stop thinking and forget about worry, allow the nose breathing to be natural, smooth, and slender, as though it were there and yet as though it were not there.

閉氣者，非閉噎其氣也，乃神定氣和，絕思忘慮，便鼻息悠悠，若有若無。

This document reassures us that regulating the breathing is not to hold it, but to regulate it until it can be natural, smooth, and slender.

The Secret of Cultivating Original Qì Internally, by Huànzhēn
《幻真先生內服元氣訣》(Huànzhēn Xiānshēng Nèifú Yuánqì Jué)

If there is a sudden uncomfortable feeling in cultivation, or occasional sickness, then immediately go to a secret room. Follow the method of breathing to cultivate the Qì. Once it is abundant, stop and regulate it, and swallow. Think of the place which is in pain, seal your breath, and place your whole mind there, using the Yì to attack the sick place. When inhalation reaches its limit, then utter it. After complete uttering, again swallow. Continue and follow the same method to attack. When the breathing becomes urgent, then stop. After breathing has been regulated, again attack. It may take twenty to fifty times; attack the painful place until sweating and turning a red color, then stop. If there is no improvement, then practice it every midnight or early morning. Practice day and night and use the Yì to attack. It does not matter if the sickness is at the head, face, hands, or feet, just attack wherever there is a problem.

> 忽有修養乖宜，偶生疾患，宜速于密室，依服氣法，布足訖則調氣咽之，念所苦之處，閉氣想注，以意攻之。氣極則吐之，訖，復咽。相繼依前攻之，氣急則止，氣調復攻，或二十至五十，攻覺所苦處，汗出通潤即止。如未損，即每日夜半，或五更晝日頻作，以意攻及。若病在頭面、手足，但有疾之處則攻之。

Sicknesses here means common uncomfortable feeling, such as the beginning of catching cold, joint pain, internal pain caused by Qì and blood stagnation, or minor injury. Normally, these problems can be corrected through meditation.

First build up Qì in the False Lower Dāntián through Abdominal Breathing, or in the Real Lower Dāntián through Embryonic Breathing. Then inhale smoothly and slenderly, and swallow (Yàn, 咽) the saliva while using your Yì to lead the Qì to the painful place. Hold the breath until it reaches its limit, and then exhale slowly, using the mind to lead the Qì away from the painful place. Repeat these processes continuously. If you feel your breathing becoming urgent, return to normal breathing until it is comfortable once more. Then repeat the whole process. You may have to do it many times, but it doesn't matter, keep doing it until you start to sweat and become flushed and red, then stop. If it does not ease the pain, repeat day and night until the pain has gone.

The Important Secret Song of Embryonic Breathing
《胎息秘要歌訣》(Tāixí Mìyào Gējué)

> *If the body is injured or gets sick suddenly, or regularity is abnormal (feeling uncomfortable), condense your Yì, and return to a leisure room (separate and secret room). Strip the body, and lie down on the bed. Face up as though sleeping, and hold firm (place both hands at the Lower Dāntián). Knock your teeth and burn incense. After swallowing thirty-six times, the Qì in the Dāntián passes the normal stage. Follow the Xīn to lead Qì continuously. Lead it to the injured place. It is adequate when it sweats. This saves the effort of searching for medical prescriptions.*
>
> 忽然身染疾，非理有損傷。斂意歸閒室，脫身臥本床。仰眠兼握固，扣齒與焚香。三十六咽足，丹田氣越常。隨心連引導，損處最為良。汗出以為度，省求廣利方。

To place the hands at the Lower Dāntián area is to "Hold Firm" (Wògù, 握固). Then the mind is in the Dāntián, and the Qì is stored efficiently. Knocking the Teeth (Kòuchǐ, 扣齒) wakes up the brain and raises the spirit. Burn incense (Fénxiāng, 焚香) to calm and focus the mind. Other descriptions of training methods are the same as in the previous document.

These two documents about using meditation for self-healing are translated for your reference. The most important way to achieve successful healing is through practice and accumulated experience. Through constant practice and pondering, you soon grasp the secret key of healing.

References

1. 《道德經・五十五章》：〝骨弱筋柔而握固。〞

2. 《諸病源候論・風身體手足不隨候》：〝握固者，以兩手各自以四指把手姆指。〞

3. 《道門通教必用集》：〝握固以大指掐中指指節，四指齊收于心。〞

4. 指行佛家氣功時，手的姿勢。其作用有二：一精神思維活動專注于手印，持之以恒，獲得禪定。二調節手形成印後，精神思維活動專注于呼吸，達到最高境界，〝即身成佛。〞

5. 《陀羅尼集經》：〝誦咒有身印等種種印法，若作手印，誦諸咒法，易得成驗。〞

6. 《慧林音義》：〝結跏趺坐，略有兩種。一曰吉祥，二曰降魔。凡坐皆先以右趾押左股，後以左趾押右股。此即左押右。手亦左在上，名曰降魔坐。諸禪宗多傳此座。依持明藏教瑜珈法門，即傳吉祥為上，降魔座有時而用。其吉祥座，先以左趾押右股，后以右趾押左股，令兩足掌仰于二股之上，手亦右壓左，安仰跏趺之上，名曰吉祥坐。如來昔在菩提樹下，成正覺時，身安吉祥之座，手作降魔之印，故如來常安此座，轉妙法輪。〞

7. 《赤風髓》：〝訣在閉兌目，半垂簾，赤龍頭胝上齶。〞

8. 《崔公入藥鏡》注：〝銀河阻隔，陰陽之相會，必借鵲橋而渡。人之舌，喻為鵲橋。練功時，舌舐上齶，有溝通陰陽之作用。〞

9. 《道德經・十章》：〝專氣致柔，能嬰兒乎？〞

10. 《性命圭旨全書・亨集》：〝專氣致柔神久留，往來真息自悠悠。綿綿迤邐歸元氣，不汲靈泉常自流。〞

11. 〝吐唯細細，納唯綿綿〞

12. 《道言淺近》：〝調息要調真息息〞，〝凝神調息，只要心平氣和。〞

13. 《性命圭旨全書・蟄藏氣穴，眾妙歸根》：〝調息要調真息息，煉神須煉不神神。〞

14. 《性命圭旨・大小鼎爐說》：〝黃庭為鼎，氣穴為爐。黃庭正在氣穴上，縷絡相連，乃人身百脈交會之處。〞元氣氤氳二穴之間，謂之〝小鼎爐。〞〝乾位為鼎，坤位為爐。〞即泥丸宮為鼎，下丹田為爐，謂之〝大鼎爐。〞

15. 《金仙証論》：〝采藥運周天者，當從氣穴坤爐而起火，升乾首以為鼎，降坤腹以為爐。即古人所謂乾坤為鼎器者是也。見神氣之起伏，而鼎氣在是矣。注：乾在上為鼎，坤在下為爐。有神氣即有爐鼎，無神氣即無爐鼎。〞

16. 《道鄉集》：〝何謂文火？若守若存，勿亡勿助。〞

17. 《性天風月通玄記・師徒傳道》：〝靜中一動火正燃，此時正好煉大還。采時謂之藥，藥中有火焉。若問武火，大舉巽風；若問文火，胎息綿綿。〞

18. 眼觀鼻，鼻觀心。

19. 孔子曰：〝知止而后有定，定爾后能靜，靜而后能安，安爾后能慮，慮爾後能得。〞

20. 性命圭旨全書・玉液煉形法則》：〝欲除生滅心，必自無念始。〞

21. 道德經・十六章》：〝致虛極，守靜篤。〞

22 《性命圭旨全書・天人合發，采藥歸壺》：〝心中無物為虛，念頭不起為靜，致虛而至于極，守靜而至于篤。陰陽自然交媾，陰陽一交而陽精產矣。〞

23. 《道鄉集》：〝有心觀竅，無心觀妙等語。乃道之功用也。有欲以觀竅，又為無心觀妙之用。無心以觀妙，又為有心觀竅之體。要知有欲觀竅有為也，神返氣自回之時也。無欲觀妙無為也，無人無我，無山川草木，混混然不知不覺之時代也。〞指〝致虛極，守靜篤。〞之意識活動的寧靜，靜而后一陽生，萌發奇妙生機。

24. 意不在氣，在氣則滯。

25. 河車：運載水火之工具。河車搬運水火，由尾閭至泥丸，一撞三關。三車：羊車：尾閭關到夾脊關，其行緩慢。鹿車：夾脊關到玉枕關，其行宜速。牛車：玉枕關到泥丸關，力大方能過關。

26. 《道德經・一章》：〝常無欲，以觀其妙。〞

27. 《道德經・十六章》：〝致虛極，守靜篤。〞

28. 《諸真聖胎神用訣・徐神公胎息訣》：〝夫神者，虛無之用。〞

29. 《六祖壇經》：〝菩提本無樹，明鏡亦非台，本來無一物，何處惹塵埃。〞

30.《本草綱目》：〝腦為元神之府。〞

31.《脈望》：〝腦為上田，元神所居之宮，人能握元神，棲于本宮，則金氣自升，真息自定，所謂一竅開而百竅齊開，大關通則百關盡通也。〞

32.《參同契發揮》：〝隨真息之往來，任真氣之生降，自朝至暮，元神常棲于泥丸也。〞

33.《道德經・六章》：〝谷神不死，是謂玄牝。玄牝之門，是謂天地根，綿綿若存，用之不勤。〞

34.《武當修真圖》：〝明堂下，兩眉連線中點上方。有神光出，而曰天目。〞

35.《云笈七簽》：〝兩眉間為泥丸之玉門。〞指印堂穴。

36.《周易參同契》：〝真人至妙，若有若無，仿佛大淵，乍沉乍浮，退而分佈，各守境偶。〞

37.《論衡・超奇》：〝天稟元氣，人受元精。〞

38.《古文參同契》：〝元氣之積厚而精英者稱為元精。〞

39.《性命圭旨全書》：〝煉精者，煉元精，抽坎中之元陽也，元精固則交感之精自不泄漏。〞

40. *Chinese Qìgōng Dictionary* (中國氣功辭典), by Lǚ, Guāng-Róng (呂光榮), 人民衛生出版社, Běijīng, 1988.

PART IV

Questions and Future Human Possiblities

CHAPTER 9

Questions and Future Human Possiblities

Many Qìgōng practices were kept secret in the past and their theories and methods passed down at random. Only recently have many of them been revealed to the general public, so practitioners can learn the secrets of other styles. Even so, because of the long years of secrecy, many available documents remain incomplete or unconfirmed. To compile them and formalize a systematic theory is very difficult. During the course of my study and research, many questions have arisen, the answers to which seem accurate but need scientific verification. Some questions are beyond the scope of any test which could be carried out with current scientific equipment.

Some questions arise due to my limited understanding of Qìgōng training, others from advances in modern science. In the course of my continuing research, many will be answered. I also await answers from other Qìgōng masters. Many questions need to be investigated through experiments involving modern equipment. Some may remain unanswered, since I firmly believe that nobody could achieve the very high level of Qìgōng practice attained by earlier masters.

Personally, I hope these questions help stimulate interest in Western scientific society, and lead to further research. Although the material sciences continue to develop rapidly, our spiritual sciences remain in the same state of stagnation as centuries ago.

About Essence

1. Chinese medicine and Qìgōng society tell us that one's Original Essence is stored in the kidneys. How is it stored?
2. Why is it stored there instead of in other organs? We need a theoretical explanation and experimental proof for this.
3. If Original Essence is stored in the kidneys, what about those people who have only one kidney? Will they die earlier? Will the Original Essence stored in the single kidney be enough for life? Will its conversion to Qì be reduced?

4. How could we tell a person whose Original Essence is strong from someone whose Essence is weak? Normally, it is judged from one's spirit of vitality and state of health, but there is no standard for this. Is there any scientific way of doing so?
5. Could we see Original Essence? Is it material? Is it the source of hormones? Could we see it in a dead body?
6. Does Original Essence comprise the genes or the hormones? Many sources lead me to believe that genes and hormones are what the ancient Chinese called Original Essence, or at least that they are closely related.
7. Could the quantity of Original Essence be increased and its quality improved through modern technology?
8. Could the stimulation of semen production be done in a modern way? For example, through minor electrical stimulation? Would this cause problems, since the one being stimulated need not regulate his mind?
9. Could the stimulation of semen production through modern technology achieve the same purpose of longevity? Could this be done for an old man without causing problems, such as a heart attack?
10. Could technology enhance the conversion of Essence to Qì, such as using an electromagnetic field to lead Qì from the Real Lower Dāntián to the brain?
11. Could artificial hormones benefit the body as much as the Essence generated inside the body? What side effects would there be?
12. What biochemical reaction occurs during the conversion of Essence to Qì? If we knew this, could we enhance it with modern technology?
13. Could we use modern technology to transfer Essence from one person to another, like a blood transfusion?
14. Is it true that Water Qì is converted from Original Essence? How is this done? If Original Essence consisted of the body's hormones, then it could not be converted into Qì. The function of hormones is to regulate the body's metabolism by regulating the biochemical reactions in the body. They act as catalysts which ensure that biochemical reactions occur smoothly, without actively participating in them. Perhaps Original Essence refers to fat being converted to Qì.

About Qì

1. Is the traditional concept of Human Qì the same as bioelectromagnetic energy, or is it a synthesis of various types of energy? Many practitioners are not convinced that Human Qì is merely bioelectromagnetic energy circulating in the body. Many Qìgōng phenomena cannot be explained satisfactorily by this hypothesis. For example, how does a Qìgōng master hold a burning coal in his hand without being burned?
2. How do we standardize the measurement of Qì? A unit system is necessary. Many different types of equipment have been designed to measure it in terms of thermal energy (heat), infrared radiation, and electricity. Since Human Qì has not been defined, there is no specific equipment which we are convinced is the most accurate method for measuring it. However, if it is proven that Qì is human electromagnetic energy, then we could use an electrical unit system to measure it.
3. Since the general definition of Qì is universal energy, how do we relate all kinds of different energy into one, if that were possible? To me, there is no absolute way to relate them. The unit system used to measure heat cannot measure electricity. It may be better to designate Qì, referring for example to Heat Qì or Electric Qì.
4. When Qì is transferred from one person to another, what, other than heat and bioelectricity, is transferred? I have often wondered how one person could be more effective in transferring his Qì than another. There must be some extra force transferred emotionally to help the patient build up EMF to cure himself internally. What is this force? Brain waves, emotional touch, or self-confidence, perhaps?
5. If Qì is bioelectricity, how could modern technology increase its circulation in the body and achieve the same results as with Qìgōng practice? It was not possible to generate electromagnetic fields in ancient times, but very easy to do so today. There should be a way to use external fields to increase circulation, regulate Qì, and clean the marrow. Naturally, we must proceed with caution to determine the side effects. How could an external field duplicate the mental calmness necessary for enlightenment? Even if circulation could be improved, without a disciplined mind there would be fewer benefits. Might other problems arise if people become exceptionally powerful without the discipline of control?
6. How do clouds and fog affect Qì circulation? Low clouds generate an electric field which affects the human energy field. Does fog do this as well? When

you are in fog, do the charges surround you uniformly? Can this affect your Qì circulation?

7. Is there any modern way to stimulate and raise fasciae for Qì storage? Would this cause problems if we could not generate enough Qì to keep them full?
8. Since Qì and the brain are closely related, could we adjust the Qì nourishment of the brain to cure mental illness?

About Spirit (Shén)

1. How do we define spirit? Is it a form of energy? Could a spirit have its own thoughts? If so, how?
2. How do we define spirit and mind? The relationship between them is very confusing. Is Shén generated from mind? If Shén must be generated from mind, how can it exist after physical death? If it can, does this Shén have a mind and can it think independently? How do they relate to brainwaves? Can Shén be measured?
3. Can the spirit and soul exist even if there is no physical life form? It is believed in Chinese religions that the spirit and soul exist even after death. Are spirit and soul in energy form? Are they part of the non-human natural energy, or are they the residues of human energy?
4. Is it true that there is another dimension or world not known to science, yet which can be reached by the spirit or soul? There are many stories of people dying and then coming back. They often say they were outside their physical bodies and could see it. The Chinese believe that the world we live in is the Yáng World (Yángjiān, 陽間), and when a person dies, his spirit enters the Yīn World (Yīnjiān, 陰間). According to the theory of Yīn and Yáng, Yáng must be balanced by Yīn. Could this Yīn world be reached, other than by energy or spirit?
5. Are events recorded in the spiritual world? Could this spiritual memory be erased? I believe what happens in nature influences its energy, and this influence is recorded in nature. I believe once human science has reached a certain level, we will be able to trace past events through spiritual memory.
6. Is a thought energy or matter? How could it travel from one end of the universe to the other instantaneously? Could it penetrate the past or the future?
7. Is the mind the "God" (Tàijí or Dào) of the human universe (small heaven and earth)? If so, could we then use the model of the human universe to understand the grand universe? Isn't mankind derived from the grand universe, with all spiritual and energy structures being similar to that of the grand universe?

8. How does a human spirit communicate with that of another human or animal? Through the vibrations of the Spiritual Valley? From the structure of the brain, can we regard every brain as a radio transmitter and receiver? Could this spirit communicate with the natural spirit in the same way?
9. Could one person affect another's thinking through brainwave correspondence?
10. Could modern technology increase the flow of bioelectricity to the brain to activate more brain cells? Would there be any side effects? Nowadays, many bodybuilders use electricity to speed the growth of their muscles and develop the body in a short time. Later they discover that the inner body cannot produce enough bioelectricity to support the muscles, so they degenerate faster than normal. Would we encounter this problem if we activated brain cells in the same way?
11. Could we open the gate of the Upper Dāntián, the third eye, through external electrical stimulation? What would happen if we opened it quickly, without enough Qì internally to support this wandering spirit? Would we go crazy?
12. When we reach a higher level of spiritual enlightenment, will we then be able to communicate with aliens from outer space? If they are thousands of years ahead of us scientifically, they should have reached a higher spiritual level, so we should be able to contact them somehow.
13. Is the spiritual dimension a new dimension in which we can travel much faster than the speed of light? Would that be how UFOs travel to earth?
14. How important a role will the human spirit play in human history when science leaves its present stage of infancy and enters the stage of its youth?
15. What is the scientific explanation for the halo around the head, or the glow around the body, of a meditator? Though I try to explain it as air de-ionization generated by the body's electrical charge, an experiment needs to be conducted to determine whether this is true.
16. How is spirit generated in a newborn baby? Where does it originate? Does it start when the baby begins to think? Does it exist only in humans?
17. Does a newborn child need a preexisting spirit? Some religions say that it does, in order to form a complete human. If so, where does this spirit come from? From those who died before? If a newborn baby needs this preexisting spirit, then how does the population keep increasing? Where do the new spirits originate? Do they come from the sun, or from universal energy? Could spirits from other planets immigrate to the earth and be born into human bodies?
18. What are the differences between spirit and soul? Since there is no exact translation from Chinese into English, I would like the exact differences and definitions of these words.

19. How do we generate a "spiritual baby" in Qìgōng training? In the Qìgōng tradition, to reach enlightenment you must train until you give birth to this spiritual baby. Only when it has grown to be independent can your spirit survive, and live forever. Is this true? Scientifically, how could this be possible? Could modern science explain it, or is it still beyond what today's science can grasp? If we believe that a highly developed mind could speed up the process of evolution, then it might be able to reach many other things still beyond human understanding.
20. Do the spirits of enlightened people who have died continue to exist? If so, can they help the living? If the answer is yes, do you agree that spirit and soul can exist even after death? When you pray, do you actually receive help from God or the spirits of the dead, or are you helping yourself by building your self-confidence?
21. Does a spirit make its own decisions or is it affected by natural Qì? Can a spirit think? How could it help a living person? Through brainwave communication? Or is the spirit only some human energy residue roaming around in the energy world and being affected by surrounding energy forces?
22. When someone communicates with animals, is this brainwave correspondence? I once saw a woman on a live TV show who seemed able to communicate with all kinds of dogs. The information she learned was verified by the owners. If this were real, would it be brainwave communication? Do the brains of animals and man function on the same frequency band, or just partially overlap?
23. Could a highly concentrated mind make an object move without touching it? What would be the principle behind this? How could brainwave energy become strong enough to do this? Are miracles done with brainwaves or through the spiritual dimension?
24. Could the spirit really leave the body and travel, or is it only that the brainwaves sense something and match its frequency so that you can be aware of it? When someone is hypnotized, he can sense many things beyond his ordinary capability. Is this similar to what happens when a person seems to leave his body during meditation?
25. Could modern technology create an electromagnetic wave whose wavelength is equivalent to the human brainwave? Our technology seems to have progressed that far already. If so, could a brainwave machine generate a wave to affect our thinking and judgment? That would truly be brainwashing. Could we create a machine to generate brainwave white noise, to act as a shield

against such a weapon? Could the wars of the future be fought using brainwave machines?

26. If it is possible to make a brainwave machine, could we determine what frequencies are associated with crime, and somehow block them? Is it possible to really brainwash criminals? Of course, if such a machine fell into the hands of criminals, they would have a powerful tool for evil. Could we accept the moral responsibility for changing an individual's brainwaves?
27. Could a good Qìgōng meditator avoid being controlled and affected by a brainwave machine? Personally, I believe that one who regulates his mind effectively would be able to avoid the effects, but how long would he be able to do so?
28. What is the bandwidth of the brainwave? What existing materials could shield them out? Metal is usually a good insulator against radio waves, but could it also keep out brainwaves? If not, is there any material which could be used to shield against them?
29. What is the relationship between spirit (Shén) and brainwaves? I personally believe that when your Shén is high, your brainwaves are stronger, and probably more focused and sensitive in different wavelengths. Is this true?
30. Since our spirit is so closely related to Qì or the energy field, how much has our spirit been affected by energy pollution such as radio waves?

About Channels, Vessels, and Cavities

1. How did the ancients find out about the Qì channels, vessels, and cavities? How did they locate them with such accuracy? How did they discover they could use them to cure illness?
2. How do blocked channels interfere with the Qì flow? This is a simple question, but one without an easy answer. It will take the most advanced technology to find out exactly how the Qì channels become blocked. Is it caused by an accumulation of fat which significantly reduces electric conductivity, or by some defect in the electrically conductive tissues?
3. How do the channels conduct Qì? How much stimulation can make it move? If Qì is bioelectric energy, then the question is, how much EMF can make the energy move, and where is it?
4. How do the vessels store Qì? If Qì is bioelectric energy, then is a Qì vessel like a battery or a capacitor, which can store and release energy as necessary?
5. What do the Qì channels and vessels actually look like? If they are areas where electrical conductivity is different, then experiments should determine how they are shaped.

6. How could we design a machine sensitive enough to accurately locate all the Qì channels and cavities? This would be very helpful for acupuncture practice.
7. Why are there four vessels in the legs and none in the arms? Is it because people use their legs more than their arms? I believe the vessels in the legs evolved to supply extra Qì to the legs and help regulate them more efficiently.
8. Are there any other vessels which have not yet been discovered? It is possible that there are other, smaller vessels in the body which remain undiscovered. For example, I believe there should be extra vessels in the arms, to serve much the same purposes as those in the legs.
9. What actually happens when we open a channel (gate) in Qìgōng practice? Does the channel recover its conductivity? What is the best way to do this?
10. Could we use modern bioelectric technology to open the channels and smooth the Qì circulation?
11. Could we use technology to fill up the Qì reservoirs? If they are bioelectric capacitors, we might be able to use external electromagnetic methods to refill them. We would then have enough Qì to nourish the whole body and slow down the aging process significantly.
12. What actually happens when an experienced Qìgōng master helps a student open his channels? Does he really transport his Qì into the student's body to do the job, or does he only offer stimulation and confidence to the student, allowing him to open them by himself?
13. Exactly what are cavities? Do all cavities have higher electric conductivity, and do they differ in capacity? Is increased electrical conductivity the only factor for locating cavities, or did the ancients have additional criteria?
14. Why are there cavities? Do they just circulate Qì to the skin surface to nourish it and regulate Qì channels, or are there any other purposes than these?
15. How does acupuncture actually correct the Qì flow? We need a more complete explanation through modern experimentation and scientific study.
16. The *Sùwèn* (素問), or *Book of Plain Questions,* said our lives run in cycles of 7 years for women and 8 years for men. When the book was written, boys reached puberty around the age of 16, and girls around 14. Now that puberty comes 2 to 4 years earlier, have the cycles changed? Did they have objective reality, or were they more philosophical ideas?

About Mutual Qì Nourishment

1. Two people can practice together to balance their Qì through mutual Qì nourishment. The one with the stronger Qì gives his Qì, while the weaker one gains it. Two people with weak Qì can help each other build it up. In this kind of mutual Qì nourishment, each must be able to coordinate with the other in every aspect, especially in breathing. Emotionally, they must be willing to share with each other. In this kind of practice, is it inevitable that they will fall in love? If so, isn't it contrary to the principle of meditation that the mind should be calm and peaceful, without emotional disturbance? If not, how are they able to touch and share Qì with each other?
2. When two people practice mutual Qì nourishment, do they actually share Qì, or do they stimulate each other's minds to enhance the brain's EMF and thereby increase their own Qì circulation, or both?
3. Love is a natural way of promoting mutual Qì nourishment and helping the other one recover from illness. Could this be a form of Qìgōng?
4. Is sexual activity the ultimate natural way of mutual Qì nourishment? Sex is a natural human desire. Through regular sexual activity, a person achieves mental calmness and peace, and releases the pressure generated by emotional disturbance. Could this be a form of Qìgōng practice?
5. When a man ejaculates, he loses Qì to the woman. How does this happen? Is this why women live longer? If she has reached a higher level of Qìgōng, could the man receive Qì instead of losing it?
6. How is it that Essence and Qì are lost during ejaculation? In certain Qìgōng practices, men avoid ejaculation. How is Qì transmitted under such circumstances?
7. If sex is beneficial for Qìgōng practice, why did all Buddhist monks and many of the Daoists hide in the mountains to avoid sexual contact? Were they afraid that sex and love would destroy the calm and peaceful mind they were cultivating?
8. Why did the Daoists develop so many techniques which used sexual activity for Qì nourishment? Could these techniques have been developed by those whose minds could not be calm? Or did they want, on the one hand to reach enlightenment, and the other hand to enjoy a natural, normal human life?

About Health and Longevity

1. Could we use external electromagnetic stimulation to cure sickness in the same way that Qìgōng and acupuncture reinstate normal bioelectric circulation? Qìgōng cures many kinds of cancer. Could this be achieved with modern electric and magnetic technology?
2. Could the immune system be strengthened through electromagnetic stimulation to cure AIDS and cancer? The immune system is related closely to the body's bioenergy system. Could we increase the EMF of the brain and strengthen the bioenergetic circulation in the body?
3. Is it dangerous to use electricity and magnetism in acupuncture when we do not understand Qì science completely? So far, there is no conclusive report on the use of electricity and magnetism in acupuncture, even though they are widely used. Are they safe for general practice, or do we need more research?
4. Is practicing Qìgōng to obtain a longer life the correct goal? I believe that if someone really wants a much longer life, he needs to leave society to avoid emotional disturbance. However, when he does this, he loses the ordinary meaning of human life. I believe the correct purpose of Qìgōng practice is to achieve a healthy body and mind, while still experiencing life. You extend your lifespan somewhat because you are healthy, and you are still able to experience life.
5. What is the meaning of life? Could Qìgōng help humanity understand it? Does a long life mean more to you than a happy one? If you want both, what should you do? Qìgōng practice has helped me understand nature, and myself. It has stopped me wondering and being confused. Do you expect the same?
6. Could we use modern technology to reach the same goal as Marrow Washing training and obtain a longer life without sacrificing our emotions? I feel certain that once we understand exactly how Marrow Washing training works, we will be able to use modern technology to quickly reach the same goal.

About Qì and Modern Living

1. Could we use ice to maintain the body's Qì balance during the summer? It was not possible to research this before refrigerators were invented. In summertime, when the heart is on fire (Yáng), could placing ice in the palm of your hand cool the heart, or would it quench the heart fire too quickly and cause problems? What if we were to use alcohol instead of ice?

2. How does working night shifts affect one's Qì circulation? In ancient times, few people worked at night, so there are no documents available today which discuss this. Since the time of day has to be taken into account when giving acupuncture treatments, would being on night shift affect the treatment?
3. How is Qì circulation affected when you travel several time zones in a short time? Does jet lag indicate that the body's Qì is disturbed?

About the Human Magnetic Field

1. Theoretically, there are two magnetic poles in the human body, matching those formed by the Earth's magnetic field. Do these two poles reverse when you move from the Northern to the Southern Hemisphere?
2. The Earth's magnetic field starts at the South Magnetic Pole and goes to the North Magnetic Pole. Since a person's South Magnetic Pole seems to be on the head if one is in the Northern Hemisphere, does this mean his brain constantly receives energy nourishment? If the human magnetic poles are reversed in the Southern Hemisphere, does this mean that the brains of people there constantly lose nourishment?
3. Does this explain why the most highly developed technology has been created in the Northern Hemisphere?
4. If those in the Southern Hemisphere have their south magnetic poles in the Lower Dāntián, do they have more energy, and does this help them live longer?
5. When people are sick, could they speed their recovery by flying to the equator, where the effect of the Earth's magnetic field is minimized? I believe many illnesses are caused or worsened by disturbances in the body's electromagnetic field. The earth energy can worsen the situation, since your body loses its natural balance. Could you remove this hindrance by moving to the Equator?
6. We are surrounded by energy fields, both natural and man-made. Could we insulate a room against them to help people convalesce? Would this also be a good place to meditate?

Others

1. Are there specific spots on earth where natural energy is especially beneficial for Qìgōng? Many practitioners believe there are places where Heaven or Earth Qì nourishes your Qì and speeds up your training. Is this true? Would these areas be good for hospitals?

2. What happens when we are exposed to a strong electromagnetic field for a long time? How does it affect the body? Could it energize our vital force and improve our health?
3. Since ancient times, Qìgōng practitioners have claimed that there is a practice which makes the body light. Is this true? Is this beyond scientific explanation?
4. The Chinese have used jade for generations to regulate Qì in their bodies or to absorb excess Qì. Has this ever been investigated scientifically?
5. Could we use electromagnetic means to increase the Qì on the scalp to prevent hair loss or increase its growth?
6. Meditators talk about absorbing energy from the earth through the feet. Is this different from magnetic energy?
7. Could a highly trained Qìgōng practitioner predict the future, or is this simply a matter of judgment, combined with experience and wisdom? Some Qìgōng masters are said to read your mind and even predict your future. I believe it is possible to read minds through brainwave correspondence, but predicting the future needs more than this. Intelligence and wisdom are needed, and a lot of experience. One's personality is the main factor in success, and it can be read in the face and even in the palms. Is this how the future is read, or is there another way?
8. How does the material of your clothing affect your health? Natural materials such as cotton and wool dissipate some energy to the surrounding environment. Most artificial materials generate a Qì shield which does not allow your Qì to exchange with nature. This affects your body's electromagnetic field and perhaps even disturbs your Qì circulation. This needs to be investigated.
9. How does the weather affect our moods? Moods may be caused by the electric fields generated between low clouds and the ground. These strong, natural electric fields affect your body's electromagnetic field and may cause sickness or emotional disturbance.
10. Is there a way to energize the muscles to a higher level via external electromagnetic stimulation, or must we rely on traditional practices? If it were possible, would it be fair in competitive sports such as boxing or football? Could it be safe for bodybuilders to use electrical stimulation of the muscles?
11. Would there be any danger in these experiments? We don't understand the human body very well, and we are such delicate and complicated creatures. Naturally, many experiments could be performed on other animals first, but since the inner energy field is closely related to emotions, it is probable that most need to be conducted directly on humans.

12. Why do many Qìgōng practitioners hide themselves in caves for their cultivation? Is it because a cave shields one from external energy disturbances, such as electromagnetic fields or ions in the clouds?
13. Have there been several human civilizations on earth in the past, before the beginning of our recorded history? If there were, what happened? Did they destroy each other? How many cycles of civilization have there been? Is there some truth to the legend of Atlantis?
14. Will our human civilization survive or will we destroy ourselves, or be destroyed by natural disasters like those which came before us?
15. Will the development of our spiritual science ever match that of our material science? Although material science has advanced to a level capable of leading us to self-destruction, our spiritual development remains disappointingly stagnant.
16. While we frantically search for the origin of the material world, we have ignored the origin of our spiritual world. What is the root of our spiritual being?
17. We are increasingly playing the role of God in material science. Will we attempt to play the role of God in spiritual science as well?
18. Since the study of science such as mathematics and physics is a type of meditation, will humanity be able to open our third eye in the next few generations?
19. Did people from an earlier civilization go to Mars? Did Mars once have a similar climate to that on earth? If so, what happened? Did the settlers destroy each other, and the planet with them?
20. Will the 21st century be a spiritual century?
21. If modern medical science progresses to a point which allows humans to live for centuries, will we gain new understanding of the meaning of human life?
22. Would we obtain a harmonious life if we could live for several hundred years while still wasting this time searching for wealth and glory, whose importance gets instilled in us from an early age? Would we find new meaning in life?
23. Could we reach the stage of Wúwéi (無為) in human society? Wúwéi means doing nothing and regulating without regulating, ruling without ruling, a matrix without order. To achieve this, we would need to communicate telepathically. Would the whole of mankind need to open the third eye?
24. If we had been visited by intelligent aliens, this would mean their understanding of spiritual and material science would be far more advanced then our own. Have they opened their third eyes? Have they experienced a similar historical pattern as that of the human race?

25. If aliens had any intention of invading and taking over the earth, why would they have waited until now? Human technology is advancing rapidly. If they had intended to take over the earth, they could easily have done so in the past.
26. Were aliens in the past taken for Gods in the West or Immortals in the East? If our technology advanced to a level which allowed us to visit other undeveloped planets, would the local population consider us Gods?
27. If there were aliens among us, would they help us? Is it important for us to learn everything the hard way so we can gradually evolve spiritually by ourselves? If we were helped by intelligent aliens, would we appreciate it? Or would we be greedy and take their help for granted? We have not protected nature, which provides for us. We simply take it for granted and destroy it.
28. How could we help each other to wake up and start building a spiritual connection with nature?

These are some questions I have. I have found some answers during forty years of study, but many of them need to be verified. You also have many unanswered questions in your mind. You should not ignore them, but continue searching for the answers. This is the way and the meaning of our lives.

CHAPTER 10

Conclusion

If we attempt to comprehend any profound philosophy, we must first be calm. When the mind is calm and clear, judgment becomes logical and accurate. Through thousands of years of meditation and profound thought, science has developed. Unfortunately, most of this effort has been on developing material science, while spiritual development has been widely ignored. Since the eighteenth century, the gap between these two has increased rapidly. Most people seek glory, power, and wealth, becoming bogged down in the emotional bondage of material satisfaction, while the Yīn spiritual side has been degraded.

To save humanity, we need to spend more effort contemplating spirituality instead of concentrating solely on material science. The various religious organizations must recognize their role and teach their followers the correct methods of meditation and spiritual development. This requires them to make revolutionary changes in policy. They must teach their followers that meditation is for self-awakening and enlightenment, not for worship. If they continue to educate their followers to worship and follow blindly, then we follow the same destructive paths as we have in the past, remaining in the domain of spiritual abuse.

Meditation has been widely practiced in the East. Often these meditators lived in obscurity in the mountains. Through meditation, they comprehended the Dào of mankind and of nature. I believe the documents written by these pioneers are amongst the most precious treasures mankind possesses. That is why I continue to study and translate them into English. Unfortunately, my progress has been very slow. I sincerely hope that an organization with a good financial foundation can sponsor and host the conversion of these ancient Eastern philosophical texts into English. If this study were introduced into every level of education I believe it would be very successful in gradually changing Western society's view on spirituality.

I would like you to keep a few things in mind in the course of your study and research. These are:

Avoid prejudice. Any culture and tradition which has survived must have had some benefits to offer. Perhaps some of them do not fit in with our view of the world today, but they still deserve our respect. If you deny your past, you pull out your root. You should not be stubborn and claim that traditional culture is absolutely correct, or that a foreign culture must be better than your own. What you should do is keep the good of your own tradition and absorb the best of the foreign.

Be objective in your judgment. You should consider everything from the viewpoint of both sides to analyze it objectively. Your emotional responses should be taken into account, but should not dominate your judgment.

Be scientific. Although many things still cannot be explained by science, you should always judge scientifically. New sciences are constantly being developed. Phenomena which could not be tested before, should be examined with modern techniques.

Be logical. Whenever you read or study, always ask "Is it logical and does it make sense?" Contemplate and understand, instead of blindly believing.

Do not ignore prior experience. Prior experience which has been passed down is the root of research. You should always be sincere and respectful when you study the past. From it, you come to understand the present. By understanding the present, you create the future. The accumulation of experience is the best teacher. You should respect the past, be cautious about the present, and challenge the future.

China has more than seven thousand years of culture. There have been many incredible accomplishments, of which Qìgōng is only one. There has never been such open communication between different cultures as there is today. It is our responsibility to encourage the general public to accept, study, and research other cultures. In this way, humanity can adopt the good aspects of each and live in a more peaceful and meaningful way.

Qìgōng is part of traditional Chinese medical science. It has sought to achieve calm, peace, and happiness for thousands of years. I believe this aspect of Chinese culture can help Westerners, especially in spiritual training. Further publications need to be encouraged, and scholastic and scientific study, research, and testing need to be conducted, especially by universities and medical organizations. We should not fear to face the truth and challenge old beliefs and ways of thinking.

I predict that the study of Chinese medical science and internal, meditative Qìgōng will produce great results in the next few decades. I invite you to join me and become a pioneer in this new field in the Western world.

Acknowledgments

Thanks to Tim Comrie for photography and typesetting, to Kyle McCauley for general help and to Erik Elsemans, David Silver, Roger Whidden, and Leslie Takao for proofing the manuscript and contributing valuable suggestions. Thanks to Tony Richard Chee for the drawings and cover design. Special thanks to Keith Brown for the first edit, and to David Silver for the final edit. Special thanks to Dr. Thomas G. Gutheil for the foreword.

Thanks to Johnny Houx for proofreading this new edition, to Doran Hunter for copyediting, and Axie Breen for the cover design and illustration enhancements.

Appendix A

Translation and Glossary of Chinese Terms

Ài 愛 Love, kindness.

Ānlú 安爐 To install a furnace, by establishing abundant Qì at the Real Lower Dāntián (Zhēn Xiàdāntián, 真下丹田), using Embryonic Breathing (Tāixí, 胎息).

Ànmó 按摩 Press and rub. Together they mean massage.

Āntiān Lèmìng 安天樂命 Peace with heaven and delight in your destiny.

Bāchù 八觸 The Eight Touches, which are sensations often felt during Qìgōng practice, such as heat, touch, or heaviness.

Bāduànjǐn 八段錦 Eight Pieces of Brocade. A Wàidān Qìgōng (外丹氣功) practice said to have been created by Marshal Yuè, Fēi (岳飛) during the Southern Sòng Dynasty (1127–1280 CE, 南宋).

Bāguà 八卦 Eight Divinations, also called Eight Trigrams. In Chinese philosophy, the eight basic variations in the *Yìjīng* (易經, *Book of Changes*) designated as groups of solid and broken lines.

Bāguàzhǎng 八卦掌 Eight Trigrams Palm. One of the internal martial styles, believed to have been created by Dǒng, Hǎi-Chuān (董海川) between 1866 and 1880 CE.

Báiháo 白毫 Tiny white beams of spiritual light, emitted from the head or third eye.

Báihè 白鶴 White Crane. A well known southern Chinese martial style which originated in the Shàolín Temple (少林寺).

Bǎihuì (Gv-20) 百會 Hundred Meetings. An important acupuncture cavity located at top of the head on the Governing Vessel (Dūmài, 督脈). Also called Tiānlínggài 天靈蓋 Heavenly Spiritual Cover.

Bǎihuì Hūxī 百會呼吸 Bǎihuì Breathing, also called Spiritual Breathing (Shénxí, 神息).

Bǎirì Zhújī 百日築基 One Hundred Days to Build the Foundation. In *Yìjīnjīng* (易筋經) and *Xǐsuǐjīng* (洗髓經), the training of the first hundred days is the most important because it lays the foundation for further progress.

Bāmài 八脈 The Eight Extraordinary Vessels. These are considered to be Qì reservoirs, which regulate the Qì in the primary Qì channels.

Bào 抱 Embrace, hold together, stick together, enfold, harbor, or cherish.

Bāoxī (2852–2737 BCE) 包羲 An ancient ruler of China.

Bàoyī 抱一 Embracing the state of oneness. To keep the spirit (or mind) and Qì at the central energy line, and unify spirit and Qì at the Real Lower Dāntián (Zhēn Xiàdāntián, 真下丹田).

Bàoyuán 抱元 Embrace the origin. That means to keep your spirit at its residence, the Mud Pill Palace (Níwángōng, 泥丸宮), and keep the Qì at the Real Lower Dāntián (Zhēn Xiàdāntián, 真下丹田).

Bì 閉 To close, namely to close and hold up the Huìyīn (Co-1, 會陰), or to hold the breath.

Biǎnquè 扁鵲 A well-known physician who wrote the book *Nànjīng* (難經, *Classic on Disorders*) during the Chinese Qín and Hàn Dynasties (255 BCE–220 CE, 秦・漢).

Bìhù 閉戶 See Mìngmén (Gv-4, 命門), definition 1.

Bóyáng 伯陽 A nickname of Lǎozi (老子).

Bǔ 補 Nourishment.

Bùtiáo Értiáo 不調而調 Regulating without regulating. The stage of doing nothing (Wúwéi, 無為), when regulating is no longer necessary, and all regulating processes cease.

Cǎiyào 采藥 Picking up the herb. A Daoist term that means to receive the generated Qì.

Chán 禪

1. Buddhist term for meditation, from Sanskrit "Dhyana." Means to regulate the Xīn (心) until it is calm and steady.

2. Buddhist practices, which include cultivating, refining, and studying Buddhahood.

3. Chinese school of Mahayana Buddhism that asserts enlightenment can be attained through meditation, self-contemplation, and intuition. Called "Zen" in Japan.

Cháng 長 Long.

Chángqiáng (Gv-1) 長強 Long strength. The acupuncture name for the coccyx. Called Wěilǘ (尾閭, tailbone) in Daoist society. See also Shuǐhuǒ Zhījì (水火之際).

Chángquán 長拳 Long fist or long sequence. Chángquán includes all northern Chinese long-range martial styles. Tàijíquán (太極拳) is called Chángquán because its sequence is long.

Chángzài 常在 The name of the spleen's spirit, which is related to the soul.

Chànǚ 奼女 The shy lady (mother), implying Qì.

Chǎnyào 產藥 Produce the herb (Qì).

Chén 沈 Sink.

Chēng, Gīn-Gsào (1911 to 1976) 曾金灶 Dr. Yáng, Jwìng-Mǐng's White Crane master.

Chéngfó 成佛 Achieving Buddhahood.

Chéntǔ 塵土 Dust. According to Buddhism, secular society is filled with emotions and desires, regarded as emotional mud or dust.

Ch'i 氣 See Qì.

Ch'i Kung 氣功 See Qìgōng.

Chílǎo Huánjī Yùndòng 遲老還機運動 Qìgōng exercises to slow aging and return the function to a healthy state.

Chin Na 擒拿 See Qínná.

Chónglóu 重樓 Multi-towers, means layers of stories, which refers to the throat area.

Chōngmài 衝脈 Thrusting Vessel. One of the Eight Extraordinary Vessels (Bāmài, 八脈).

Chōngqì 充氣 To accumulate Qì in the Real Lower Dāntián (Zhēn Xiàdāntián, 真下丹田).

Chòupínáng 臭皮囊 Smelly skin bag, a Buddhist term for the human body.

Chùgǎn 觸感 Touch Feel, also called Moving Touch (Dòngchù, 動觸). A sensation which occurs in meditation.

Chūnqiū 春秋 Spring and Autumn. One of the Chinese warring periods (722 to 484 BCE) (戰國).

Confucius 孔子 See Kǒngzǐ (孔子)

Cuō 撮 To condense, focus, or concentrate. It means to concentrate the mind and Qì.

Dà Dǐnglú 大鼎爐 Large tripod and furnace. The final stage of conceiving a Spiritual Embryo (Shéntāi, 神胎) is to unite the Shén with the Qì at the Huángtíng (黃庭) cavity. The head is a tripod while the Huángtíng is a furnace.

Dàdìng 大定 Great Steadiness. Profound steadiness of body and mind.

Dàfǎn 大返 Great Return. To return the human temperament to the natural state.

Dàhuándān 大還丹 Large Returning Elixir. The meditation which is used to lead Qì up to nourish the brain for spiritual enlightenment.

Dàimài 帶脈 Girdle Vessel. One of the Eight Extraordinary Vessels (Bāmài, 八脈).

Dàimàixí 帶脈息 Girdle Vessel Breathing. Also known as Skin Breathing (Fūxí, 膚息) or Body Breathing (Tǐxí, 體息).

Dámó 達摩 Also known as Bodhidharma. The Indian Buddhist monk credited with creating the Yìjīnjīng (易筋經) and Xǐsuǐjīng (洗髓經) at the Shàolín monastery (少林寺) during the Liáng Dynasty (502–557 CE, 梁朝). Formerly a minor prince in southern India. His last name was Sardili (剎地利).

Dān 丹 Elixir.

Dāndǐng Dàogōng 丹鼎道功 The Elixir Cauldron Way of Qìgōng. A form of Daoist Qìgōng training.

Dānjiā 丹家 Elixir Family, meaning Daoist Qìgōng society.

Dānlú 丹爐 Elixir Furnace. Abdominal area (False Lower Dāntián) which produces elixir.

Dāntián 丹田 Elixir Field. Locations in the body which store and generate Qì in the body. The Upper (Shàng Dāntián, 上丹田), Middle (Zhōng Dāntián, 中丹田), and Lower (Xià Dāntián, 下丹田) Dāntiáns are located respectively in the brain, at the sternum (Jiūwěi, Co-15, 鳩尾), and just below the navel.

Dāntián Hūxī 丹田呼吸 Dāntián Breathing.

Dānyuán 丹元 The name of the heart's spirit. It contains the Líng (靈) and maintains its activities.

Dào 道 The Way, or Natural Way.

Dào Dé Jīng 道德經 *Classic on the Virtue of the Dào*. Written by Lǎozi (老子) during the Zhōu Dynasty (1122–255 BCE, 周朝).

Dàojiā 道家 Daoist School, or Scholar Daoism. Created by Lǎozi (老子) when he wrote *Dào Dé Jīng* (道德經) during the Zhōu Dynasty (1122–255 BCE, 周朝). See also Dàojiào (道教).

Dàojiā Hūxī 道家呼吸 Daoist breathing, also called Reverse Abdominal Breathing (Fǎn Fùhūxī or Nì Fùhūxī, 反腹呼吸・逆腹呼吸).

Dàojiào 道教 Daoist Religion. During the Hàn Dynasty (58 CE, 漢朝), Zhāng, Dào-Líng (張道陵) combined Scholar Daoism (Dàojiā 道家) with Buddhism to create Religious Daoism (Dàojiào, 道教).

Dàowài Cǎiyào 道外採藥 To pick the herb outside the Dào (道). A form of Daoist Qìgōng training.

Dǎoyǐn 導引 Direct and lead. Another name for Qìgōng.

Dāqiáo (Dā Quèqiáo) 搭橋（搭鵲橋）To build the (magpie) bridge. See Quèqiáo (鵲橋).

Dàzhōutiān 大周天 Grand Cyclic Heaven or Grand Circulation, called Macrocosmic Meditation in Indian Yoga. After a Nèidān practitioner completes Small Circulation (Xiǎozhōutiān, 小周天), he circulates Qì throughout the body or exchanges it with nature.

Dàzhuī (Gv-14) 大椎 Big vertebra. Acupuncture cavity on the Governing Vessel (Dūmài, 督脈).

Dǎzuò 打坐 Engaging in Sitting. Daoist term for meditation.

Dé 德 The manifestation of the Dào or the activities of nature.

Dì 地 The Earth. Along with Heaven (Tiān, 天) and Man (Rén, 人), one of the Three Natural Powers (Sāncái, 三才).

Dǐ 抵 To press up. The tongue presses up against the palate of the mouth.

Dì 蒂 The stalk of a fruit or flower, connecting to the root of life.

Dì Wǔxīn Hūxī 第五心呼吸 Fifth Gate Breathing, also called Bǎihuì Breathing (百會呼吸), or Upper Dāntián Breathing (Shàng Dāntián Hūxī, 上丹田呼吸).

Diǎnmài 點脈 Mai means the blood vessel (Xuěmài, 血脈) or the Qì channel (Qìmài, 氣脈). Diǎnmài means to press the blood vessel or Qì channel.

Diànqì 電氣 Diàn means electricity, so Diànqì means electrical energy. In China, a word is often placed before "Qì" to identify the different kinds of energy.

Diǎnxuè 點穴 Cavity Press. Qínná (擒拿) techniques that attack acupuncture cavities to immobilize or kill an opponent.

Diào 掉 Shake.

Dìlǐshī 地理師 Dìlǐ (地理) means geomancy, and Shī (師) means teacher. Therefore Dìlǐshī is a master who analyzes geographic locations according to the formula in the *Yìjīng* (易經, *Book of Changes*) and the energy distribution in the Earth. Also called Fēngshuǐshī (風水師).

Dìng 定 To stabilize or firm. The goal is to reach steadiness, the firmness of the body, mind, and spirit.

Dǐnglú 鼎爐 Furnace Tripod, also called Elixir Furnace (Dānlú, 丹爐). A Daoist term.

Dìngshén 定神 To stabilize the spirit. To keep the spirit at one place (usually the Shàng Dāntián at the Third Eye). An exercise for regulating Shén (神, spirit) in Qìgōng.

Dìngxīn 定心 To stabilize the mind from emotional disturbance.

Dìqì 地氣 Earth Qì.

Dòng 動 Moving.

Dòngchù 動觸 Moving Touch, or Touch Feel (Chùgǎn, 觸感). A sensation in meditation.

Dōngmiánxí 冬眠息 Hibernation Breathing.

Dòuniú 斗牛 Big Dipper. Condensing the Shén at the Upper Dāntián.

Duānpǐn 端品 Straighten the behavior. Keep good habits.

Dūmài 督脈 Governing Vessel. One of the Eight Extraordinary Vessels (Bāmài, 八脈).

Éméi Shān 峨嵋山 Famous mountain in Sìchuān province (四川).

Ézhōng (M-HN-2) 額中 The acupuncture name for the center of the forehead, above the midpoint of the eyebrows, also called Míngtáng (明堂).

Fǎlún 法輪 Wheel of Law. Buddhist translation of Indian term Dharmachakra. The common name for Buddhism.

Fǎn Fùhūxī 反腹呼吸 Reverse Abdominal Breathing. A Qìgōng breathing method, also called Reverse Breathing (Fǎn Hūxī, 反呼吸) or Daoist breathing (Dàojiā Hūxī, 道家呼吸).

Fǎn Hūxī 反呼吸 Reverse breathing. Also called Fǎn Fùhūxī (反腹呼吸).

Fǎnjīng Bǔnǎo 返精補腦 To return the Jīng to nourish the brain, a special Daoist Qìgōng term. Also called Huánjīng Bǔnǎo (還精補腦).

Fǎntóng Hūxī 返童呼吸 Back to Childhood Breathing, also called Abdominal Breathing. A Nèidān practice through which one regains control of the muscles in the lower abdomen.

Fēishēng 飛升 Spiritual Ascending. Separation of the spiritual body from the physical body.

Fēngchí (GB-20) 風池 Wind Pond. An acupuncture cavity on the Gall Bladder Primary Channel.

Fēngfǔ (Gv-16) 風府 Wind's Dwelling. Acupuncture cavity on the Governing Vessel. Also see Yùzhěn (玉枕).

Fēnglù 風路 Wind Path. Also called Nìxíng (逆行, Reversed Path). The reverse of the Fire Path (Huǒlù, 火路) of Small Circulation.

Fēngshuǐ 風水 Wind-Water. Geomancy. Divination of natural energy relationships in a location, especially the interrelationships of wind and water, hence the name.

Fēngshuǐshī 風水師 Wind-Water Teacher. Master of divination. Also called Dìlǐshī (地理師).

Fěnsuì Xūkōng 粉碎虛空 To crush the nothingness. Daoist training for enlightenment which destroys the illusion connecting the physical world and the spiritual plane.

Fénxiāng 焚香 Burning incense.

Fó 佛 The stage of enlightenment of truth, the stage of Buddhahood.

Fójiā (Fójiào) 佛家 (佛教) Buddhist family or religion. Jiào (教) means religion.

Fójiā Hūxī 佛家呼吸 Buddhist Breathing or Normal Abdominal Breathing (Zhèn Fùhūxī, 正腹呼吸).

Fú 符 1. To accord, match, harmonize, coordinate, or cooperate.

2. See Fúshuǐ (符水).

Fú 浮 Float.

Fúqì 伏氣 Tame the Qì. To govern Qì at will.

Fùshì Hūxī 腹式呼吸 Abdominal Way of Breathing. As you breathe, the muscles in the lower abdomen control the diaphragm. Also called Back to Childhood Breathing (Fǎntóng Hūxī, 返童呼吸).

Fúshuǐ 符水 Fú water, the magic water for curing diseases.

Fūxí 膚息 Skin breathing. A Nèidān Qìgōng (內丹氣功) breathing practice.

Gāowán Yùndòng 睪丸運動 Testicle exercises. Qìgōng exercises.

Gōng (Kung) 功 Energy or hard work.

Gōngfū (Kung Fu) 功夫 Energy Time. Any study, learning, or practice which requires patience, energy, and time to accomplish. Chinese martial arts require a great deal of time and energy, so they are commonly called Gōngfū.

Gù 固 To solidify and to firm.

Guān 觀 To look, observe, pay attention. To feel and to sense.

Guānniàn 觀念 Observing the Thoughts.

Guānxīn 觀心 Observing the Xīn. Pay attention to the activities of the Emotional Mind.

Guānyuán 關元 Key Origin. Lower Dāntián, where Pre-birth Qì, or Original Qì, is converted from Original Essence (Yuánjīng, 元精).

Guānyuán (Co-4) 關元 Hinge at the Source. An acupuncture cavity on the Conception Vessel.

Guānzhǐ 觀止 Observation is stopped and no longer necessary. Once you have regulated your Emotional Mind, then no more regulating is necessary. The observation of Xīn stops by itself.

Gǔdào 穀道 Grain path, anus.

Guǐ 鬼 Ghost. When you die, if your spirit is strong, your soul's energy does not decompose and return to nature. This soul energy is a ghost.

Guǐqì 鬼氣 The Qì residue of a dead person or ghost.

Guīxí 龜息 Turtle breathing. A turtle lives long because it breathes deep and slowly. This breathing leads Qì to the skin surface and to the marrow.

Gùjīng 固精 To solidify the Essence. A Qìgōng exercise for firming the Essence.

Gǔshén 谷神 Valley Spirit.

Gǔshén 固神 Regulate the Shén (神), firm and strengthen the spirit at its residence.

Guó 國 Country.

Hǎidǐ 海底 Sea Bottom. Martial arts name for the Huìyīn (Co-1, 會陰), or perineum.

Hàn (206 BCE–221 CE) 漢 A Chinese dynasty.

Hán, Chìng-Táng (1900–1976) 韓慶堂 A well-known Chinese martial artist, especially in Táiwān, and Dr. Yáng Jwìng-Mǐng's Long Fist grandmaster.

Hé 和 Harmony or peace.

Héchē 河車 River Vehicles. The means of transporting Qì in Small Circulation Meditation.

Hèn 恨 Hate.

Hēng 哼 A Yīn Qìgōng sound that is the opposite of the Yáng Hā (哈) sound. This sound leads the Qì inward to the bone marrow. It can also be used for attack when only partial manifestation of power is desired. One of two sounds used in Tàijíquán (太極拳).

Hénggémó 橫膈膜 Diaphragm.

Hòutiānqì 後天氣 Post-birth Qì or Post-Heaven Qì. This is converted from the Essence of food and air, and classified as Fire Qì, since it makes your body Yáng.

Hǔ 虎 Tiger.

Huá 滑 Slippery.

Huáhào 華皓 The name of the spirit of the lungs. Associated with the nose which takes in air (insubstantial material) and fills the body with life.

Huǎn 緩 Slow.

Huánjīng Bǔnǎo 還精補腦 To Return the Essence to Nourish the Brain. A Daoist Qìgōng process wherein Qì produced from Essence is led to nourish the brain. Also called Fǎnjīng Bǔnǎo 返精補腦.

Huángpó 黃婆 Old Yellow Lady. The matchmaker who brings Yīn and Yáng together.

Huángtíng 黃庭 Yellow Yard.

1. The area at the solar plexus where Fire and Water Qì blend to generate a spiritual embryo (Shéntāi, 神胎). Also called Jade Ring (Yùhuán, 玉環) Zhōnggōng (中宮, Central Palace)

2. Can also refer to the Middle Dāntián (Zhōng Dāntián, 中丹田).

3. Can also refer to Tiāngǔ (天谷, Heavenly Valley).

Huátuó 華佗 A famous doctor during the Jìn Dynasty (晉朝) during the 3rd century CE.

Huǐguò 悔過 Confess.

Huìnéng 慧能 Sixth Chán (禪) ancestor during the Táng Dynasty (713–907 CE, 唐朝). He changed some meditation methods and philosophy, and was long considered a traitor.

Huìyīn (Co-1) 會陰 Meet Yīn. The perineum, an acupuncture cavity on the Conception Vessel.

Hún 魂 The Soul. Commonly used with the word Líng (靈), which means spirit. Daoists believe one's Hún (魂) and Pò (魄) originate with his Original Qì (Yuánqì, 元氣), and separate from the physical body at death.

Huǒlù 火路 Fire Path. The regular path of Small Circulation which follows the natural Qì circulation of the body. Also called Shùnxíng (順行, Following the Natural Path).

Huǒqì 火氣 Fire Qì or Post-Heaven Qì. From the Middle Dāntián. Makes the body Yáng.

Huóqì 活氣 Living Qì or Vital Qì. When something is alive, it has Vital Qì.

Jiǎ Xiàdāntián 假下丹田 False Lower Dāntián. Called Qìhǎi (Co-6, 氣海, Qì ocean) in Chinese medicine. Daoists believe that the Lower Dāntián in front of the abdomen is not the Real Dāntián or center of gravity.

Jiǎguān 假觀 Observation of falseness or illusion.

Jiájí 夾脊 Squeeze the Spine. See Língtái (靈臺).

Jiān 堅 Hard or strong.

Jiànggōng 絳宮 Crimson Palace. The space under the heart, or Middle Dāntián. A term often used as an alternative for heart (Xīn, 心). The Middle Dāntián provides you with Post-birth Qì converted from food and air.

Jiāzuò 跏坐 To sit with crossed legs. A special Buddhist meditation term.

Jiéjiā Fūzuò 結跏趺坐 Buddhist term for sitting with crossed legs.

Jiétāi 結胎 Conceive the embryo.

Jiětuō 解脫 Liberate yourself from spiritual bondage.

Jīn, Shào-Fēng 金紹峰 Dr. Yáng, Jwìng-Mǐng's White Crane grandmaster.

Jīndān 金丹 Golden Elixir. Precious Qì.

Jīndān Dàdào 金丹大道 Golden Elixir Large Way. Major Daoist Qìgōng training. The elixir is produced in the body and used to extend life.

Jīndiàn 金殿 Golden Palace. The lungs or brain. Also called Jīnshì (金室).

Jīng 經 Channels or meridians. Twelve organ-related rivers which circulate Qì throughout the body.

Jìng 靜 Calm and silent.

Jīng 精 Essence. The most refined part of anything. What is left after something has been refined and purified. In Chinese medicine, Jīng can mean semen, but it generally refers to the basic substance of the body enlivened by the Qì and Shén.

Jīngliàn 精煉 To refine or purify a liquid to a high quality.

Jīngliáng 精良 Pure and Good. Excellent quality.

Jīngmíng 精明 Keen and clever.

Jīngōng 金公 Golden Male. Original Essence (Yuánjīng, 元精).

Jǐngqì 景氣 Qì scenery or Qì view, a feeling generated in meditation by the Qì.

Jīngqì 精氣 Essence Qì or semen Qì, converted from Original Essence (Yuánjīng, 元精).

Jīngshén 精神 Essence Spirit. Spirit of Vitality, raised by Qì but restrained by Yì (意).

Jīnguān 金關 Golden Gate. Upper Dāntián.

Jīngxì 精細 Pure and Fine. Delicate and painstaking.

Jīngzǐ 精子 Son of Essence. A man's most refined essence. The sperm.

Jìngzuò 靜坐 To sit quietly in meditation.

Jīnniǎo 金鳥 Golden Bird. Original Spirit (Yuánshén, 元神).

Jīnpǐn 金品 Golden Material. Spiritual Embryo.

Jīnquè 金闕 Golden Palace. The space under the heart. The Middle Dāntián.

Jīnshì 金室 Golden Residence. Upper Dāntián or the lungs. Also called Jīndiàn (金殿).

Jīnzhōngzhào 金鐘罩 Golden Bell Cover. A high level of Iron Shirt training.

Jiǔgōng 九宮 Nine Palaces. A Daoist name for the brain.

Jiǔnián Miànbì 九年面壁 Nine years Facing the Wall. The last stage of Xǐsuǐjīng (洗髓經) training for enlightenment or Buddhahood.

Jiūwěi (Co-15) 鳩尾 Wide Pigeon's Tail. An acupuncture cavity at the lower sternum on the Conception Vessel. Called Xīnkǎn (心坎, Heart Pit) by martial society.

Jīxíng 積行 Accumulate good deeds. Doing good things for others.

Jízhōng (Gv-6) 脊中 Middle of the Spine, an acupuncture cavity on the Governing Vessel.

Jùjīng Huìshén 聚精會神 Gathering Jīng to meet Shén. Concentration.

Jūnqiàn 君倩 A Daoist doctor during the Jìn Dynasty (265–420 CE, 晉朝). Credited with creating the Five Animal Sports (Wǔqínxì, 五禽戲) Qìgōng practice.

Kāiqiào 開竅 Opening the tricky gate. Opening the gate of the Upper Dāntián.

Kǎn 坎 Water. One of the Eight Trigrams.

Kǎngōng 坎宮 Kǎn Palace. Qìhǎi (氣海, Qì ocean) or Lower Dāntián (Xià Dāntián, 下丹田).

Kǎn-Lí 坎離 Kǎn represents water and Lí represents fire. Kǎn and Lí means to use water and fire to adjust the body's Yīn and Yáng.

Kāo, Táo 高濤 Dr. Yáng, Jwìng-Mǐng's first Tàijíquán master.

Kōngdòng 崆峒 There are three mountains called Kōngdòng, located in Hénán (河南), Jiāngxī, (江西) and Gānsù (甘肅) provinces.

Kōngguān 空觀 Observation of emptiness.

Kōngqì 空氣 The air is called Kōngqì, which means the Qì in space.

Kǒngzǐ (551–479 BCE) 孔子 Confucius. A Chinese scholar and during the Spring and Autumn Period (722–484 BCE, 春秋) whose philosophy significantly influenced Chinese culture.

Kòuchǐ 扣齒 Biting the teeth.

Kung Fu 功夫 See Gōngfū.

Kūnlún 崑崙

1. Kūnlún Shān (崑崙山) One of the highest mountains in China, located in the west.
2. Another name for Tiāngǔ (天谷, Heavenly Valley).

Lǎma 喇嘛 Tibetan priest.

Lǎodān 老聃 Lǎozi (老子).

Láogōng (P-8) 勞宮 Labor Palace. A cavity on the Pericardium Primary Channel in the center of the palm.

Lǎojūn 老君 Lǎozi (老子). Lǎojūn is the name given by his followers.

Lǎozi (604–531 BCE) 老子 The creator of *Dào Dé Jīng* (道德經) and, therefore, of Daoism (Dàojiā, 道家). Also called Lǐěr (李耳), Lǎodān (老聃), Lǎojūn (老君), or his nickname, Bóyáng (伯陽).

Lè 樂 Joy or happiness.

Léi 雷 Thunder.

Lěng 冷 Cold.

Lí 離 Fire. One of the Eight Trigrams (Bāguà, 八卦).

Lì 立 To establish.

Lǐ, Mào-Chīng 李茂清 Dr. Yáng, Jwìng-Mǐng's Long Fist master.

Lǐ, Shí-Zhēn (1518–1593 CE) 李時珍 A famous doctor and Qìgōng master who wrote a book about the eight Qì vessels, titled *Qíjīng Bāmài Kǎo* (奇經八脈考, *The Study of Strange Meridians and Eight Vessels*) in the 16th century.

Lìan 練（煉） To refine, train, or discipline.

Lìanjǐ 煉己 Train the self. Self-discipline.

Lìanjīng Huàqì 煉精化氣 To refine the Essence and convert it into Qì. A Qìgōng training process.

Lìanqì 煉氣 To train and refine. Daoist training to strengthen and increase Qì.

Lìanqì Huàshén 煉氣化神 To refine the Qì to nourish the spirit. Qìgōng training to lead Qì to nourish the brain and Shén (神, spirit).

Lìanqì Shēnghuá 煉氣昇華 To train the Qì and sublimate it. Xǐsuǐjīng (洗髓經) training to lead Qì to the Huángtíng (黃庭) or the brain.

Lìanshēn 煉身 To train the body.

Lìanshén 煉神 To train the spirit. To refine, strengthen, and focus the Shén.

Lìanshén Fǎnxū 煉神返虛 To train the spirit to return to nothingness, to attain freedom from emotional bondage. An advanced stage of enlightenment and Buddhahood training to lead the spirit to separate from the body.

Lìanshén Lìǎoxìng 煉神了性 To refine the spirit and end human nature. The final stage of enlightenment training where you keep your emotions neutral, undisturbed by human nature.

Lìanyào 煉藥 Refine or purify the herb (Qì).

Líang (502–557 CE) 梁 A Chinese dynasty.

Líang 涼 Cool.

Líanquán (Co-23) 廉泉 Modesty's Spring. An acupuncture cavity on the Conception Vessel.

Líǎo 了 The end or completion of the cultivation.

Líǎowù 了悟 The end of comprehension. Enlightenment.

Lǐěr 李耳 Lǎozi (老子).

Lígōng 離宮 Lí Palace. The heart. Lí means fire in the Eight Trigrams.

Líng 靈

1. The spirit of being, which acts upon others. Líng only exists in highly spiritual animals such as humans and apes. It represents an emotional comprehension and understanding. When you are alive, it is your intelligence and wisdom. When you die, it is the spirit of the ghost. Líng also means divine or supernatural. Together with Shén (Língshén, 靈神) it means supernatural spirit. Qì is the source which nourishes it, called Língqì (靈氣), meaning supernatural energy, power, or force.

2. Supernatural Shén is called Líng. Líng describes someone who is sharp, clever, nimble, and able to quickly empathize with others. Líng can also be a supernatural psychic capability which allows you to communicate with nature or other spiritual beings. Often, it means Divine Inspiration which allows you to comprehend and understand changes or variations in nature.

Língguāng 靈光 Supernatural divine light.

Língguǐ 靈鬼 Spiritual ghost.

Línghún 靈魂 Spiritual soul.

Língshān 靈山 Spiritual Mountain. A Buddhist term equivalent to the Spiritual Valley (Shéngǔ, 神谷) of the Daoists.

Língshén 靈神 Supernatural spirit or Divine.

Língtāi 靈胎 Spiritual embryo. See Shéntāi 神胎.

Língtái 靈臺 Spiritual Platform.

1. Acupuncture cavity (Gv-10) on the Governing Vessel. Called Jiájí (夾脊, Squeeze the Spine) by Daoists, Mìngmén (命門, Life Door) by martial arts society. Also known as Lùlúguān (轆轤關, Windlass Gate).

2. Another name for Spiritual Valley (Shéngǔ, 神谷).

Líú 流 Flow.

Líùhé Bāfǎ 六合八法 Six Combinations Eight Methods. One of the Chinese internal martial arts. Its techniques combine Tàijíquán (太極拳), Xíngyìquán (形意拳), and Bāguàzhǎng (八卦掌). This style was reportedly created by Chén, Bó (陳博) during the Sòng Dynasty (960–1280 CE, 宋朝).

Líùzǔ Shuō Chuánfǎ 六祖說傳法 Sixth Ancestor Disrupting the Passed-Down Method. The sixth ancestor of Chán (禪), Huìnéng (慧能), who lived during the Táng Dynasty (713–907 CE, 唐朝), changed some of the meditation methods and philosophy and was long considered a traitor. Because of this, Chán divided into Northern and Southern styles.

Lìzhì 立志 To establish or build strong willpower.

Lóng 龍 Dragon.

Lónghǔ Jiāogòu 龍虎交媾 Intercourse of dragon and tiger. Implies the interaction of Yīn and Yáng.

Lóngmén (M-CA-24) 龍門 Dragon Gate. Acupuncture cavity in the groin area, in the miscellaneous category. Also called Xiàyīn (下陰, Low Yīn).

Lóngyān 龍煙 The name of the liver's spirit, which is associated with the eyes. When the liver is healthy, the eyes are bright and sharp.

Lóngyào 龍曜 The name of the gall bladder's spirit, which is associated with the liver.

Lùchē 鹿車 Deer Vehicle. The way of leading Qì from Jiájí (夾脊) to Yùzhěn (玉枕) should be fast like a deer. See also Sānchē (三車, Three Vehicles).

Lùlúguān 轆轤關 Windlass Gate. A cavity located at the center of the back, from where the shoulders turn like a windlass. See Língtái (Gv-10) (靈臺).

Luò 絡 The small Qì channels which branch out from the primary ones, and which connect to the skin and bone marrow.

Mǎ 馬 Horse.

Mài 脈 Vessel or Qì Channel. The Eight Vessels involved with transporting, storing, and regulating Qì.

Mencius (372–289 BCE, Mèngzǐ) 孟子 A famous follower of Confucius during the Chinese Warring States Period (403–222 BCE, Zhànguó, 戰國).

Mìhù 密戶 Concealed Door. See Mìngmén (Gv-4, 命門), definition 1.

Mìzōng 密宗（秘宗） Secret style. Chinese term for Tibetan Qìgōng because it is kept secret from outsiders.

Mián 綿 Soft.

Miànbì 面壁 Face the wall.

Mìng 命 Life. Refers to the physical body.

Míngtiāngǔ 鳴天鼓 To Beat the Heavenly Drum. One of the Eight Pieces of Brocade (Bāduànjǐn, 八段錦) exercises in which one taps the head, which is regarded as heaven, with the fingertips.

Míngxīn Jiànxìng 明心見性 Understand your Xīn to see your human nature.

Mìngmén 命門 Life Door.

1. Acupuncture cavity (Gv-4) on the Governing Vessel on the lower back (between L2 and L3). Also called Bìhù (閉戶, Closed Door) and Mìhù (密戶, Concealed Door).

2. In Martial society, term for Língtái (Gv-10) (靈臺) area between the shoulder blades.

3. In Qìgōng society, can mean the two kidneys.

4. In Daoist society, often means navel or Qìhǎi (Co-6, 氣海), and implies the Lower Dāntián.

Míngtáng 明堂 The space between the two eyebrows and one inch inward.

Mǔ 母 Mother.

Mùmǔ 木母 Wood Mother. Refers to the liver.

Mǔzǐ Xiànghé 母子相合 Mutual Harmonization of Mother and Son. Qì is referred to as mother and the spirit as the son. When the spirit is led down to unite with the Qì at the Real Lower Dāntián, it is called Mǔzǐ Xiànghé, the state of Embryonic Breathing.

Mǔzǐ Xiāngyī 母子相依 Mutual Dependence of Son and Mother.

Nǎohù (Gv-17) 腦戶 Brain's Household. An acupuncture cavity on the Governing Vessel. Also see Yùzhěn (玉枕).

Nèidān 內丹 Internal Elixir. A form of Qìgong in which Qì (elixir) is built up in the body and spread out to the limbs.

Nèigōng 內功 Internal Gōngfū. All training in which the mind leads the circulation of Qì, either for manifestation or enlightenment.

Nèiqì 內氣 Lower Level Qì, also called Inner Qì (Xiàcéngqì, 下層氣).

Nèishèn 內腎 Internal Kidneys. In Chinese medicine and Qìgōng, the real Kidneys. Wàishèn (外腎, External Kidneys) refers to the testicles.

Nèishì Gōngfū 內視功夫 To look inside to determine your state of health and the condition of your Qì.

Nì Fùhūxī 逆腹呼吸 Reverse Abdominal Breathing. Also called Fǎn Fùhūxī (反腹呼吸) or Daoist Breathing (Dàojiā Hūxī, 道家呼吸).

Niàn 念 Idea. The thoughts which linger in your mind and are hard to get rid of.

Níng 凝 To concentrate, condense, refine, focus, and strengthen.

Níngshén 凝神 To condense or focus the spirit. Once you can keep your spirit in one place, you condense it into a tiny spot to make it stronger.

Niúchē 牛車 Bull Vehicle. When leading the Qì from Yùzhěn (玉枕) to Níwán (泥丸, Bǎihuì), the Qì movement should be strong as a bull. See also Sānchē (三車, Three Vehicles).

Niúláng 牛郎 Cowherd. See Niúlángzhīnǚ (牛郎織女).

Niúlángzhīnǚ 牛郎織女 A Chinese romantic legend in which the Cowherd (Niúláng, 牛郎) falls in love with the Weaving Lady (Zhīnǚ, 織女), but their union is forbidden. They are kept apart by the River of Heaven and allowed to meet only once a year, when the Magpie Bridge connects the two sides of the river. See also Quèqiáo (鵲橋).

Níwán 泥丸 A Daoist name for the crown, brain, or Upper Dāntián.

Níwángōng 泥丸宮 Mud Pill Palace. Qìgōng term for the brain or Upper Dāntián. Mud pills refer to the pineal and pituitary glands.

Nìxíng 逆行 Reversed Path. See Fēnglù (風路, Wind Path).

Nù 怒 Anger.

Nuǎn 暖 Warm.

Péng, Zǔ 彭祖 A legendary Qìgōng practitioner during the period of Emperor Yáo (2356–2255 BCE, 堯), who was said to have lived for 800 years.

Pénglái Xiāndǎo 蓬萊仙島 Pénglái Immortal Island. An island in the East Sea where the immortals resided, according to Chinese legend.

Pìn 牝 Female Animals, or Mothers.

Píng 平 Peace and harmony.

Píngcháng Hūxī 平常呼吸 Normal regular breathing.

Pò 魄 Vigorous life force. The Po is considered to be the inferior animal soul. It is the sentient animal life which is an innate part of the body. At death, it returns to the earth with the rest of the body. When someone is in high spirits and gets vigorously involved in some activity it is said he has Pòlì (魄力), which means he has vigorous strength or power.

Qì 氣 The general definition of Qì is universal energy, including heat, light, and electromagnetic energy. A narrower definition refers to the energy circulating in human or animal bodies. A current popular model is that Qì in the body is bioelectricity.

Qì Xuě 氣血 Qì Blood. According to Chinese medicine, Qì and blood cannot be separated, and the two words are commonly used together.

Qiángjiān (Gv-18) 強間 Between Strength. Acupuncture cavity on the Governing Vessel located, along with Tiānmù (天目), at the exit of the Spiritual Valley.

Qìànmó 氣按摩 Qì massage. One of the high levels of massage techniques in which a massage doctor uses his own Qì to remove Qì stagnation in the patient's body. Also called Wàiqì Liáofǎ (外氣療法), which means "healing with external Qì."

Qiānshàn 遷善 Shift into goodness. Change from bad to good.

Qiào 竅 The changes or variations of nature.

Qiàomén 竅門 A secret way of learning and practicing.

Qìgōng (Chì Kūng) 氣功 Gōng (功) means Gōngfū (功夫). Qìgōng is the study and training of Qì.

Qìhǎi (Co-6) 氣海 Qì Ocean. An acupuncture cavity on the Conception Vessel, about two inches below the navel. See also Jiǎ Xiàdāntián (假下丹田).

Qìhuàlùn 氣化論 *Theory of Variations of Qì*. An ancient book on changes in natural energy.

Qǐhuǒ 起火 To start the fire. Build up Qì at the Lower Dāntián (Xià Dāntián, 下丹田).

Qíjīng 奇經 Extraordinary Vessels or Strange Meridians. Qì vessels that function like reservoirs, regulating the distribution and circulation of Qì in the body.

Qíjīng Bāmài 奇經八脈 Strange Channels Eight Vessels. The Eight Extraordinary Vessels. Called strange because they are not well understood, and some do not exist in pairs.

Qín and Hàn Dynasties (255 BCE–223 CE) 秦、漢 Two dynasties in Chinese history.

Qīng 輕 Light.

Qīng Dynasty (1644–1912 CE) 清朝 The last Chinese dynasty.

Qīngchéng 青城 A mountain in Sìchuān province (四川省).

Qīngxiūpài 清修派 Peaceful Cultivation Style. A branch of Daoist Qìgōng.

Qínná (Chín Ná) 擒拿 Seize Control. Gōngfū which emphasizes grabbing techniques to control the opponent's joints, while attacking certain acupuncture cavities. One of the four main fighting categories in Chinese martial arts. The four categories are kicking (Tī, 踢), striking (Dǎ, 打), wrestling (Shuāi, 摔), and controlling (Qínná, 擒拿). Qínná specializes in controlling the enemy through misplacing the joint (Cuògǔ, 錯骨), dividing the muscle/tendon (Fēnjīn, 分筋), sealing the breath (Bìqì, 閉氣), and cavity press (Diǎnxuè, 點穴).

Qīqíng Líuyù 七情六慾 The seven passions and six desires. The seven passions are happiness (Xǐ, 喜), anger (Nù, 怒), sorrow (Āi, 哀), joy (Lè, 樂), love (Ài, 愛), hate (Hèn, 恨), and desire (Yù, 慾). The six desires are the six sensory pleasures derived from the eyes, ears, nose, tongue, body, and mind.

Qìshì 氣勢 Shi means the way something looks or feels. Qìshì is the feeling of Qì as it expresses itself. For example, the spiritual state or morale of an army is called its energy state.

Quèqiáo 鵲橋 Magpie bridge. Either of two methods of connecting the Conception and Governing Vessels. The tongue is the Upper Magpie Bridge (Shàng Quèqiáo, 上鵲橋), while the Huìyīn is the Lower Magpie Bridge (Xià Quèqiáo, 下鵲橋). See also Niúlángzhīnǚ (牛郎織女).

Qūjiāng 曲江 Curved Rivers. Intestines, Real Lower Dāntián.

Rè 熱 Hot.

Rèqì 熱氣 Heat Qì.

Rén 仁 Humanity, kindness, or benevolence. When Dào and Dé are applied in human society, it is benevolence (Rén, 仁) and righteousness (Yì, 義).

Rén 人 Person or Mankind. Along with Heaven (Tiān, 天) and Earth (Dì, 地), one of the Three Powers (Sāncái, 三才).

Rènmài 任脈 Conception Vessel. One of the Eight Extraordinary Vessels.

Rénqì 人氣 Human Qì.

Rénshì 人事 Human Relations. Human events, activities, and relationships.

Rénzhōng (Gv-26) 人中 Acupuncture cavity on the Governing Vessel at the Philtrum over the upper lip. Also called Shuǐgōu (水溝), meaning water ditch.

Ruǎn 軟 Soft.

Rùdào 入道 Enter the Dào. Means getting involved in Daoist study and practice.

Rùdìng 入定 Enter the state of mental and physical steadiness.

Rùguān 入觀 Enter the observation. The mind is calm and clear, which allows you to enter a profound state of observation and analysis.

Rújiā 儒家 Confucian family. Followers of Confucian precepts.

Rùjǐng 入景 Enter the scenery. Various phenomena one may experience in profound meditation.

Rùmó 入魔 Enter the devil. Falling into fantasy or illusion due to wrong feeling or perception.

Ruòcún 若存 As if it were existing.

Sānbǎo 三寶 Three Treasures. Refers to Jīng (Essence, 精), Qì (energy, 氣), and Shén (spirit, 神). Also called Sānběn (三本, Three Foundations) and Sānyuán (三元, Three Origins).

Sānběn 三本 See Sānbǎo (三寶).

Sāncái 三才 Three Powers. Refers to Heaven (Tiān, 天), Earth (Dì, 地), and Humanity (Rén, 人).

Sānchē 三車 Three Vehicles. Three ways of leading Qì in the course of Small Circulation practice: Yángchē (羊車, Sheep vehicle), Lùchē (鹿車, Deer Vehicle), and Niúchē (牛車, Bull Vehicle).

Sàngōng 散功 Energy Dispersion. Premature degeneration of the body where Qì cannot effectively energize it, generally caused by excessive training.

Sānguān 三關 Three Gates in Small Circulation. They are Wěilǘ (尾閭), Jiájí (夾脊), and Yùzhěn (玉枕).

Sānguān 三觀 Three observations in Buddhist meditation: 1. Observing Emptiness (Kōngguān, 空觀)—to observe the emptiness of all natural laws and events, 2. Observing Falseness (Jiǎguān, 假觀)—to observe the falseness of all natural laws, 3. Observing Double Reflections (Zhōngguān, 中觀)—to observe between the two.

Sānhuā Jùdǐng 三花聚頂 Three flowers reach the top. One of the final goals of Qìgōng, whereby the Three Treasures are led to the top of the body to nourish the spirit at the Upper Dāntián.

Sānjiào 三教 Three Schools. Refers to Buddhism (Fójiā, 佛家), Daoism (Dàojiā, 道家), and Confucianism (Rújiā, 儒家).

Sānjiè 三界 Three Worlds. 1. The world of desires, 2. The world of colors (material world), 3. The world of no color (extreme calmness through meditation).

Sānmèiyìn 三昧印 See Sānmódì (三摩地).

Sānmódì 三摩地 From Sanskrit "Samadhi,"a special Indian Buddhist term which means steadiness of the mind and body (Dìng, 定). Also called Sānmèiyìn (三昧印). The Buddhist name for Small Circulation. Also called Yīn-Yáng Xúnhuán Yī Xiǎozhōutiān, (陰陽循環一小周天, Yīn-Yáng Circulation Small Heavenly Cycle) in Daoist society.

Sānnián Bǔrǔ 三年哺乳 Three years of nursing.

Sānqì Guīyuán 三氣歸元 The three Qì (essence, Qì, and spirit) return to their origins.

Sānyīnjiāo (Sp-6) 三陰交 Three Yīn Junction. Acupuncture cavity on the spleen channel. The junction of the three Yīn channels, namely spleen, liver, and kidneys.

Sānyuán 三元 See Sānbǎo (三寶).

Sè 澀 Harsh.

Sēngbīng 僧兵 Monk Soldiers. Shàolín martial monks.

Shàngcéngqì 上層氣 Upper Level Qì. Also called Wàiqì (c, External Qì).

Shàng Dāntián 上丹田 Upper Dāntián in the brain at the Third Eye, the residence of Shén.

Shàng Dāntián Hūxī 上丹田呼吸 Upper Dāntián Breathing. Spiritual Breathing (Shénxí, 神息).

Shàng Quèqiáo 上鵲橋 See Quèqiáo (鵲橋).

Shàngè 上顎 Palate of the mouth.

Shānzhōng (Co-17) 膻中 The central area between the nipples. Some Qìgōng practitioners consider Shānzhōng to be the Middle Dāntián. Its acupuncture name is Penetrating Odor.

Shàolín 少林 Young Woods. A Buddhist temple in Hénán, famous for its martial arts.

Shèjīng 攝精 Absorb the essence.

Shēn 深 Deep.

Shén 神 Spirit.

1. The conscious functioning of mind and thought, residing at the Upper Dāntián (Shàng Dāntián, 上丹田).

2. When a spirit becomes divine, it is called Shén.

Shénbù Shǒushè 神不守舍 The Spirit is not kept at its Residence.

Shēngmén 生門 Life Door. Implies navel.

Shēngmìng Zhīběn 生命之本 The root of our lives.

Shēngqì 生氣 To produce Qì.

Shèngtāi 聖胎 Holy embryo. See Shéntāi (神胎).

Shéngǔ 神谷 Spirit Valley. See Tiāngǔ (天谷, Heavenly Valley).

Shénguī 神龜 Spiritual Turtle.

Shénhún 神魂 The spirit of a dying person, between Shén and Hún.

Shénjiāo 神交 Spiritual communication.

Shénmíng 神明 Spiritually divine or enlightened beings.

Shénqì Xiànghé 神氣相合 Mutual Harmony or Unification of Shén and Qì. The final regulating of Shén.

Shènshū (B-23) 腎俞 Kidney's Admittance or Kidney Hollow. Two acupuncture cavities on the bladder channels. They are the immediate entrance and exit of kidney Qì to the outside through the back.

Shéntāi 神胎 Spiritual embryo. Also called Língtāi (靈胎, Spiritual embryo), Shèngtāi (聖胎, Holy embryo), Shényīng (神嬰, Spiritual baby), or Yīngér (嬰兒).

Shénxí 神息 Spirit breathing. The stage of Qìgōng training where the spirit is coordinated with the breathing.

Shénxí Xiāngyī 神息相依 Mutual Dependence of Spirit and Breathing.

Shénxiān 神仙 Xiān originates with Shén, sometimes called Shénxían, or immortal spirit.

Shēnxīn Pínghéng 身心平衡 Body and heart/mind are balanced.

Shényīng 神嬰 Spiritual baby. See Shéntāi 神胎.

Shénzhì 神志 The mind generates the will, which keeps the Shén firm. The Chinese commonly write Shén and Zhì (will) together as Shénzhì, because they are so closely related.

Shénzhì Bùqīng 神志不清 The spirit and the will (generated from Yì) are not clear. The mind is confused and unsteady.

Shēnzhù (Gv-12) 身柱 Body Pillar. An acupuncture cavity on the Governing Vessel.

Shíèr Dìzhī 十二地支 The Twelve Terrestrial Branches, the traditional Chinese divisions of the day: Zǐ (子, 11 pm to 1 am, Rat), Chǒu (丑, 1 to 3 am, Ox), Yīn (寅, 3 to 5 am, Tiger), Mǎo (卯, 5 to 7 am, Hare), Chén (辰, 7 to 9 am, Dragon), Yǐ (巳, 9 to 11 am, Snake), Wǔ (午, 11 am to 1 pm, Horse), Wèi (未, 1 to 3 pm, Sheep), Shēn (申, 3 to 5 pm, Monkey), Qiú (酉, 5 to 7 pm, Cock), Shù (戌, 7 to 9 pm, Dog) and Hài (亥, 9 to 11 pm, Boar).

Shíèrjīng 十二經 The Twelve Primary Qì Channels in Chinese medicine.

Shíèrjīng Luò 十二經絡 The Twelve Primary Qì Channels and Their Branches.

Shíèrshí 十二時 Twelve Timings. See Shíèr Dìzhī (十二地支).

Shìjiè 世界 The world.

Shíqīzhūixià (M-BW-25) 十七椎下 An acupuncture cavity located below the 17th vertebra.

Shítiāngān 十天干 The Ten Celestial Stems. The Chinese use The Ten Celestial Stems together with the Twelve Terrestrial Branches (Shíèr Dìzhī, 十二地支) to form a cycle of sixty. From this, they distinguish the different natural cycles of the year. The Ten Celestial Stems are: Jiǎ (甲), Yǐ (乙), Bǐng (丙), Dīng (丁), Wù (戊), Jǐ (己), Gīng (庚), Xīn (辛), Rèn (壬), and Guǐ (癸).

Shíyuè Huáitāi 十月懷胎 Ten months of pregnancy. The stage in Yìjīnjīng training during which the spiritual embryo is nourished.

Shǒu 守 To keep and protect.

Shǒu Juéyīn Xīnbāoluòjīng 手厥陰心包絡經 Arm Absolute Yīn Pericardium Primary Qì Channel. One of the twelve primary Qì channels.

Shǒu Shàoyáng Sānjiāojīng 手少陽三焦經 Arm Lesser Yáng Triple Burner Primary Qì Channel. One of the twelve primary Qì channels.

Shǒu Shàoyīn Xīnjīng 手少陰心經 Arm Lesser Yīn Heart Primary Qì Channel. One of the twelve primary Qì channels.

Shǒushén 守神 To focus the mind on the spirit. Qìgōng meditation training.

Shǒu Tàiyáng Xiǎochángjīng 手太陽小腸經 Arm Greater Yáng Small Intestine Primary Qì Channel. One of the twelve primary Qì channels.

Shǒu Tàiyīn Fèijīng 手太陰肺經 Arm Greater Yīn Lung Primary Qì Channel. One of the twelve primary Qì channels.

Shǒu Yángmíng Dàchángjīng 手陽明大腸經 Arm Yáng Brightness Large Intestine Primary Qì Channel. One of the twelve primary Qì channels.

Shǒuyìn 手印 Hand stamp. Hand forms that assist meditation. "Stamp" here means to press.

Shūtóu 梳頭 Combing the Hair. A Qìgōng practice following a motion similar to sweeping back the hair.

Shuāngxiū 雙修 Dual Cultivation. A Qìgōng training method in which Qì is exchanged with a partner to balance the Qì of both. It also means dual cultivation of the body and the spirit.

Shuāngzhào 雙照 The observation of double reflections, or relative comparison. A Buddhist terminology which implies comparison with the opposite position.

Shuǐgōu 水溝 Water Ditch. Another name for Rénzhōng (Gv-26, 人中) acupuncture cavity.

Shuǐhuǒ Zhījì 水火之際 The Junction of Water and Fire. Wěilǘ (尾閭, tailbone) is where Qì enters either the Water Path or Fire Path. It is called Chángqiáng (Gv-1, 長強, long strength) in acupuncture.

Shuǐlù 水路 Water Path. Path in which Qì is led up through the Thrusting Vessel to the brain for nourishment. Can calm down physical excitement. Also the path of spiritual enlightenment cultivation.

Shuǐqì 水氣 Water Qì. Qì created from Original Essence, which can calm the body.

Shùnxíng 順行 Following the Natural Path. See Huǒlù (火路, Fire Path).

Sìdà 四大 Four Larges: Earth (Dì, 地), Water (Shuǐ, 水), Fire (Huǒ, 火), and Air/Wind (Fēng, 風).

Sìdà Jiēkōng 四大皆空 Four Larges are Empty. A stage of Buddhist training where all four elements (Earth, Water, Fire, and Air) are absent from the mind, so that one is completely indifferent to worldly temptations.

Sǐqì 死氣 Dead Qì. The Qì remaining in a dead body. Also called ghost Qì (Guǐqì, 鬼氣).

Sìzìjué 四字訣 Four Secret Words: Cuō (撮, condensing or concentrating), Dǐ (抵, pressing up), Bì (閉, closing) and Xī (吸, drawing in).

Sòng and Yuán Dynasties (960–1367 CE) 宋、元 Two dynasties in Chinese history.

Suànmìngshī 算命師 Calculate Life Teacher. A fortune teller who calculates your future and destiny.

Suǐqì 髓氣 Marrow Qì.

Tǎ 塔 Pagoda.

T'ai Ch'i Chuan 太極拳 See Tàijíquán.

Tàijí 太極 Grand Ultimate. The invisible force which causes Wújí (無極, no extremity) to derive into Yīn and Yáng, and into which Yīn and Yáng resolve. Also called Xuánpìn (玄牝).

Tàijíquán 太極拳 Grand Ultimate Fist. A Chinese internal martial style based on the theory of Tàijí.

Táipěi Xiàn 台北縣 A county in the north of Táiwān.

Táiwān 台灣 An island to the southeast of mainland China. Also called Formosa.

Táiwān University 台灣大學 A well known university in Táipěi (Táiběi).

Tāixí 胎息 Embryonic Breathing. A Qìgōng breathing technique which stores Qì in the Lower Real Dāntián.

Tāixí Jìngzuò 胎息静坐 Embryonic Breathing Meditation.

Tàixū 太虛 Grand Emptiness. The great nature of the universe (Dào, 道).

Tàizǔquán 太祖拳 A southern style of Chinese external martial arts.

Tamkang (Dànjiāng) 淡江 A university in Táiwān.

Táng Dynasty (713–907 CE) 唐朝 One of the Chinese dynasties.

Tàngyǎn 燙眼 Iron the Eyes. A Qìgōng practice which keeps the eyes in a healthy condition.

Tiān 天 Heaven or Sky. Along with Earth (Dì, 地) and Man (Rén, 人), one of the Three Powers (Sāncái, 三才). In ancient China, people believed Heaven to be the most powerful force in the universe.

Tiānchíshuǐ 天池水 Heavenly Water. Saliva.

Tiāndì 天地 Heaven and Earth. Qìgōng term for the physical body.

Tiāngǔ 天谷 Heavenly Valley. The space between the two hemispheres of the brain. It has many other names, such as Spiritual Valley (Shéngǔ, 神谷), Yellow Yard (Huángtíng, 黄庭), Mud Pill Palace (Níwángōng, 泥丸宫) or Kūnlún (崑崙).

Tiānhéshuǐ Nìliú 天河水逆流 Reversed Flow of the Heavenly River Water. To lead Qì up from Huìyīn (Co-1, 會陰) to Bǎihuì (Gv-20, 百會).

Tiānlínggài 天靈蓋 Heavenly Spiritual Cover. See Bǎihuì (Gv-20, 百會).

Tiānmù 天目 Heaven Eye. Called Yìntáng (M-HN-3, 印堂, Seal Hall) in acupuncture, and the "Third Eye" by Western society. Also called Tiāntíng (天庭, Heavenly Yard), Tiānyǎn (天眼, Heaven Eye), and Yùmén (玉門, Jade Gate). The Chinese believe that prior to our evolution into humans, our race possessed an additional sense organ in our forehead.

This third eye provided a means of spiritual communication between one another, and with the natural world. As we evolved and developed means to protect ourselves from the environment, and as societies became more complex and human vices developed, this third eye gradually closed and disappeared.

Tiānqì 天氣 Heaven Qì. Commonly refers to the weather, which is governed by Heaven Qì.

Tiānrén Héyī 天人合一 Heaven and Man Unified as One. A high level of Qìgōng meditation in which one can communicate with the Qì of Heaven.

Tiānshí 天時 Heavenly timing. The repeated natural cycles generated by the heavens, such as seasons, months, days, and hours.

Tiānshān 天山 Sky Mountain. The name of a mountain in Xīnjiāng province (新疆省).

Tiāntíng 天庭 Heavenly Yard. See Tiānmù (天目).

Tiāntū (Co-22) 天突 Heaven's Prominence. Acupuncture cavity on the Conception Vessel. This cavity connects with the Dàzhuī cavity (Gv-14, 大椎) on the back, and they are regarded as a pair of corresponding cavities.

Tiānyǎn 天眼 Heaven Eye. See Tiānmù (天目).

Tiáo 調 A gradual regulating process, resulting in that which is regulated achieving harmony with others.

Tiáoqì 調氣 To regulate the Qì.

Tiáoshén 調神 To regulate the spirit.

Tiáoshēn 調身 To regulate the body.

Tiáoxí 調息 To regulate the breathing.

Tiáoxīn 調心 To regulate the Emotional Mind.

Tiěbùshān 鐵布衫 Iron shirt. Gōngfū training which toughens the body externally and internally.

Tiěshāzhǎng 鐵砂掌 Iron Sand Palm. A special martial arts conditioning for the palms.

Tǐxí 體息 Body Breathing. Also called Skin Breathing (Fūxí, 膚息). This Qìgōng breathing technique enables you to lead Qì to the skin surface, to strengthen Guardian Qì.

Tōngsānguān 通三關 Pass through Three Gates. The Three gates are Wěilǘ (尾閭), Jiájí (夾脊), and Yùzhěn (玉枕).

Tuīná 推拿 To push and grab. Chinese massage for healing and treating injuries.

Tǔnà 吐納 Qìgōng is commonly called Tǔnà, which means to "utter and admit." This implies expelling and admitting the air through the nose in respiration.

Tuóyuè 槖籥 Bellows. A tube used to fan the fire in a furnace.

Wàidān 外丹 External Elixir. External Qìgōng exercises to build up Qì in the limbs and lead it into the center of the body for nourishment.

Wàijiā 外家 External Family. Those schools which practice external styles of Chinese martial arts.

Wàiqì 外氣 External Qì. Also called Upper Level Qì (Shàngcéngqì, 上層氣).

Wàiqì Líáofǎ 外氣療法 External Qì Healing. See Qìànmó (氣按摩).

Wàishèn 外腎 External Kidneys. Chinese define the testicles or ovaries as "External kidneys," as opposed to "Internal kidneys" (Nèishèn, 內腎), which are the kidneys defined by Western medicine.

Wǎnzhuǎn 宛轉 Soft, gradual, and gentle.

Wěilǘ 尾閭 Coccyx. See Chángqiáng (Gv-1, 長強).

Wèiqì 衛氣 Guardian Qì or Protective Qì. The Qì at the surface of the body forms a shield to protect the body from negative external influences such as cold.

Wògù 握固 To hold and firm.

Wǔ 午 Noon (11 am to 1 pm). See Shíèr Dìzhī (十二地支) and Zǐwǔ Líúzhù 子午流注.

Wǔdāng Mountain 武當山 Located in Húběi province (湖北省).

Wújí 無極 No Extremity. The state of undifferentiated emptiness before beginning.

Wúniàn 無念 The mind of no mind, or the thought of no thought.

Wǔqì Cháoyuán 五氣朝元 Five Qì Return to their Origins. When Qì has been regulated to its normal original level in the five Yīn organs, it is called Wǔqì Cháoyuán. The five internal organs are the heart, lungs, liver, spleen, and kidneys.

Wǔqínxì 五禽戲 Five Animal Sports. A set of medical Qìgōng practice created by Jūnqiàn (君倩) during the Jìn Dynasty (265–420 CE, 晉朝). It imitates the movements of the tiger, deer, bear, ape, and bird. Others say it was created by Dr. Huátuó (華佗).

Wǔshù 武術 Martial Techniques. A common name for Chinese martial arts. Many other terms are used, including Wǔyì (武藝, martial arts), Wǔgōng (武功, martial Gōngfū), Guóshù (國術, national techniques) and Gōngfū (功夫, energy-time). Because Wǔshù has been modified in mainland China over recent decades into gymnastic martial performance, many traditional Chinese martial artists have given up this name, to avoid confusing modern Wǔshù with traditional Wǔshù. Recently, mainland China has attempted to bring modern Wǔshù back to its traditional roots and practice.

Wǔtiáo 五調 Five regulating methods in Qìgōng practice, namely regulating the body, the breathing, the mind, the Qì, and the spirit.

Wútiáo Értiáo 無調而調 The regulating of no regulating. All actions are so natural that no more regulating is necessary.

Wúwéi 無為 Doing Nothing. Regulating without regulating.

Wúxīn 無心 When there is no Emotional Mind generated, it is called Wúxīn.

Wǔxīn Hūxī 五心呼吸 A Nèidān Qìgōng practice in which one uses the mind in coordination with breathing to lead Qì to the center of the palms, feet, and head.

Wǔxíng 五行 Five Elements. Metal (Jīn, 金, Lungs, Fall), Wood (Mù, 木, Liver, Spring), Water (Shuǐ, 水, Kidneys, Winter), Fire (Huǒ, 火, Heart, Summer), and Earth (Tǔ, 土, Spleen, Four Seasons).

Wùxìng 悟性 To comprehend the temperament. One requirement for spiritual cultivation.

Wùzhēn 悟真 To comprehend the truth. Implies reaching spiritual enlightenment.

Xí 息 Breathing.

Xǐ 喜 Joy, delight, and happiness.

Xī 吸 To draw in or to suck in. Leading Qì up the spine together with inhalation.

Xì 細 Slender.

Xià Dāntián 下丹田 Lower Elixir Field. See also Xià Zhēndāntián (下真丹田, Real Lower Elixir Field) and Jiǎ Xiàdāntián (假下丹田, False Lower Elixir Field).

Xià Quèqiáo 下鵲橋 See Quèqiáo (鵲橋).

Xià Zhēndāntián 下真丹田 Real Lower Elixir Field, or the second brain. Called the Enteric Nervous System in current Western medical science.

Xiān 仙 An Immortal. One who has attained enlightenment or Buddhahood and whose spirit can separate from and return to his physical body at will.

Xiānrén 仙人 Those who have reached spiritual immortality or enlightenment.

Xiāntāi 仙胎 Immortal Embryo.

Xiāntiānqì 先天氣 Pre-birth Qì or Pre-Heaven Qì. Also called Dāntiānqì (丹田氣). The Qì which is converted from Original Essence and stored in the Lower Dāntián. Considered to be Water Qì, it calms the body.

Xiāntiān Zhīzhēn 先天之真 Pre-Heaven Truth. The truthful mind before birth.

Xiào 孝 Filial Piety.

Xiǎo Dǐnglú 小鼎爐 Small Tripod and Furnace. Huángtíng (黃庭) is a tripod, while the Real Lower Dāntián is a furnace.

Xiǎotōng 小通 Small smoothness. The smooth circulation of Qì.

Xiǎozhōutiān 小周天 Small Cyclic Heaven or Small Circulation. Called Microcosmic Orbit in Yoga, or Turning the Wheel of Natural Law (Zhuǎnfǎlún, 轉法輪) by Buddhist society. A Nèidān Qìgōng (內丹氣功) training in which Qì is generated at the Dāntián (丹田) and then moved through the Conception and Governing Vessels.

Xiǎozhōutiān Jìngzuò 小周天靜坐 Small Circulation Meditation. See Xiǎozhōutiān (小周天).

Xiàyīn 下陰 Low Yīn. The groin. Called Lóngmén (M-CA-24, 龍門, Dragon Gate) in Chinese medicine.

Xiè 洩 Releasing.

Xíhuǒ 熄火 Cease the fire.

Xǐliǎn 洗臉 Washing the face. A practice in which both hands brush downward on the face.

Xīn 心 Heart. The mind generated from emotional disturbance, desire.

Xìn 信 Trust.

Xìng 性 Human nature or temperament.

Xínggōng 行功 To carry out the Gōng. To train.

Xìngmìng Shuāngxiū 性命雙修 Dual Cultivation of Human Nature and Life. Originally a Buddhist, though now predominantly a Daoist, approach to Qìgōng, it emphasizes the cultivation of both spirituality and the physical body.

Xíngqì 行氣 Transporting or circulating the Qì.

Xíngyìquán (Xíngyì) 形意拳 Shape-Mind Fist. An internal style of Gōngfū in which the mind determines the shape or movement of the body. Its creation is attributed to Marshal Yuè, Fēi (岳飛) during the Chinese Southern Sòng Dynasty (1127–1280 CE, 南宋).

Xīnkǎn 心坎 Heart Pit. Martial arts name for Jiūwěi (Co-15, 鳩尾, Wide Pigeon's Tail).

Xīnshén Bùníng 心神不寧 The (emotional) mind and spirit are not at peace. The mind is scattered.

Xīnxí Xiāngyī 心息相依 Heart (mind) and breathing are mutually dependent.

Xīnyuán Yìmǎ 心猿意馬 Heart Monkey Yì Horse. Xīn (heart) represents the Emotional Mind, which acts like a monkey, unsteady and disturbing. Yì is the Wisdom Mind generated from calm, clear thinking and judgment. The Yì is like a horse, powerful yet calm.

Xīnzhāi 心齋 Purified Xīn, which implies a calm, sincere mind.

Xīnzhúxiàn 新竹縣 Birthplace of Dr. Yáng, Jwìng-Mǐng in Táiwān.

Xiōngbù Hūxī 胸部呼吸 Chest breathing.

Xǐsuǐgōng 洗髓功 Marrow and Brain Washing Qìgōng practice. See *Xǐsuǐjīng* (洗髓經).

Xǐsuǐjīng 洗髓經 *Marrow and Brain Washing Classic*. Describes Qìgōng training to lead Qì to the marrow to cleanse it, or to the brain to nourish the spirit for enlightenment. Regarded as the key to longevity and spiritual enlightenment. See also Dámó (達摩).

Xiūqì 修氣 Cultivate the Qì. Buddhist Qìgōng training to protect, maintain, and refine.

Xiūshēn 修身 Cultivating the physical body.

Xíxīn 息心 To cease the activity of Xīn is called Xíxīn.

Xíyuán 息緣 To cease the affinity which connects with secular affairs is called Xíyuán.

Xū 虛 Emptiness, nothingness.

Xuán 玄 marvelous, incredible, or mysterious. It also means original (Yuán, 元).

Xuánguān 玄關 Tricky Gates. Key places in Qìgōng training.

Xuánmíng 玄冥 The spirit of the kidneys. It produces sperm so a baby can be born.

Xuánpìn 玄牝 The marvelous and mysterious Dào, mother of creation of millions of objects.

Xūmí 須彌 The Daoist term for the human spiritual being in the fullness of human virtue.

Xúndàozhě 尋道者 Dào seeker. One who studies the truth of the Dào.

Xùqì 蓄氣 Store the Qì to an abundant level.

Xūwú 虛無 Nothing.

Yǎmén (Gv-15) 啞門 Door of Muteness. An acupuncture cavity on the Governing Vessel.

Yán 言 Speaking or negotiating.

Yǎng 養 To nourish, increase, raise up, or to cultivate.

Yǎng 癢 Itching.

Yáng 陽 One of the two poles (Liǎngyí, 兩儀). The other is Yīn. In Chinese philosophy, the active, positive, masculine Pole is classified as Yáng. In Chinese medicine, Yáng means excessive, overactive, or overheated. The Yáng (or outer) organs are the Gall Bladder, Small Intestine, Large Intestine, Stomach, Bladder, and Triple Burner.

Yáng, Jwìng-Mǐng 楊俊敏 Author of this book.

Yáng Style Tàijíquán 楊氏太極拳 A style of Tàijíquán created by Yáng, Lù-Chán (楊露禪, 1799–1872 CE).

Yángchē 羊車 Sheep Vehicle. The way to lead Qì from Wěilǘ to Jiájí. The Qì movement should be slow. See also Sānchē (三車, Three Vehicles).

Yánghuǒ 陽火 Yáng Fire. The way of increasing the body's fire so it becomes more Yáng.

Yángjiān 陽間 Yáng World. The material world in which we live.

Yǎngqì 養氣 Nourishing and protecting the Qì.

Yángqiāomài 陽蹺脈 Yáng Heel Vessel. One of the Eight Extraordinary Vessels (Bāmài, 八脈).

Yǎngshén 養神 Yǎng means to raise, nourish, and maintain. Shén means spirit. Yǎngshén is the main Buddhist approach to regulating the Shén.

Yángshén 陽神 When Shén manifests Qì into action, it is powerful. Though Shén itself is considered Yīn, it is called Yángshén.

Yǎnguānbí 眼觀鼻 To use the eyes to look at the tip of the nose. To pay attention to the breathing.

Yángwéimài 陽維脈 Yáng Línking Vessel. One of the Eight Extraordinary Vessels (Bāmài, 八脈).

Yǎngyīng 養嬰 Nursing the baby.

Yànxí 晏息 Meditation or profound breathing.

Yáo (2356 BCE) 堯 Ancient Chinese emperor said to have lived to be 800 years old.

Yī 一 Oneness, singularity.

Yì 義 Justice, righteousness.

Yī 猗 Ripple.

Yì 意 Mind. (Pronounced "ee") Specifically, the mind generated by clear thinking and judgment, which can make you calm, peaceful, and wise.

Yìjīng 易經 *The Book of Changes*. A book of divination written during the Zhōu Dynasty (1122–255 BCE, 周朝).

Yìjīnjīng 易筋經 *The Muscle/Tendon Changing Classic*. Describes Wàidān Qìgōng training for strengthening the physical body. See also Dámó (達摩).

Yīn 陰 In Chinese philosophy, this is the passive, negative, feminine Pole. In Chinese medicine, Yīn means deficient. The Yīn organs are the Heart, Lungs, Líver, Kidneys, Spleen, and Pericardium.

Yīnfú 陰符 Yīn magic water. The way to enhance the body's water, so its Yáng can be made more Yīn.

Yīngér 嬰兒 Baby (son), which implies the Spiritual Embryo (Shéntāi, 神胎).

Yìnggōng 硬功 Hard Gōngfū. Any martial training which emphasizes strength and power.

Yíngqì 營氣 Managing Qì. The Qì which manages the functions of the body and its organs.

Yíngzhōu 瀛洲 A legendary mountain in the East Sea where the Chinese immortals dwell.

Yīnhé 陰核 Yīn center. The weak Yīn which exists within the great Yáng. This Yīn stabilizes the Yáng's manifestation.

Yīnjiān 陰間 Yīn world. The spirit world after death is considered Yīn.

Yīnjiāo (Co-7) 陰交 Yīn junction. Acupuncture point on the Conception Vessel (Rènmài, 任脈), and junction of Conception Vessel and Thrusting Vessel (Chōngmài, 衝脈). Considered a paired cavity with Mìngmén (Gv-4, 命門, Lífe's Door), located between L2 and L3 vertebrae.

Yínjiāo (Gv-28) 齦交 Gum Junction. An acupuncture cavity at the mouth, on the Governing Vessel.

Yǐnqì 引氣 To lead the Qì.

Yīnqiāomài 陰蹺脈 Yīn Heel Vessel. One of the Eight Extraordinary Vessels (Bāmài, 八脈).

Yīnshén 陰神 Yīn Spirit. The Yīn center of the Upper Dāntián.

Yīn-Yáng Xúnhuán Yī Xiǎozhōutiān 陰陽循環一小周天 A Yīn-Yáng Circulation Small Heaven Cycle. Daoist name for Small Circulation. See also Sānmódì (三摩地).

Yìntáng (M-HN-3) 印堂 Seal Hall. See Tiānmù (天目).

Yīnwéimài 陰維脈 Yīn Línking Vessel. One of the Eight Extraordinary Vessels (Bāmài, 八脈).

Yìqì Xiànghé 意氣相合 Harmonization of the Yì and Qì.

Yǐshén Yùqì 以神馭氣 Use spirit to govern and manage the Qì.

Yìshǒu Dāntián 意守丹田 Keep your Yì at your Lower Dāntián (Xià Dāntián, 下丹田). In Qìgōng training, you keep your mind at the Lower Dāntián to accumulate Qì. When you circulate it, you always lead it back to your Lower Dāntián at the end of practice.

Yǐyì Yǐnqì 以意引氣 Use the Yì to lead the Qì.

Yǒngquán (K-1) 湧泉 Gushing Spring. An acupuncture cavity on the Kidney Primary Qì Channel.

Yǒngquán Hūxī 湧泉呼吸 Yǒngquán breathing. The mind leads Qì to the Yǒngquán (K-1, 湧泉) cavities on the bottom of the feet.

Yōu 悠 Continuous.

Yù 慾 Desire or lust.

Yuánjīng 元精 Original Essence. The fundamental, original essential substance inherited from your parents. It is converted into Original Qì (Yuánqì, 元氣).

Yuánqì 元氣 Original Qì. Created from the Original Essence (Yuánjīng, 元精) inherited from your parents.

Yuánshén 元神 Original Spirit. The spirit you already had when you were born.

Yuē 曰 To speak.

Yuè, Fēi 岳飛 A Chinese hero of the Southern Sòng Dynasty (1127–1280 CE, 南宋). Said to have created Bāduànjǐn (八段錦), Xíngyìquán (形意拳), and Yuè's Yīngzhǎo (岳家鷹爪).

Yùhuánxuè 玉環穴 Jade ring cavity. See Huángtíng (黃庭).

Yùmén 玉門 Jade Gate. See Tiānmù (天目).

Yún 勻 Uniform.

Yùtáng 玉堂 Jade Hall. Implies the palate of the mouth.

Yùtù 玉兔 Jade Rabbit. Implies Original Essence (Yuánjīng, 元精).

Yùzhěn 玉枕 Jade Pillow. Daoist name for acupuncture cavity Nǎohù (Gv-17, 腦戶, Brain's Household), as well as for Fēngfǔ (Gv-16, 風府, Wind's Dwelling). The area of these cavities is the third gate of Small Circulation.

Zāijiēpài 栽接派 Plant-and-Graft Style. A style of Daoist Qìgōng training.

Zen 禪 See Chán (禪).

Zhāng, Dào-Líng 張道陵 Combined scholarly Daoism (Dàojiā, 道家) with Buddhist philosophies to create Religious Daoism (Dàojiào, 道教) during the Eastern Hàn Dynasty (25–220 CE, 東漢).

Zhànguó 戰國 Warring States Period in Chinese history (403–222 BCE).

Zhēn Xiàdāntián 真下丹田 Real Lower Dāntián, the main Qì reservoir or bioelectric battery in the body.

Zhèng Fùhūxī 正腹呼吸 Abdominal Breathing, commonly called Buddhist Breathing (Fójiā Hūxī, 佛家呼吸).

Zhèngniàn 正念 Righteous mind or thought.

Zhèngqì 正氣 Righteous Qì. When one is righteous, he is said to have righteous Qì which evil Qì cannot overcome.

Zhēnniàn 真念 The real righteous mind or thought.

Zhēnrén 真人 Real Person or Truthful Person. A Daoist.

Zhēnrú 真如 Real Buddhahood.

Zhēnxí 真息 The real breathing or true breathing. Breathing that has been regulated to a deep and profound level. It implies Embryonic Breathing.

Zhēnyī 真一 Real One, Real Singularity, or Real Oneness. One, or Singularity refer to one's main energy Pole comprising the spiritual center and the Qì center.

Zhǐ 止 Stop.

Zhǐguān 止觀 To stop the observation, which implies stopping the observation of the activities of the Xīn.

Zhīnǚ 織女 Weaving Lady. See Niúlángzhīnǚ (牛郎織女).

Zhòng 重 Heavy.

Zhōng 忠 Loyalty.

Zhōng Dāntián 中丹田 The Middle Dāntián located at the Shānzhōng (膻中) area at the center between the nipples.

Zhōnggōng 中宮 Central Palace.

1. Huángtíng (黃庭) area (solar plexus) between Middle and Real Lower Dāntiáns.
2. The Middle Dantian (Zhōng Dāntián, 中丹田).

Zhōngguān 中觀 Observation of neutral (neither empty nor illusory). That means to observe events from a neutral point of view.

Zhōngjí (Co-3) 中極 Middle Summit. An acupuncture cavity on the Conception Vessel.

Zhōngwǎn (Co-12) 中脘 Middle Cavity. Solar plexus. An acupuncture cavity on the Conception Vessel.

Zhǒngxí 踵息 Sole breathing.

Zhōu 周 To be complete, perfect, or round.

Zhù 注 Tendency. Also means major flow or pouring.

Zhuǎnfǎlún 轉法輪 Turning the Wheel of Natural Law. A Buddhist term for Small Circulation.

Zhuāngzhōu 莊周 Zhuāngzi. A Daoist scholar during the Warring States Period (403–222 BCE). He wrote a book called *Zhuāngzi* (莊子).

Zhuāngzi 莊子 See Zhuāngzhōu (莊周)

Zhújī 築基 Build a foundation.

Zǐ 子

1. Son.
2. Midnight (11 pm to 1 am). See Shíèr Dìzhī (十二地支) and Zǐwǔ Líúzhù (子午流注).

Zìjué 自覺 Self-awareness.

Zìshì 自識 Self-recognition.

Zìtuō 自脫 Freedom from emotional or spiritual bondage.

Zìwù 自悟 Self-awakening.

Zǐwǔ Líúzhù 子午流注 Zǐ (子) refers to the period around midnight (11 pm to 1 am), and Wǔ (午) refers to midday (11 am to 1 pm). Líúzhù (流注) means the tendency to flow. The term refers to a schedule of Qì circulation showing which channel has the predominant Qì flow at any particular time, as well as where the predominant Qì flow is in the Conception and Governing Vessels. See also Shíèr Dìzhī (十二地支).

Zìxǐng 自醒 Self-awakening.

Zǒuhuǒ 走火 Walk into the Fire. To lead one's Qì into the wrong path. Dangerous.

Zǒuhuǒ Rùmó 走火入魔 Walk into the Fire and Enter the Devil. If you lead your Qì into the wrong path, it is called Walking into the Fire. If your mind is led into confusion, it is called Entering the Devil.

Zú Juéyīn Gānjīng 足厥陰肝經 Leg Absolute Yīn Liver Primary Qì Channel. One of the twelve primary Qì channels.

Zú Shàoyáng Dǎnjīng 足少陽膽經 Leg Lesser Yáng Gall Bladder Primary Qì Channel. One of the twelve primary Qì channels.

Zú Shàoyīn Shènjīng 足少陰腎經 Leg Lesser Yīn Kidney Primary Qì Channel. One of the twelve primary Qì channels.

Zú Tàiyáng Pángguāngjīng 足太陽膀胱經 Leg Greater Yáng Bladder Primary Qì Channel. One of the twelve primary Qì channels.

Zú Tàiyīn Píjīng 足太陰脾經 Leg Greater Yīn Spleen Primary Qì Channel. One of the twelve primary Qì channels.

Zú Yángmíng Wèijīng 足陽明胃經 Leg Yáng Brightness Stomach Primary Qì Channel. One of the twelve primary Qì channels.

Zuòchán 坐禪 Meditation is called Zuòchán by Buddhists, which means to sit for Chán.

Index

About the Author

Yáng, Jwìng-Mǐng, PhD (楊俊敏博士)

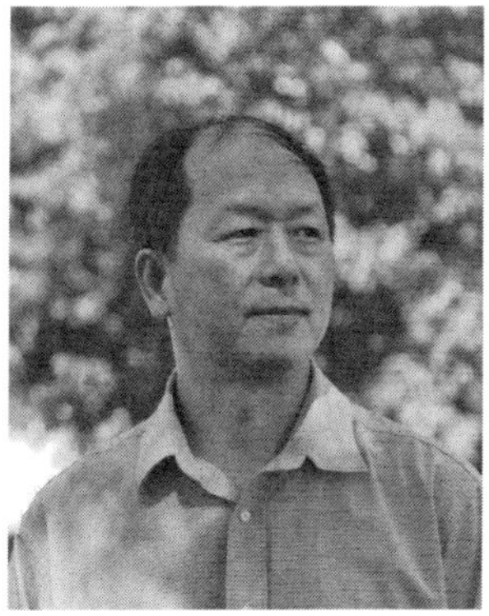

Dr. Yáng, Jwìng-Mǐng was born on August 11, 1946, in Xīnzhúxiàn (新竹縣), Táiwān (台灣), Republic of China (中華民國). He started his Wǔshù (武術) (Gōngfū or Kūng Fū, 功夫) trainingat the age of fifteen under Shàolín White Crane (Shàolín Báihè, 少林白鶴) Master Chēng, Gīn-Gsào (曾金灶). Master Chēng originally learned Tàizǔquán (太祖拳) from his grandfather when he was a child. When Master Chēng was fifteen years old, he started learning White Crane from Master Jīn, Shào-Fēng (金紹峰) and followed him for twenty-three years until Master Jīn's death.

In thirteen years of study (1961–1974) under Master Chēng, Dr. Yáng became an expert in the White Crane style of Chinese martial arts, which includes both the use of bare hands and various weapons, such as saber, staff, spear, trident, two short rods, and many others. With the same master he also studied White Crane Qìgōng (氣功), Qín Ná or Chín Ná (擒拿), Tuīná (推拿), and Diǎnxué massage (點穴按摩) and herbal treatment.

At sixteen, Dr. Yáng began the study of Yáng Style Tàijíquán (楊氏太極拳) under Master Kāo, Táo (高濤). He later continued his study of Tàijíquán under Master Lǐ, Mào-Chīng (李茂清). Master Lǐ learned his Tàijíquán from the well-known Master Hán, Chìng-Táng (韓慶堂). From this further practice, Dr. Yáng was able to master the Tàijí bare-hand sequence, pushing hands, the two-man fighting sequence, Tàijí sword, Tàijí saber, and Tàijí Qìgōng.

When Dr. Yáng was eighteen years old, he entered Tamkang College (淡江學院) in Taipei Xiàn to study physics. In college, he began the study of traditional Shàolín Long Fist (Chángquán or Cháng Chuán, 少林長拳) with Master Lǐ, Mào-Chīng at the Tamkang College Guóshù Club (淡江國術社), 1964–1968, and eventually became an assistant instructor under Master Lǐ. In 1971, he completed his MS degree in physics at the National Táiwān University (台灣大學) and then served in the Chinese Air Force of the Republic of China from 1971 to 1972. In the service, Dr. Yáng taught physics at the Junior Academy of the Chinese Air Force (空軍幼校) while also teaching Wǔshù (武術). After being honorably discharged in 1972, he returned to Tamkang College to teach physics and resumed study under Master Lǐ, Mào-Chīng. From Master Lǐ, Dr. Yáng learned Northern Style Wǔshù, which includes both bare hand and kicking techniques, and numerous weapons.In 1974, Dr. Yáng came to the United States to study mechanical engineering at Purdue University. At the request of a few students, Dr. Yáng began to teach Gōngfū, which resulted in the establishment of the Purdue University Chinese

Kūng Fū Research Club in the spring of 1975. While at Purdue, Dr. Yáng also taught college-credit courses in Tàijíquán. In May of 1978, he was awarded a PhD in mechanical engineering by Purdue.

In 1980, Dr. Yáng moved to Houston to work for Texas Instruments. While in Houston, he founded Yáng's Shàolín Kūng Fū Academy, which was eventually taken over by his disciple, Mr. Jeffery Bolt, after Dr. Yáng moved to Boston in 1982. Dr. Yáng founded Yáng's Martial Arts Academy in Boston on October 1, 1982.

In January of 1984, he gave up his engineering career to devote more time to research, writing, and teaching. In March of 1986, he purchased property in the Jamaica Plain area of Boston to be used as the headquarters of the new organization, Yáng's Martial Arts Association (YMAA). The organization expanded to become a division of Yáng's Oriental Arts Association, Inc. (YOAA).

In 2008, Dr. Yáng began the nonprofit YMAA California Retreat Center. This training facility in rural California is where selected students enroll in a five to ten-year residency to learn Chinese martial arts.

Dr. Yáng has been involved in traditional Chinese Wǔshù since 1961, studying Shàolín White Crane (Báihè), Shàolín Long Fist (Chángquán), and Tàijíquán under several different masters. He has taught for more than forty-six years: seven years in Táiwān, five years at Purdue University, two years in Houston, twenty-six years in Boston, and more than eight years at the YMAA California Retreat Center. He has taught seminars all around the world, sharing his knowledge of Chinese martial arts and Qìgōng in Argentina, Austria, Barbados, Botswana, Belgium, Bermuda, Brazil, Canada, China, Chile, England, Egypt, France, Germany, Holland, Hungary, Iceland, Ireland, Italy, Latvia, Mexico, New Zealand, Poland, Portugal, Saudi Arabia, Spain, South Africa, Switzerland, and Venezuela.

Since 1986, YMAA has become an international organization, which currently includes more than fifty schools located in Argentina, Belgium, Canada, Chile, France, Hungary, Iran, Ireland, Italy, New Zealand, Poland, Portugal, South Africa, Sweden, the United Kingdom, Venezuela, and the United States.

Many of Dr. Yáng's books and videos have been translated into many languages, including French, Italian, Spanish, Polish, Czech, Bulgarian, Russian, German, and Hungarian.

Books by Dr. Yáng, Jwìng-Mǐng

Analysis of Shàolín Chín Ná, 2nd ed. YMAA Publication Center, 1987, 2004

Ancient Chinese Weapons: A Martial Artist's Guide, 2nd ed. YMAA Publication Center, 1985, 1999

Arthritis Relief: Chinese Qìgōng for Healing & Prevention, 2nd ed. YMAA Publication Center, 1991, 2005

Back Pain Relief: Chinese Qìgōng for Healing and Prevention, 2nd ed. YMAA Publication Center, 1997, 2004

Bāguàzhǎng: Theory and Applications, 2nd ed. YMAA Publication Center, 1994, 2008

Comprehensive Applications of Shàolín Chín Ná: The Practical Defense of Chinese Seizing Arts. YMAA Publication Center, 1995

Essence of Shàolín White Crane: Martial Power and Qìgōng. YMAA Publication Center, 1996

How to Defend Yourself. YMAA Publication Center, 1992

Introduction to Ancient Chinese Weapons. Unique Publications, Inc., 1985

Meridian Qìgōng, YMAA Publication Center, 2016

Northern Shàolín Sword, 2nd ed. YMAA Publication Center, 1985, 2000

Qìgōng for Health and Martial Arts, 2nd ed. YMAA Publication Center, 1995,1998

Qìgōng Massage: Fundamental Techniques for Health and Relaxation, 2nd ed. YMAA Publication Center, 1992, 2005

Qìgōng Meditation: Embryonic Breathing. YMAA Publication Center, 2003

Qìgōng Meditation: Small Circulation, YMAA Publication Center, 2006

Qìgōng, the Secret of Youth: Dá Mó's Muscle/Tendon Changing and Marrow/Brain Washing Qìgōng, 2nd ed. YMAA Publication Center, 1989, 2000

Root of Chinese Qìgōng: Secrets of Qìgōng Training, 2nd ed. YMAA Publication Center, 1989, 1997

Shàolín Chín Ná. Unique Publications, Inc., 1980

Shàolín Long Fist Kūng Fū. Unique Publications, Inc., 1981

Simple Qìgōng Exercises for Health: The Eight Pieces of Brocade, 3rd ed. YMAA Publication Center, 1988, 1997, 2013

Tài Chí Ball Qìgōng: For Health and Martial Arts. YMAA Publication Center, 2010

Tài Chí Chuán Classical Yáng Style: The Complete Long Form and Qìgōng, 2nd ed. YMAA Publication Center, 1999, 2010

Tài Chí Chuán Martial Applications, 2nd ed. YMAA Publication Center, 1986, 1996

Tài Chí Chuán Martial Power, 3rd ed. YMAA Publication Center, 1986, 1996, 2015

Tài Chí Chuán: Classical Yáng Style, 2nd ed. YMAA Publication Center, 1999, 2010

Tài Chí Qìgōng: The Internal Foundation of Tài Chí Chuán, 2nd ed. rev. YMAA Publication Center, 1997, 1990, 2013

Tài Chí Secrets of the Ancient Masters: Selected Readings with Commentary. YMAA Publication Center, 1999

Tài Chí Secrets of the Wǔ and Lǐ Styles: Chinese Classics, Translation, Commentary. YMAA Publication Center, 2001

Tài Chí Secrets of the Wú Style: Chinese Classics, Translation, Commentary. YMAA Publication Center, 2002

Tài Chí Secrets of the Yáng Style: Chinese Classics, Translation, Commentary. YMAA Publication Center, 2001

Tài Chí Sword Classical Yáng Style: The Complete Long Form, Qìgōng, and Applications, 2nd ed. YMAA Publication Center, 1999, 2014

Tàijí Chín Ná: The Seizing Art of Tàijíquan, 2nd ed. YMAA Publication Center, 1995, 2014

Tàijíquan Theory of Dr. Yáng, Jwìng-Mǐng: The Root of Tàijíquan. YMAA Publication Center, 2003

Xíngyìquán: Theory and Applications, 2nd ed. YMAA Publication Center, 1990, 2003 Yáng Style Tài Chí Chuán. Unique Publications, Inc., 1981

Videos by Dr. Yáng, Jwìng-Mǐng

Advanced Practical Chín Ná in Depth, YMAA Publication Center, 2010

Analysis of Shàolín Chín Ná. YMAA Publication Center, 2004

Bāguàzhǎng (Eight Trigrams Palm Kūng Fū). YMAA Publication Center, 2005

Chín Ná in Depth: Courses 1–4. YMAA Publication Center, 2003

Chín Ná in Depth: Courses 5–8. YMAA Publication Center, 2003

Chín Ná in Depth: Courses 9–12. YMAA Publication Center, 2003

Five Animal Sports Qìgōng. YMAA Publication Center, 2008

Knife Defense: Traditional Techniques. YMAA Publication Center, 2011

Meridian Qìgōng. YMAA Publication Center, 2015

Neigong. YMAA Publication Center, 2015

Northern Shàolín Sword. YMAA Publication Center, 2009

Qìgōng Massage. YMAA Publication Center, 2005

Saber Fundamental Training. YMAA Publication Center, 2008

Shàolín Kūng Fū Fundamental Training. YMAA Publication Center, 2004

Shàolín Long Fist Kūng Fū: Basic Sequences. YMAA Publication Center, 2005

Shàolín Saber Basic Sequences. YMAA Publication Center, 2007

Shàolín Staff Basic Sequences. YMAA Publication Center, 2007
Shàolín White Crane Gōng Fū Basic Training: Courses 1 & 2. YMAA Publication Center, 2003
Shàolín White Crane Gōng Fū Basic Training: Courses 3 & 4. YMAA Publication Center, 2008
Shàolín White Crane Hard and Soft Qìgōng. YMAA Publication Center, 2003
Shuāi Jiāo: Kūng Fū Wrestling. YMAA Publication Center, 2010
Simple Qìgōng Exercises for Arthritis Relief. YMAA Publication Center, 2007
Simple Qìgōng Exercises for Back Pain Relief. YMAA Publication Center, 2007
Simple Qìgōng Exercises for Health: The Eight Pieces of Brocade. YMAA Publication Center, 2003
Staff Fundamental Training: Solo Drills and Matching Practice. YMAA Publication Center, 2007
Sword Fundamental Training. YMAA Publication Center, 2009
Tài Chí Ball Qìgōng: Courses 1 & 2. YMAA Publication Center, 2006
Tài Chí Ball Qìgōng: Courses 3 & 4. YMAA Publication Center, 2007
Tài Chí Chuán: Classical Yáng Style. YMAA Publication Center, 2003
Tài Chí Fighting Set: 2-Person Matching Set. YMAA Publication Center, 2006
Tài Chí Pushing Hands: Courses 1 & 2. YMAA Publication Center, 2005
Tài Chí Pushing Hands: Courses 3 & 4. YMAA Publication Center, 2006
Tài Chí Qìgōng. YMAA Publication Center, 2005
Tài Chí Sword, Classical Yáng Style. YMAA Publication Center, 2005
Tài Chí Symbol: Yīn/Yáng Sticking Hands. YMAA Publication Center, 2008
Tàijí 37 Postures Martial Applications. YMAA Publication Center, 2008
Tàijí Chín Ná in Depth. YMAA Publication Center, 2009
Tàijí Saber: Classical Yáng Style. YMAA Publication Center, 2008
Tàijí Wrestling: Advanced Takedown Techniques. YMAA Publication Center, 2008
Understanding Qìgōng, DVD 1: What is Qìgōng? The Human Qì Circulatory System. YMAA Publication Center, 2006
Understanding Qìgōng, DVD 2: Key Points of Qìgōng & Qìgōng Breathing. YMAA Publication Center, 2006

Understanding Qìgōng, DVD 3: Embryonic Breathing. YMAA Publication Center, 2007

Understanding Qìgōng, DVD 4: Four Seasons Qìgōng. YMAA Publication Center, 2007

Understanding Qìgōng, DVD 5: Small Circulation. YMAA Publication Center, 2007

Understanding Qìgōng, DVD 6: Martial Arts Qìgōng Breathing. YMAA Publication Center, 2007

Xíngyìquán: Twelve Animals Kūng Fū and Applications. YMAA Publication Center, 2008

Yáng Tài Chí for Beginners. YMAA Publication Center, 2012

YMAA 25-Year Anniversary. YMAA Publication Center, 2009

BOOKS FROM YMAA

101 REFLECTIONS ON TAI CHI CHUAN
108 INSIGHTS INTO TAI CHI CHUAN
A WOMAN'S QIGONG GUIDE
ADVANCING IN TAE KWON DO
ANALYSIS OF SHAOLIN CHIN NA 2ND ED
ANCIENT CHINESE WEAPONS
ART AND SCIENCE OF STAFF FIGHTING
THE ART AND SCIENCE OF SELF-DEFENSE
ART AND SCIENCE OF STICK FIGHTING
ART OF HOJO UNDO
ARTHRITIS RELIEF, 3D ED.
BACK PAIN RELIEF, 2ND ED.
BAGUAZHANG, 2ND ED.
BRAIN FITNESS
CHIN NA IN GROUND FIGHTING
CHINESE FAST WRESTLING
CHINESE FITNESS
CHINESE TUI NA MASSAGE
COMPLETE MARTIAL ARTIST
COMPREHENSIVE APPLICATIONS OF SHAOLIN CHIN NA
CONFLICT COMMUNICATION
DAO DE JING: A QIGONG INTERPRETATION
DAO IN ACTION
DEFENSIVE TACTICS
DIRTY GROUND
DR. WU'S HEAD MASSAGE
ESSENCE OF SHAOLIN WHITE CRANE
EXPLORING TAI CHI
FACING VIOLENCE
FIGHT LIKE A PHYSICIST
THE FIGHTER'S BODY
FIGHTER'S FACT BOOK 1&2
FIGHTING ARTS
FIGHTING THE PAIN RESISTANT ATTACKER
FIRST DEFENSE
FORCE DECISIONS: A CITIZENS GUIDE
INSIDE TAI CHI
JUDO ADVANTAGE
JUJI GATAME ENCYCLOPEDIA
KARATE SCIENCE
KATA AND THE TRANSMISSION OF KNOWLEDGE
KRAV MAGA COMBATIVES
KRAV MAGA FUNDAMENTAL STRATEGIES
KRAV MAGA PROFESSIONAL TACTICS
KRAV MAGA WEAPON DEFENSES
LITTLE BLACK BOOK OF VIOLENCE
LIUHEBAFA FIVE CHARACTER SECRETS
MARTIAL ARTS OF VIETNAM
MARTIAL ARTS INSTRUCTION
MARTIAL WAY AND ITS VIRTUES
MEDITATIONS ON VIOLENCE
MERIDIAN QIGONG EXERCISES
MINDFUL EXERCISE
MIND INSIDE TAI CHI
MIND INSIDE YANG STYLE TAI CHI CHUAN
NATURAL HEALING WITH QIGONG
NORTHERN SHAOLIN SWORD, 2ND ED.
OKINAWA'S COMPLETE KARATE SYSTEM: ISSHIN RYU
PRINCIPLES OF TRADITIONAL CHINESE MEDICINE
PROTECTOR ETHIC
QIGONG FOR HEALTH & MARTIAL ARTS 2ND ED.
QIGONG FOR TREATING COMMON AILMENTS
QIGONG MASSAGE
QIGONG MEDITATION: EMBRYONIC BREATHING
QIGONG GRAND CIRCULATION
QIGONG MEDITATION: SMALL CIRCULATION
QIGONG, THE SECRET OF YOUTH: DA MO'S CLASSICS
REDEMPTION
ROOT OF CHINESE QIGONG, 2ND ED.
SAMBO ENCYCLOPEDIA
SCALING FORCE
SELF-DEFENSE FOR WOMEN
SHIN GI TAI: KARATE TRAINING
SIMPLE CHINESE MEDICINE
SIMPLE QIGONG EXERCISES FOR HEALTH, 3RD ED.
SIMPLIFIED TAI CHI CHUAN, 2ND ED.
SOLO TRAINING 1&2
SPOTTING DANGER BEFORE IT SPOTS YOU
SPOTTING DANGER BEFORE IT SPOTS YOUR KIDS
SPOTTING DANGER BEFORE IT SPOTS YOUR TEENS
SUMO FOR MIXED MARTIAL ARTS
SUNRISE TAI CHI
SURVIVING ARMED ASSAULTS
TAE KWON DO: THE KOREAN MARTIAL ART
TAEKWONDO BLACK BELT POOMSAE
TAEKWONDO: A PATH TO EXCELLENCE
TAEKWONDO: ANCIENT WISDOM
TAEKWONDO: DEFENSE AGAINST WEAPONS
TAEKWONDO: SPIRIT AND PRACTICE
TAI CHI BALL QIGONG: FOR HEALTH AND MARTIAL ARTS
THE TAI CHI BOOK
TAI CHI CHIN NA, 2ND ED.
TAI CHI CHUAN CLASSICAL YANG STYLE, 2ND ED.
TAI CHI CHUAN MARTIAL POWER, 3RD ED.
TAI CHI CONCEPTS AND EXPERIMENTS
TAI CHI CONNECTIONS
TAI CHI DYNAMICS
TAI CHI FOR DEPRESSION
TAI CHI IN 10 WEEKS
TAI CHI PUSH HANDS
TAI CHI QIGONG, 3RD ED.
TAI CHI SECRETS OF THE ANCIENT MASTERS
TAI CHI SECRETS OF THE WU & LI STYLES
TAI CHI SECRETS OF THE WU STYLE
TAI CHI SECRETS OF THE YANG STYLE
TAI CHI SWORD: CLASSICAL YANG STYLE, 2ND ED.
TAI CHI SWORD FOR BEGINNERS
TAI CHI WALKING
TAIJIQUAN THEORY OF DR. YANG, JWING-MING
FIGHTING ARTS
TRADITIONAL CHINESE HEALTH SECRETS
TRADITIONAL TAEKWONDO
TRAINING FOR SUDDEN VIOLENCE
TRIANGLE HOLD ENCYCLOPEDIA
TRUE WELLNESS SERIES (MIND, HEART, GUT)
WARRIOR'S MANIFESTO
WAY OF KATA
WAY OF SANCHIN KATA
WAY TO BLACK BELT
WESTERN HERBS FOR MARTIAL ARTISTS
WILD GOOSE QIGONG
WINNING FIGHTS
XINGYIQUAN

AND MANY MORE . . .

VIDEOS FROM YMAA